MENTAL IMAGERY

MENTAL IMAGERY

Edited by

Robert G. Kunzendorf

University of Lowell
Lowell, Massachusetts

FCH Learning Centre
University of Gloucestershire
Swindon Road
Cheltenham GL50 4AZ
Tel: 01242 532913

PLENUM PRESS • NEW YORK AND LONDON

Library of Congress Cataloging-in-Publication Data

American Association for the Study of Mental Imagery. Conference
  (11th : 1989 : Washington, D.C.)
   Mental imagery / edited by Robert Kunzendorf.
      p.   cm.
   "Proceedings of the Eleventh and Twelfth Annual Conferences of the
American Association for the Study of Mental Imagery, held June
15-18, 1989, in Washington, D.C., and June 14-17, 1990, in Lowell
and Boston, Massachusetts"--T.p. verso.
   Includes bibliographical references.
   Includes index.
   ISBN 0-306-43825-9
   1. Imagery (Psychology)--Congresses.   I. Kunzendorf, Robert G.
II. American Association for the Study of Mental Imagery.
Conference (12th : 1990 : Lowell, Mass. and Boston, Mass.)
III. Title.
   [DNLM: 1. Cognition--congresses. 2. Imagination--congresses.
3. Mental Processes--congresses. 4. Symbolism (Psychology)-
-congresses.   BF 367 A512m 1989]
BF367.A43   1991
DNLM/DLC
for Library of Congress   91-4605
                                                              CIP

Proceedings of the Eleventh and Twelfth Annual Conferences of the
American Association for the Study of Mental Imagery, held June 15–18,
1989, in Washington, D.C., and June 14–17, 1990, in Lowell and
Boston, Massachusetts

ISBN 0-306-43825-9

© 1991 Plenum Press, New York
A Division of Plenum Publishing Corporation
233 Spring Street, New York, N.Y. 10013

Printed in the United States of America

For my mother,
and in memory
of my father

PREFACE

The current book presents select proceedings from the Eleventh Annual Conference of AASMI (The American Association for the Study of Mental Imagery) in Washington, DC, 1989, and from the Twelfth Annual Conference of AASMI in Lowell and Boston, MA, 1990. This presentation of keynote addresses, research papers, and clinical workshops reflects a broad range of theoretical positions and a diverse repertoire of methodological approaches. Within this breadth and diversity, however, four aspects of the nature of imagery stand out: its *mental* nature, its *private* nature, its *conscious* nature, and its *symbolic* nature.

The mental nature of imagery--i.e., its epistemological aspect--is explored in the book's first section of articles by Marcia Johnson, Laura Snodgrass, Leonard Giambra and Alicia Grodsky, Vija Lusebrink, Selina Kassels, Helane Rosenberg and Yakov Epstein, M. Elizabeth D'Zamko and Lynne Schwab, and Laurence Martel. These first eight articles fall, essentially, into various domains of cognitive psychology, including the psychology of art and educational psychology.

In the second section, the private nature of imagery is studied by Ernest Hartmann, Nicholas Spanos, Benjamin Wallace, Deirdre Barrett, John Connolly, James Honeycutt, Dominique Gendrin, and James Honeycutt and J. Michael Gotcher. These studies, which fall within the realm of personality and social psychology, bring to light the fact that many very public interpersonal behaviors reflect very private images. Such behaviors range from interpersonal rapport with a hypnotist, to rapport with a forensic jury.

In the third section of articles, imagery's conscious nature and its physiological manifestations are jointly examined by Robert Kunzendorf, R. Kunzendorf *et al.*, Paul Bakan, John Schneider *et al.*, Deirdre Brigham and Philip Toal, Nicholas Brink, Bonney Schaub *et al.*, and Dan Smith. Throughout this examination, these eight articles explore various theories of the mysterious relationship between conscious experience and neural events, and various applications of the important relationship between conscious imagination and bodily responses.

In the fourth and final section, the symbolic nature of imagery in psychopathology and psychotherapy is explored by Jerold Gold, Donald Levis, Lewis Mehl, Nicholas Brink, Archa Mati, Daniel Tomasulo, Valerie Hookham, and Jacqueline Sallade. Of course, imagery's symbolic nature is also explored in some cognitive studies, like those by Snodgrass and Martel, just as imagery's private nature is emphasized in some clinical studies. But generally, clinical psychology draws attention to imagery's symbolic aspect, just as psychophysiology draws attention to its conscious nature, and social psychology to its private nature.

Within the four sections of this book, a common focus on imagery--symbolic, conscious, private, mental imagery--unites all of the studies. Indeed at AASMI conferences, unlike most psychological meetings, therapists and researchers listen to and talk to each other. Accordingly, as editor of these AASMI proceedings, I hope that readers appreciate how the study of imagery can bring such very different psychologists together, even as the whole of psychology becomes increasingly fractionated.

In conclusion, I thank all authors for their contributions to the last two AASMI conferences and to this publication of select proceedings. In addition, I gratefully acknowledge the support of Anees Sheikh and Nick Spanos from AASMI's Board, John Hurtado and Claire Hoffman from the University of Lowell, and Melanie Yelity and Gregory Safford from Plenum.

Robert G. Kunzendorf
September 25, 1990

CONTENTS

COGNITIVE STUDIES AND APPLICATIONS OF MENTAL IMAGES

PRIVATE IMAGES BEHIND PERSONALITY TRAITS AND INTERPERSONAL DYNAMICS

COGNITIVE STUDIES AND APPLICATIONS OF MENTAL IMAGES

REFLECTION, REALITY MONITORING, AND THE SELF

Marcia K. Johnson, Ph.D.

Department of Psychology
Princeton University
Princeton, NJ 08544

For some time now, I have been investigating the problem of reality monitoring--how people discriminate, when remembering, between information that had a perceptual source and information that was self-generated from thought, imagination, fantasy, or dreams (Johnson, 1977; Johnson, Taylor, & Raye, 1977). This question has many intriguing facets. It makes contact with fundamental philosophical issues of epistemology; it is a stimulating theoretical puzzle in itself; it is critically important for our everyday functioning in the world. It also has a certain science fiction quality about it that is disconcerting but compelling. If, as the analysis of reality monitoring that I will describe suggests, our ideas of reality and fantasy originate from imperfect attributional processes, who knows what might be true?

These philosophical, theoretical, practical, and science fiction aspects of reality monitoring could easily sustain my interest but, as it turns out, there has been an added attraction: Exploring the problem of reality monitoring has profoundly shaped my thinking about memory and cognition in general. The ideas about memory that have evolved from these efforts with colleagues and students to understand reality monitoring are summarized in a cognitive architecture that we call MEM-- a Multiple-Entry, Modular memory system (Johnson, 1983, 1990; in press; Johnson & Hirst, in press; Johnson & Multhaup, in press). Drawing on these earlier papers, I will briefly describe MEM and then some of our work on reality monitoring that grows out of the idea that records of reflective (or "self-generated") operations provide cues to the origin of information in memory. In the last section I will consider this "self" that does the generating, and discuss some implications of the MEM framework for how the idea of a "self" might arise and be maintained.

MULTIPLE-ENTRY MODULAR (MEM) MEMORY SYSTEM

According to MEM, memory is the result of processes that are organized at the most global functional level into perceptual and reflective systems. The perceptual system records information that is the consequence of perceptual processes such as seeing and hearing. The reflective system records information that is the consequence of internally-generated processes such as planning, comparing, speculating and imagining.

The perceptual system consists of two subsystems, P-1 and P-2, and the reflective system consists of two subsystems, R-1 and R-2 (Figure 1a). Each of these, in turn, includes component subprocesses. Suggestions for what some of these component subprocesses might be are given in Figures 1b and 1c. Subprocesses of P-1 might include *locating* stimuli, *resolving* stimulus configurations, *tracking* stimuli, and *extracting* invariants from perceptual arrays (e.g., cues specifying the rapid expansion of features in the visual field). P-1 processes develop connections or associations involving perceptual information of which we are often unaware, such as the cues in a speech signal that specify a particular vowel, or the aspects of a moving stimulus that specify when it is likely to reach a given point in space. Learning in the P-1

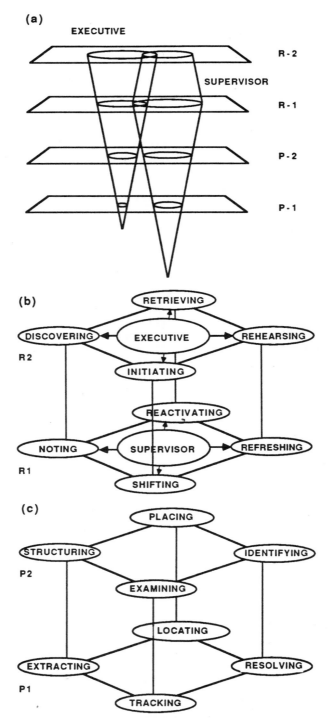

Figure 1. A multiple-entry, modular memory system:
(a) configuration of subsystems;
(b) component subprocesses of R-1 and R-2;
(c) component subprocesses of P-1 and P-2.

subsystem allows us to do things such as adjust to a person's foreign accent, or to anticipate the trajectory of a baseball. Subprocesses of P-2 might include *placing* objects in spatial relation to each other, *identifying* objects, *examining* or perceptually investigating stimuli, and *structuring* or abstracting a pattern of organization across temporally extended stimuli (e.g., syntactic structure). P-2 processes are involved in learning about the phenomenal perceptual world of objects such as chairs and balls, and events such as seeing a person sit down in a chair or catch a ball.

In contrast to perceptual processes, reflective processes occur independent of sensory stimulation. They may sometimes be initiated by perception, but reflective processes allow one to go beyond external cues. They are generative; they allow us to manipulate information and memories, anticipate events, imagine possible alternatives, compare these alternatives, and so forth. R-1 processes and R-2 processes differ in the complexity of the tasks they can handle. For example, R-1 processes would be sufficient for anticipating a picnic, but R-2 processes would be necessary for planning one.

Both R-1 and R-2 involve component processes that allow people to sustain, organize, and revive information. Some of these component processes in R-1 are *noting* relations, *shifting* attention to something potentially more useful, *refreshing* information so that it remains active and one can easily shift back to it, and *reactivating* information that has dropped out of consciousness. Component processes in R-2 include *discovering, initiating, rehearsing,* and *retrieving* (see Johnson, 1990, and Johnson & Hirst, in press, for a discussion of these component processes).

The R-1 and R-2 subsystems also include control and monitoring component processes. For R-1 these are collectively referred to as *supervisor* processes and for R-2 as *executive* processes. Supervisor and executive processes set up goals and agendas and monitor or evaluate outcomes with respect to these agendas (Miller, Galanter, & Pribram, 1960; Nelson & Narens, 1990; Stuss & Benson, 1986). Furthermore, they recruit other reflective component processes for these purposes. There is more effort, will, or control (e.g., Hasher & Zacks, 1979; Norman & Shallice, 1986; Shiffrin & Schneider, 1977) associated with executive than with supervisor processing. The difference between supervisor and executive processes is something like the difference between "tactical" and "strategic" control, or the difference between habitual and deliberate reflective processes. For example, under the guidance of an R-1 intention to *listen attentively to a story* told by your dinner companion, you might generate tacit implications of sentences, notice relations between one part of the story and an earlier part you are reminded of, and so forth. Under guidance of an R-2 agenda to *critically evaluate the story,* you might generate objections to the logic of events in the story, actively retrieve other stories for comparison, and so forth. Normal cognitive functioning draws on different component processes of reflection as needed. Disruption of various combinations of component processes results in various patterns of cognitive deficit (Johnson & Hirst, in press).

P-1, P-2, R-1, and R-2 activities go on simultaneously and they produce corresponding changes in memory. These changes are the representations of experience. At some future time, exactly which of these records are activated will depend on the kind of task probing memory (i.e., according to the encoding specificity principle, Tulving, 1983). A task in which you had to identify random syllables spoken by your dinner companion that a devious psychologist embedded in white noise would draw primarily on representations formed by P-1. A recognition task in which you had to discriminate pictures of people who were and were not at the dinner party should draw primarily on representations formed in P-2. Recall of your dinner companion's story would draw on R-1 and R-2 records.

Under ordinary circumstances, subsystems interact with each other, although exactly how they interact needs further investigation. During remembering, representations from one subsystem may directly activate related representations from another, or interactions between perceptual and reflective memory may take place through supervisor and executive components. For example, an agenda initiated by the R-2 executive, such as *look for a restaurant,* might activate relevant perceptual schemas from perceptual memory (e.g., look for building with ground level window, tables visible, menu in window). It might also activate reflective plans adapted to the current situation (e.g., check the restaurant guide for this part of town).

In Figure 1a, supervisor and executive processes are depicted as cones passing through planes representing different subsystems. The sizes of the ellipses at the intersects of cones and planes reflect the relative degree of involvement of supervisor and executive processes in each subsystem's activities. Typically, executive functions have greater access to reflective memory than to perceptual memory, and greater access to P-2 than to P-1 subsystems. An especially important aspect of reflection is that the supervisor and executive processes in R-1 and R-2 can recruit and monitor each other, as depicted by their overlap in Figure 1a. For example, an R-2 agenda to *check the restaurant guide* can initiate an R-1 goal to *note the number of stars by each entry*. Interaction between R-1 and R-2 provides a mechanism for sequencing subgoals. It also gives rise to the phenomenal experience of reflecting on reflection which, as I will discuss later, is intrinsic to our sense of self. In addition, access to information about one's own cognitive operations provides a salient cue for identifying oneself as the origin of information (Johnson, Raye, Foley, & Foley, 1981).

I have used the MEM framework to organize empirical facts obtained from cognitive-behavioral studies (Johnson, 1983). It also has prompted and been shaped by our research on anterograde amnesia (Hirst, Johnson, Kim, Phelps, Risse, & Volpe, 1986; Hirst, Johnson, Phelps, & Volpe, 1988; Johnson & Kim, 1985; Johnson, Kim, & Risse, 1985; Weinstein, 1987; see also Johnson, 1990), as well as our work on reality monitoring (Johnson & Raye, 1981; Johnson, 1988a,b, in press), and we have used it to discuss the relation between cognition and emotion (Johnson & Multhaup, in press). Several behavioral dissociations support the idea that the division between perceptual and reflective memories may capture functional organizations within the nervous system as well. For example, an argument can be made that memory for reflective processing develops later than memory for perceptual processing (e.g., Flavell, 1985; Moscovitch, 1985; Perlmutter, 1984; Schacter & Moscovitch, 1984); and that P-2 develops later than P-1 and R-2 later than R-1. Moreover, memories for reflective processing appear to be disrupted more easily by stress, depression, aging, and the use of alcohol and other drugs than are memories for perceptual processes (Craik, 1986; Eich, 1975; Hasher & Zacks, 1979; 1984; Hashtroudi & Parker, 1986). Furthermore, the breakdown in memory functioning found in patients with anterograde amnesia appears to fall disproportionately on reflective memory (Johnson, 1983, 1990; Johnson & Hirst, in press; see also chapters in Cermak, 1982).

A system like MEM is an extremely powerful cognitive architecture. For example, guided by learning in the perceptual subsystems, we can hit a tennis ball and at the same time reflectively think about a strategy for playing the game. As I mentioned before, the interaction between R-1 and R-2 permits sequencing of subgoals to perform complex tasks such as going on picnics and writing research papers. The availability of both perceptual and reflective subsystems allows us to build up a veridical representation of the world through P-1 and P-2 processes and yet to imagine, or reflectively generate, worlds as they might be.

But the same reflective processes that underlie our planfulness and creativity produce a crucial dilemma for us. Reflection generates events that take place only in thought and imagination. So, how do we know the life we remember is the product of actual experiences rather than only experiences we have thought, fantasized, or dreamed?

REALITY MONITORING

Reality monitoring is the term Carol Raye and I suggested for the processes involved in discriminating memories that originated from perception from those that arose from thought, imagination, fantasy, dreams and other self-generated processes (Johnson & Raye, 1981; Johnson, 1985; in press). Reality monitoring failures occur when people confuse the origin of information, misattributing something that was reflectively generated to perception or vice versa. According to this view, reality is not directly given in remembering, but is an attribution that is the outcome of judgment processes. To understand reality monitoring confusions we have to consider both the phenomenal characteristics of memories and the decision processes people apply to them.

We proposed that memories for perceived and imagined events differ in average value along a number of dimensions. Memories originating in perception typically have more perceptual information, (e.g., color, sound), more contextual information such as time and place, and more meaningful detail, whereas memories originating in thought typically have more accessible information about cognitive operations--that is, about those perceptual and reflective processes that took place when the memory was established. Judgment processes monitored by R-1 capitalize on these differences. That is, differences between externally and internally derived memories in average value along these dimensions or attributes form one basis for deciding the origin of a memory. For example, one would be likely to decide that a memory with very little cognitive operations information and a great deal of perceptual information was externally derived (Johnson, Raye, Foley, & Foley, 1981; Johnson, Raye, Wang, & Taylor, 1979).

In contrast, R-2 processes control a second type of decision process based on reasoning:

This may include, for example, retrieving additional information from memory and considering whether the target memory could have been perceived (or self-generated) given these other specific memories or general knowledge (e.g., Johnson, Foley, Suengas, & Raye, 1988). For example, I might have a memory of a challenging question asked by a colleague during a talk I gave (and my perfect answer), but correctly attribute this to imagination on the basis of knowledge I have that he was out of town when I gave the talk. In addition, judgments will be affected by people's opinions or by "metamemory" assumptions about how memory works.

For normally functioning adults, most reality monitoring is guided by R-1 supervisor processes; that is, reality monitoring typically takes place rapidly, in a nondeliberative fashion, based on the qualitative characteristics of memories that are activated (e.g., amount or type of perceptual detail). The generally slower, more deliberate retrieval of supporting memories and initiation of reasoning processes (e.g., Does this seem plausible given other things I know?) are R-2 functions and are engaged less often. Among other things, R-2 processes allow us to look back on ideas we initially accepted and question them.

Using this framework, consider the various ways in which reality monitoring could break down (Johnson, in press): Disrupted reality monitoring would result from any circumstance that decreases differences between phenomenal qualities of perceived and imagined events such as unusually vivid imagery or reduced cognitive operations associated with imagined information. Difficulty in retrieving relevant supporting information would also cause problems in reality monitoring, as would any disruption in R-1 or R-2 judgment processes, including more lax criteria (e.g., requiring less perceptual information to decide something had been perceived). In addition, reduced motivation to engage in reality monitoring would result in more confusions between fact and fantasy. Thus any one of these factors, or any combination, would reduce the accuracy of reality monitoring. Furthermore, we should be able to characterize clinically significant disruptions of reality monitoring such as occur in hallucinations (Bentall, 1990; Horowitz, 1978), delusions (Johnson, 1988a), confabulation (Johnson, in press), and hypnosis (Hilgard, 1977; Kihlstrom, 1987; Kunzendorf, 1986), in terms of the various factors suggested by this framework.

Most of our laboratory studies have been directed at exploring the viability of this framework for reality monitoring in normally functioning individuals. For example, one straightforward prediction is that the more imaginations are like perceptions in perceptual detail, the more subjects should confuse imaginations with perceptions. In one experiment testing this hypothesis (Johnson, Raye, Wang, and Taylor, 1979), we varied the number of times subjects saw pictures and the number of times they imagined each picture. Later, we asked subjects how many times they saw each picture. The more often subjects saw pictures, the higher their frequency judgments. More important, the more often subjects imagined the pictures, the more often they thought they had seen them. Furthermore, compared to poor imagers, good imagers were more affected by the number of times they had imagined a picture.

In another experiment on this point (Johnson, Foley & Leach, 1988), subjects imagined themselves saying some words and heard a confederate say other words. Later, subjects were asked to discriminate the words that they had thought from the words the confederate had actually said and they were quite good at this. In another condition, the procedure was the same except that subjects were asked to think in the confederate's voice; in this case subjects later had much more difficulty discriminating what they had heard from what they had thought. This study, as well as the good/poor imager study, is consistent with the idea that the more perceptual overlap there is between memories derived from perception and memories generated via imagination, the greater will be the confusion between them. (This is one reason to be careful not to make the imaginary conversations and arguments you have with people too perceptually detailed.)

REFLECTIVE COGNITIVE OPERATIONS

The perceptual quality of images is, perhaps, their most obvious and intriguing phenomenal characteristic, and certainly an aspect of them that has prompted a great deal of empirical research (e.g., Finke & Shepard, 1986; Kosslyn, 1980). The fact that perceptual detail in a memory can cause one to mistake an imagination for a perception while remembering is fundamental, but not too surprising. What has been more surprising to us is the critical importance that records of cognitive operations appear to play in reality monitoring (e.g., Johnson, Raye, Foley, & Foley, 1981; Rabinowitz, 1989). Thus, here, I want to stress an aspect of images other than their perceptual quality, namely, how they get generated. Images are under varying degrees of reflective control, and the degree of reflective control has implications for how easily they will be distinguished from percepts.

According to the reality monitoring framework, remembered cognitive operations can be a cue to the origin of a memory. If an image is generated with considerable reflection or effort, then the internally generated memory should be easier to distinguish from a memory for an external event than if the image is evoked without volition. We have done a number of studies exploring this hypothesis.

In one study (Johnson, Kahan, & Raye, 1984) based on this idea, we had people who lived together report their dreams to each other or report to each other "dreams" that they made up. Then we brought the people into the lab and had them attempt to distinguish their own reports from the reports they had heard from their partners. People experienced more confusion about the source of actual dreams than made up dreams. Our interpretation of this finding is that, compared to dreams made up under voluntary control, memories for real dreams contain less information about the cognitive operations used in the generation process, making them harder to distinguish from memories for perceived events.

The outcome of the dream study was encouraging, but studying dreams does not allow much in the way of experimental control, so we have attempted to manipulate cognitive operations in the lab. That is, our hypothesis is that memories based on normal, waking imagery will be confused with memories for perceived events, depending on how easily the images are generated. We would predict that images that are easier than others to generate would lead to greater confusion in reality monitoring.

We (Finke, Johnson, & Shyi, 1988) explored this idea using forms such as those in Figure 2. Previous studies have shown that subjects can judge symmetry more rapidly for vertically symmetrical patterns than for horizontally symmetrical patterns (e.g., Corballis & Roldan, 1975). This finding suggested to us that if we showed subjects only half of a pattern and had them imagine it as completed, they would find it easier to do this when the form is symmetrical about the vertical axis than when it is symmetrical about the horizontal axis. We confirmed this expectation in a preliminary study in which subjects were shown half forms and were instructed to imagine each half form as being completed about the axis of symmetry to make a symmetrical whole form. Once they had done so, they were to rate how easy or difficult it was to imagine completing the form. As predicted, the mean rated difficulty of completing the forms was less for vertical stimuli than for horizontal stimuli.

In the main experiment, we used the fact that vertical forms are easier to imagine as complete than are horizontal forms to test our prediction that easily generated images are more likely to be confused with perceptions than are images that are more difficult to generate. Some subjects were randomly assigned to an imagery condition, and some to a control condition. In both conditions, subjects saw stimuli in random order for five seconds each. Some of the items were forms presented in whole versions and some were presented in the incomplete versions. Subjects in both conditions were asked to rate the complexity of the forms. Control subjects

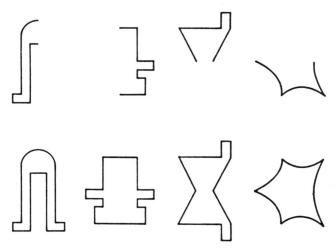

Figure 2. Example of forms used by Finke, Johnson, & Shyi, 1988.

rated each form as it was presented. Imagery subjects also rated the whole forms as presented but were instructed that if the slide contained a half form, they were to imagine it as a completed, symmetrical form, and then rate the complexity of the imagined form.

After completing their ratings, subjects received a surprise memory test. They were shown test patterns in random order consisting of whole forms they had just seen, whole forms corresponding to completions of the half forms they had just seen, and new whole forms. Subjects were asked to indicate whether each pattern had been seen as a whole, contained half of a form they had seen, or had not been shown as a whole or as a half. We explained to the imagery subjects that a form that was presented in half form but completed by imagination should be identified as a half.

First, the data were scored without regard to whether the subject remembered if the form had been presented as a half or a whole. These recognition scores are the number of correct "old" responses plus the number of correct rejections of new items, divided by the total number of test items. The overall proportion correct for this old/new discrimination score was about .72 and there were no differences among conditions. These old-new recognition results make two points. The forms were equally memorable in terms of recognition when presented vertically and when presented horizontally. Second, the performance of the imagery and control groups on old-new recognition was equivalent; hence, any differences between instructional groups in their ability to remember whether forms were presented as halves or wholes can be attributed to differences between groups in reality monitoring rather than in recognition.

To assess reality monitoring, half-whole discrimination scores were also computed. This score reflects the proportion of items identified as old that were also correctly identified as presented in half or whole form. Imagery (.75) and control (.75) subjects did not differ in their ability to discriminate half from whole forms in the horizontal condition, whereas the performance of the imagery (.67) subjects was significantly worse than that of the control (.77) subjects in the vertical condition. The most straightforward interpretation of these results is that reality monitoring is more difficult in the vertical than in the horizontal condition because images of vertically symmetrical forms are more easily constructed; thus the memory for the construction includes less information about cognitive operations. Later, in evaluating the origin of a memory, low values for cognitive operations for imagined as well as perceived events would make it difficult to distinguish them.

In a new series of experiments (Johnson, Finke, Danzer, & Shyi, in preparation), we have manipulated the ease of generation of images in a different way. Stimuli consisted of black and white patterns created by filling in squares on a five by five grid (Figure 3a). Some of the stimuli were familiar alphanumeric characters, and some were unfamiliar patterns. From these whole patterns, two incomplete versions were created. One incomplete version had three missing contiguous squares, each indicated by a dot. The other incomplete version had three missing squares randomly located throughout the figure, also indicated by dots. It should be easier to imagine the completions of familiar than unfamiliar forms, and easier to imagine forms with contiguous rather than random squares missing.

Subjects were shown some whole and some incomplete forms (equal numbers of familiar, unfamiliar, random and contiguous items) for five seconds each. Subjects in the control condition rated the complexity of the patterns as they were presented, ignoring the dots on the incomplete patterns. Subjects in the imagery condition rated the complexity of the whole patterns as presented; they imagined the incomplete patterns as whole by mentally filling in the dots and then rated the complexity of the imagined, whole pattern. This inspection phase was followed by an unexpected memory test in which only whole patterns were shown--some that were presented during the inspection phase, some that were whole versions of the incomplete patterns shown during the inspection phase, and some that were new whole patterns; subjects were asked to indicate which was which.

Again, first consider the old-new recognition. Subjects in the imagery group (.74) were actually better able to discriminate old from completely new forms than were subjects in the control group (.69). In contrast, the control group (.82) was better at discriminating whole from incomplete forms compared to the imagery group (.73). Thus, as in the last experiment, the difficulty imagery subjects had in reality monitoring cannot be attributed to an overall poorer memory for the items as indicated by old/new recognition.

We then looked at a confusion measure that reflects the proportion of items for which subjects claimed to have seen a complete pattern when an incomplete one had been presented (misattributions in Figures 3b and 3c). As you can see in Figure 3b, overall, imagery subjects were more likely to say a whole form had been presented when only half had been. Furthermore, the difference between the imagery and control groups was greater for familiar items than for unfamiliar items. This finding is consistent with the idea that familiar items were easier for the imagery group to imagine and then subsequently harder to discriminate from perceived items. In Figure 3c, imagery and control groups have been combined because for both imagery and control groups the pattern was the same -- no difference between contiguous and random conditions for familiar items, and more misattributions on contiguous than random items for unfamiliar patterns. Both imagery and control subjects were least likely to claim to have seen whole figures when the presented figure was unfamiliar and contained randomly missing squares.

In summary, several factors appear to influence the likelihood that subjects will claim to have seen an entire pattern when only a partial pattern was presented. Familiar patterns, or those with contiguous parts missing, are sometimes spontaneously filled in even without an explicit intention to make images, and then later may be misidentified as patterns actually presented whole. Explicit instructions to engage in imagery increased misattributions but less so for unfamiliar patterns. Our interpretation of this pattern is that imagery subjects were better at reality monitoring for unfamiliar than familiar patterns because unfamiliar patterns require more cognitive operations to fill in; these cognitive operations can later be used to identify oneself as the origin of the completion.

The fact that even control subjects made some misattributions in this last experiment suggests that we not only create images under voluntary control, that is, on purpose, but we also create images spontaneously, elicited by ongoing experiences as a way of filling in, or as a natural byproduct of perception and comprehension. The results of another experiment (Durso & Johnson, 1980) illustrate that such spontaneous imaginations may be the most difficult of all to later distinguish from perceptions. Subjects saw a list consisting of some words and some pictures (line drawings of common objects). Then we gave subjects a surprise test that asked them to indicate whether each item had appeared as a word or a picture (there were new items as well). We varied how the subjects processed the items initially in ways that should have affected later availability of information about cognitive operations. At acquisition, some subjects indicated the function of the referent of each item. For example, if they saw a picture of a knife (or the word knife) they might say "you *cut with* it". Still other subjects identified a particularly relevant feature of each object, for example, *blade* for knife. Other subjects had an artist time judgment task: If a picture was presented, they rated how long it took the artist to draw it. If a

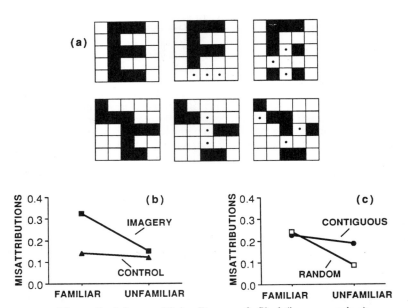

Figure 3. Johnson, Finke, Danzer, & Shyi (in preparation):
(a) Example stimuli are shown;
(b & c) Misattributions are incomplete forms that subjects claimed to have seen as complete forms.

Table 1. Mean Number of Times Subjects Said *Word* Given
the Item Was a Picture (W/P) and *Picture* Given the
Item Was a Word (P/W), Durso & Johnson, 1980.

| | Number of Confusions | |
	W/P	P/W
Function	3.42	13.25
Relevant feature	2.08	11.08
Artist time judgment	5.42	3.50

word was presented, they constructed an image of a line drawing of the referent and then rated
how long it would take the artist to draw the imagined picture.

One important difference between the first two tasks and the last one is that the artist-time
judgment task involves explicit imagery, whereas the function and relevant feature tasks are
likely to involve spontaneous, or incidental imagery. That is, in order to answer a question about
the object's relevant features, you might think of a visual representation of the object and "pick
out" a relevant feature. Explicit images are under voluntary, reflective control and thus the
memories for them should contain more information about cognitive operations than the
memories for spontaneous images. If so, people should later be better able to discriminate
memories of voluntarily constructed images from memories of pictures than they can discriminate
memories of spontaneous images from memories of pictures. The results (Table 1) were
consistent with this prediction. Consider the number of times subjects claimed to have seen a
picture when only a word was shown. In the artist time judgment task, subjects rarely said a
word had been presented as a picture. In the function and relevant feature tasks, they much more
often claimed to have seen pictures of objects that had only been named. Thus spontaneous or
incidental images were more likely to be confused with perceptions than were consciously
constructed ones.

Foley, Durso, Wilder, & Friedman (in press) recently used a similar paradigm with children
to investigate age-related reality monitoring processes. It has often been proposed that children
have a more difficult time than adults distinguishing fact from fantasy. In previous research,
however, we had not found any greater tendency for children, compared with adults, to confuse
pictures they imagined with pictures they perceived (Johnson, Raye, Hasher, & Chromiak,
1979). Foley et al. (in press) considered the possibility that we may have underestimated reality
monitoring failures in children because children might not be as successful as adults at creating
images on demand. If reality monitoring for children's *spontaneous* images were examined,
children might show more confusion than adults. Foley et al., compared 6-year old children and
adults in two tasks, one in which there were explicit imagery instructions and one in which
images would be likely to be spontaneously generated (the function condition). Children, like
adults, were more likely later to confuse spontaneous than purposeful images with perceptions;
and, as in our previous research, the amount of confusion children showed was no more than
that of adults. These results suggest that by the age of six, children are quite sensitive to the
value of cognitive operations as a cue to the origin of memories.

THE SELF

As we have seen, self-generated or reflective activity produces a record of cognitive
operations that can be used in reality monitoring. Let's consider for a few minutes this idea of
"self." Many philosophers and psychologists have tackled the concept of the self. Though not
easy to define (e.g., Bandura, 1982; Greenwald, 1982), the self is the target of a collection of
provocative questions such as: Where does the idea of a self come from (e.g., Bem, 1972;
Gergen, 1977)? Is the self a concept like any other concept or is it a special organizational
structure (e.g., Markus & Sentis, 1982)? How stable is our self-concept (Gergen, 1982)? What
are the consequences of self-awareness (Wicklund, 1982) or self-conceptions (Snyder &
Campbell, 1982)? What role does self play in consciousness (Kihlstrom, 1987; Kunzendorf,
1987) Is the self a unified entity, or, in fact, made up of dissociated selves (Beahrs, 1982;
Hilgard, 1977) or independent subsystems (Greenwald, 1982)? I think that one potentially
interesting feature of MEM is that a number of ideas about self emerge from the architecture of

the system; furthermore, which aspects of self are in the foreground depends on which aspects of MEM we are considering.

Self and Other

First consider the fundamental distinction between self and other. MEM postulates subsystems corresponding to perceptual experience and reflective activity. Reality monitoring is a set of processes that differentiate perceptually derived from reflectively generated information. How critical reality monitoring is for normal functioning becomes obvious when it breaks down markedly as in delusions (Johnson, 1988a) and confabulation (Johnson, in press). It seems reasonable to conclude that reality monitoring processes evolved along with reflective creativity and helped offset potentially dysfunctional confusion between the perceived and the imagined. The self (as originator), as distinguished from that which is perceived, arises naturally as a byproduct of this reality monitoring activity. Of course, the nature of one's experiences, especially one's interactions with others, will greatly influence how this idea of self becomes elaborated (e.g., Higgins, 1987; Markus & Nurius, 1986).

Agency and Self-Regulation

Next consider the important concept of agency. Bandura (1982) has suggested that most of the fundamental questions regarding the nature and functions of the self are concerned with the problem of human agency. "The matters of major interest center on whether, and how, people exert some influence over what they perceive and do (p. 3)." In Bandura's model, self-regulation operates through a set of subfunctions which include self-observation and judgmental processes. That is, to change how one is behaving one must observe one's own behavior and apply internal standards for evaluating it. The kind of self-regulation Bandura describes is possible in MEM because (1) the reflective system can access and evaluate perceptual information in terms of standards activated in the reflective system, and (2) the reflective system has two interacting subsystems, R-1 and R-2 that can evaluate and call on each other. Often R-1 and R-2 simply work toward the same goal, as in many problem solving situations. However, we seem to get a special sense of self-control when an R-2 agenda functions to counteract some ongoing agenda from R-1 as when, for example, an R-2 agenda to lose weight attempts to counteract an R-1 agenda to fix a sandwich. The phenomenal experience from interactive reflective activity is so powerful that, in effect, we often identify ourself with it. That is, we feel our own agency through intention, purpose, volitional action, planning, control, and so forth. These words are short-hand ways of referring to the fact that R-2 recruits and monitors R-1 and vice/versa; at the same time, they refer to the phenomenal experience resulting from this R-1/R-2 interaction.

The Self as Both Subject and Object (Self-Awareness)

Another classic problem of the self is how the self can be both subject and object (or knower and that which is known, James, 1915, cited in Markus & Sentis, p. 44). How such dual functioning is achieved in MEM is not hard to see. One R subsystem can "know" another (i.e., monitor its activities), just as R subsystems can monitor some activities of the perceptual subsystems. The overlapping supervisor and executive functions give us access to our own cognitive operations, from which we derive the phenomenal experience of thinking about ourselves thinking. Such self-awareness, like self-regulation, thus arises from the special relation between R-1 and R-2 subsystems.

Aspects or Styles of Self

We might also suppose, looking at MEM's architecture, that there would be different aspects of self or styles of self. I have been emphasizing that a sense of self arises from reflective control and monitoring of cognitive operations. This self as actor or agent might be called an *instrumental* self. I do not mean to imply, however, that this is the only way a sense of self comes about and is maintained. In addition to an instrumental self, there is another type of self that is suggested by MEM's architecture. This is an *experiential* self that arises from focusing on information from the perceptual subsystems. (The experiential self is, perhaps, something like Hume's idea that the self is nothing but a bundle of perceptions.) Especially important should be those perceptions that give rise to familiarity responses; my relatives, clothes, house, office, friends, car. These familiarity responses contribute to our sense of a temporally extended existence and, thus, to our idea of an ongoing self. A person's "autobiography" arises from both experiential activity and instrumental activity. One difference in the consequences of these two types of activities is that a primarily experiential focus might produce a sense of *fate* about what happens to us and who we are, whereas a primarily instrumental focus might produce a sense of *choice*. In any event, the idea of instrumental vs. experiential focus could characterize reasonably stable differences in self concepts across individuals, or differences in aspects of the self that are salient within the same individual at different times.

Styles of Self and Reality Monitoring

Returning now to reality monitoring, we might speculate that experiential and instrumental styles of self would be associated with characteristic differences in primary mode of reality monitoring, that is, whether R-1 or R-2 reality monitoring processes are more likely to be used. An experiential focus might be associated with using qualitative characteristics of mental experience, particularly perceptual detail or vividness as the major criteria for veridicality. An instrumental focus, in contrast, might be associated with relying more on the plausibility relations between what is remembered and what is otherwise known. Thus we might find different types of reality monitoring errors associated with differences in the types of self concept people have since such differences in self concept presumably arise from habitual modes of exercising one's cognitive architecture.

SUMMARY

According to MEM, the overall architecture of the cognitive system is an integrated configuration of perceptual and reflective processes that permits interaction as well as some degree of independence among subsystems (P-1, P-2, R-1, R-2) defined in terms of these processes. Normally, subsystems work together and account for our ability to engage in complex tasks, many of which (e.g., playing tennis, writing research papers, and responding appropriately to the feelings of others) require learning in more than one subsystem (Johnson, 1983). At the same time, the potential for MEM's subsystems to work without reference to each other (i.e., from different cues) helps explicate phenomena such as dissociations among memory measures (Johnson, 1983), variations in cognitive contributions to emotional responses (Johnson & Multhaup, in press), and selective disruption of memory such as occurs in anterograde amnesia patients (Johnson, 1990; Johnson & Hirst, in press).

Here, I have focused on one aspect of cognition that arises from the MEM architecture, namely on the possibility that information from perceptual and reflective subsystems might be confused, and on the reality monitoring processes that help offset this potential confusion (Johnson, 1988, in press; Johnson & Raye, 1981). There are two major classes of reality monitoring processes. Processes controlled by R-1 make relatively quick attributions about the origin of information based on appraising the qualitative characteristics of memories such as perceptual and contextual detail and information about cognitive operations that is available. Reality monitoring processes controlled by R-2 engage in retrieval and evaluation of additional information and consider such things as plausibility in light of antecedents, consequences, and general world knowledge. To illustrate empirical work on reality monitoring, I described research indicating that records of reflective cognitive operations later serve as evidence that we were the source of information in memory.

Finally, I suggested that the idea of a self derives from the MEM architecture via several mechanisms. A self is a byproduct of reality monitoring processes that distinguish perceptually-derived from reflectively-generated information. That is, self-as-source is a category that emerges from the reflective/perceptual dichotomy. Second, self as a phenomenal experience is associated with the mental activity of reflective control and monitoring, especially, from interactions between R-1 and R-2 in which they recruit and regulate each other. Third, this capacity for agency is embedded within an overall cognitive system that does not depend on reflective control and monitoring for all its critical activities. Consequently, in addition to an instrumental self that arises from records of reflective activity, an experiential self arises from records of what we have perceived. Thus, as in the case of other cognitive products, selves may vary in the relative contributions that perceptual and reflective processes make to their character.

REFERENCES

Bandura, A. (1982). The self and mechanisms of agency. In J. Suls (Ed.),*Psychological perspectives on the self, vol. 1*. Hillsdale, NJ: Erlbaum.

Beahrs, J. O. (1982). *Unity and multiplicity: Multilevel consciousness of self in hypnosis, psychiatric disorder and mental health*. New York: Brunner/Mazel.

Bem, D. J. (1972). Self-perception theory. In L. Berkowitz (Ed.), *Advances in experimental social psychology, vol. 6*. New York: Academic Press.

Bentall, R. P. (1990). The illusion of reality: A review and integration of psychological research on hallucinations. *Psychological Bulletin, 107*, 82-95.

Cermak, L. S. (Ed.). (1982). *Human memory and amnesia*. Hillsdale, NJ: Erlbaum.

Corballis, M. C., & Roldan, C. E. (1975). Detection of symmetry as a function of angular orientation. *Journal of Experimental Psychology: Human Perception & Performance, 1*, 221-230.

Craik, F. I. M. (1986). A functional account of age differences in memory. In F. Klix & H. Hagendorf (Eds.), *Human memory and cognitive capabilities* (pp. 409-422). Amsterdam: North Holland.

Durso, F. T., & Johnson, M. K. (1980). The effects of orienting tasks on recognition, recall, and modality confusion of pictures and words. *Journal of Verbal Learning and Verbal Behavior, 19*, 416-429.

Eich, J. E. (1975). State-dependent accessibility of retrieval cues in the retention of a categorized list. *Journal of Verbal Learning and Verbal Behavior, 14*, 408-417.

Finke, R. A., Johnson, M. K., & Shyi, G. C.-W. (1988). Memory confusions for real and imagined completions of symmetrical visual patterns. *Memory &Cognition, 16*, 133-137.

Finke, R. A., & Shepard, R. N. (1986). Visual functions of mental imagery. In K. R. Boff, L. Kaufman, & J. P. Thomas (Eds.), *Handbook of perception and human performance, vol. 2*. New York: Wiley-Interscience.

Flavell, J. H. (1985). *Cognitive development* (2nd Edition). Englewood Cliffs, NJ: Prentice Hall.

Foley, M. A., Durso, F. T., Wilder, A., & Friedman, R. (in press). Developmental comparisons of explicit vs. implicit imagery and reality monitoring. *Journal of Experimental Child Psychology*.

Gergen, K. J. (1977). The social construction of self-knowledge. In T. Mischel (Ed.), *The self: Psychological and philosophical issues*. Totowa, NJ: Rowman & Littlefield.

Gergen, K. J. (1982). From self to science: What is there to know? In J. Suls (Ed.), *Psychological perspectives on the self, vol. 1* (pp. 129-149). Hillsdale, NJ: Erlbaum.

Greenwald, A. G. (1982). Is anyone in charge? Personalysis versus the principle of personal unity. In J. Suls (Ed.), *Psychological perspectives on the self, vol. 1* (pp. 151-181). Hillsdale, NJ: Erlbaum.

Hasher, L., & Zacks, R. T. (1979). Automatic and effortful processes in memory. *Journal of Experimental Psychology, 108*, 356-388.

Hasher, L., & Zacks, R. T. (1984). Automatic processing of fundamental information: The case of frequency of occurrence. *American Psychologist, 39*, 1372-1388.

Hashtroudi, S., & Parker, E. S. (1986). Acute alcohol amnesia: What is remembered and what is forgotten. In H. D. Cappell, F. B. Glaser, Y. Israel, et. al. (Eds.), *Research advances in alcohol and drug problems, vol. 9*. New York: Plenum.

Higgins, E. T. (1987). Self-discrepancy: A theory relating self and affect. *Psychological Review, 94*, 319-340.

Hilgard, E. R. (1977). *Divided consciousness: Multiple controls in human thought and action*. New York: Wiley.

Hirst, W., Johnson, M. K., Kim, J. K., Phelps, E. A., Risse, G., & Volpe, B. T. (1986). Recognition and recall in amnesics. *Journal of Experimental Psychology: Learning, Memory, and Cognition, 12*, 445-451.

Hirst, W., Johnson, M. K., Phelps, E. A., & Volpe, B. T. (1988). More on recall and recognition in amnesia. *Journal of Experimental Psychology: Learning, Memory, and Cognition, 14*, 758-762.

Horowitz, M. J. (1978). *Image formation and cognition* (2nd Edition). New York: Appleton-Century-Crofts.

James, W. (1915). *Psychology, a briefer course*. New York: Holt.

Johnson, M. K. (1977). What is being counted none the less? In I. M. Birnbaum & E. S. Parker (Eds.), *Alcohol and human memory* (pp. 43-57). Hillsdale, NJ: Erlbaum.

Johnson, M. K. (1983). A multiple-entry, modular memory system. In G. H. Bower (Ed.), *The psychology of learning and motivation, 17* (pp. 81-123). New York: Academic Press.

Johnson, M. K. (1985). The origin of memories. In P. C. Kendall (Ed.), *Advances in cognitive-behavioral research and therapy, (Vol. 4)* (pp. 1-26). New York: Academic Press.

Johnson, M. K. (1988a). Discriminating the origin of information. In T. F. Oltmanns, & B. A. Maher (Eds.), *Delusional beliefs: Interdisciplinary perspectives* (pp. 34-65). New York: John Wiley & Sons.

Johnson, M. K. (1988b). Reality monitoring: An experimental phenomenological approach. *Journal of Experimental Psychology: General, 117*, 390-394.

Johnson, M. K. (1990). Functional forms of human memory. In J. L. McGaugh, N. M. Weinberger, & G. Lynch (Eds.), *Brain organization and memory: Cells, systems and circuits* (pp. 106-134). New York: Oxford University Press.

Johnson, M. K. (in press). Reality monitoring: Evidence from confabulation in organic brain disease patients. In G. Prigatano & D. L. Schacter (Eds.), *Awareness of deficit after brain injury*. New York: Oxford University Press.

Johnson, M. K., Finke, R. A., Danzer, A., & Shyi, G. C.-W. (in preparation). Ease of imaging and reality monitoring.

Johnson, M. K., Foley, M. A., & Leach, K. (1988). The consequences for memory of imagining in another person's voice. *Memory & Cognition, 16*, 337-342.

Johnson, M. K., Foley, M. A., Suengas, A. G., & Raye, C. L. (1988). Phenomenal characteristics of memories for perceived and imagined autobiographical events. *Journal of Experimental Psychology: General, 117*, 371-376.

Johnson, M. K., & Hirst, W. (in press). Processing subsystems of memory. In R. G. Lister & J. J. Weingartner, *Perspectives in cognitive neuroscience*. New York: Oxford University Press.

Johnson, M. K., Kahan, T. L., & Raye, C. L. (1984). Dreams and reality monitoring. *Journal of Experimental Psychology: General, 113*, 329-344.

Johnson, M. K., & Kim, J. K. (1985). Recognition of pictures by alcoholic Korsakoff patients. *Bulletin of the Psychonomic Society, 23*, 456-458.

Johnson, M. K., Kim, J. K., & Risse, G. (1985). Do alcoholic Korsakoff patients acquire affective reactions? *Journal of Experimental Psychology: Learning, Memory, and Cognition, 11*, 22-36.

Johnson, M. K., & Multhaup, K. S. (in press). Emotion and MEM. In S. A. Christianson (Ed.), *Handbook of emotion and memory*.

Johnson, M. K., & Raye, C. L. (1981). Reality monitoring. *Psychological Review, 88*, 67-85.

Johnson, M. K., Raye, C. L., Foley, H. J., & Foley, M. A. (1981). Cognitive operations and decision bias in reality monitoring. *American Journal of Psychology, 94*, 37-64.

Johnson, M. K., Raye, C. L., Hasher, L., & Chromiak, W. (1979). Are there developmental differences in reality-monitoring? *Journal of Experimental Child Psychology, 27*, 120-128.

Johnson, M. K., Raye, C. L., Wang, A. Y., & Taylor, T. H. (1979). Fact and fantasy: The roles of accuracy and variability in confusing imaginations with perceptual experience. *Journal of Experimental Psychology: Human Learning and Memory, 5*, 229-240.

Johnson, M. K., Taylor, T. H., & Raye, C. L. (1977). Fact and fantasy: The effects of internally generated events on the apparent frequency of externally generated events. *Memory & Cognition, 5*, 116-122.

Kihlstrom, J. F. (1987). The cognitive unconscious. *Science, 237*, 1445-1452.

Kosslyn, S. M. (1980). *Image and mind.* Cambridge, MA: Harvard University Press.

Kunzendorf, R. G. (1986). Hypnotic hallucinations as "unmonitored" images: An empirical study. *Imagination, Cognition and Personality, 5*, 255-270.

Kunzendorf, R. G. (1987). Self-consciousness as the monitoring of cognitive states: A theoretical perspective. *Imagination, Cognition and Personality, 7*, 3-22.

Markus, H., & Nurius, P. (1986). Possible selves. *American Psychologist, 41*, 954-969.

Markus, H., & Sentis, K. (1982). The self in social information processing. In J. Suls (Ed.), *Psychological perspectives on the self, vol. 1* (pp. 41-70). Hillsdale, NJ: Erlbaum.

Miller, G. A., Galanter, E., & Pribram, K. A. (1960). *Plans and the structure of behavior.* New York: Holt, Rhinehart & Winston.

Moscovitch, M. (1985). Memory from infancy to old age: implications for theories of normal and pathological memory. *Annals of the New York Academy of Sciences, 444*, 78-96.

Nelson, T. O., & Narens, L. (1990). Metamemory: A theoretical framework and some new findings. In G. Bower (Ed.), *The psychology of learning and motivation*.

15

Norman, D. A., & Shallice, T. (1986). Attention to action: Willed and automatic control of behavior. In R. J. Davidson, G. E. Schwartz, & D. Shapiro, *Consciousness and self-regulation* (pp. 1-18). New York: Plenum.

Perlmutter, M. (1984). Continuities and discontinuities in early human memory paradigms, processes, and performance. In R. Kail, & N. E. Spear (Eds.), *Comparative perspectives on the development of memory* (pp. 253-284). Hillsdale, NJ: Erlbaum.

Rabinowitz, J. C. (1989). Judgments of origin and generation effects: Comparisons between young and elderly adults. *Psychology and Aging, 4,* 1-10.

Schacter, D. L., & Moscovitch, M. (1984). Infants, amnesics, and dissociable memory systems. In M. Moscovitch (Ed.), *Infant memory* (pp. 173-216). New York: Plenum Press.

Shiffrin, R. M., & Schneider, W. (1977). Controlled and automatic human information processing: II. Perceptual learning, automatic attending, and a general theory. *Psychological Review, 84,* 127-190.

Snyder, M., & Campbell, B. H. (1982). Self-monitoring: The self in action. In J. Suls (Ed.), *Psychological perspectives on the self, vol. 1* (pp. 185-207). Hillsdale, NJ: Erlbaum.

Stuss, D. T., & Benson, D. F. (1986). *The frontal lobes.* New York: Raven Press.

Tulving, E. (1983). *Elements of episodic memory.* New York: Oxford University Press.

Weinstein, A. (1987). *Preserved recognition memory in amnesia.* Unpublished doctoral dissertation, State University of New York at Stony Brook.

Wicklund, R. A. (1982). How society uses self-awareness. In J. Suls (Ed.), *Psychological perspectives on the self, vol. 1* (pp. 209-230). Hillsdale, NJ: Erlbaum.

THE IMPORTANCE OF MENTAL IMAGERY IN MAP READING

Laura L. Snodgrass, Ph.D.

Psychology Department
Muhlenberg College
Allentown, PA 18104

INTRODUCTION

How do we relate what we see in a map to the world around us? A map provides a bird's eye view of an extended area with the spatial relationships presented in terms of two-dimensional euclidean geometry. As we look out into the world, we are presented with a horizontal or straight-on view of a limited area -- the extended view is usually cut off by buildings or trees or other objects, and the spatial relationships are presented in terms of perspective geometry. I am currently investigating how people translate between the bird's eye view with two dimensional euclidean geometry and the horizontal or straight-on view with perspective geometry.

Perkins (1983) points out that people are not very good perceptual geometers. In a wide variety of tasks subjects were not very accurate at judging shape, slant or other geometrical properties of visual stimuli. Intuitively, it seems unlikely that we work directly with mathematical translations of the geometry. One way that we might manipulate the information provided in a map is to work with an analog mental representation. There is abundant evidence that people make mental representations of their environments and use this stored information to navigate (Downs & Stea, 1977; Evans, Marrero, & Butler,1981; Foley & Cohen, 1984; Lieblich & Arbib, 1982; Presson & Hazelrigg, 1984). Tolman (1948) referred to the mental representation of spatial information as a "cognitive map".

One of the important questions has been whether cognitive maps are visual images. The name itself, cognitive map, implies an analogy to a real map, which is certainly a visual stimulus. Evidence that the blind have a spatial representation and are capable of the behaviors used to assess spatial knowledge indicates that the representation is not necessarily visual (Dodds, Howarth & Carter, 1982; Herman, Chatman, & Roth, 1983; Strelow, 1985). However, sighted subjects show a clear superiority in their ability to gather and use spatial information (Fletcher, 1980; Millar, 1976; Rosencranz & Suslick, 1976). Therefore, we can conclude that a visual representation is normally used. I am proposing that a visual image, similar to a cognitive map, is used to translate between a map and what we see around us.

A visual image would allow you to perform analog operations on the map. As mentioned earlier, mathematically translating between the two dimensional euclidean geometry of a bird's eye view map and the perspective geometry of the horizontal view is too complicated a process to be used in common map reading. However, the two view points can be smoothly rotated into each other. That is, if you took the bird's eye view and rotated it away from the vertical you would get the perspective view. People might be able to use the visual image to rotate between the two view points The question then is whether people can rotate a complex spatial configuration such as a map.

We know from the work of Cooper and Shepard (1973) that people can smoothly rotate mental images. Cooper (1975), Cooper and Podgorny (1976), and Shwartz (cited in Kosslyn 1980) have shown that people can rotate complex polygons. Shepard and Metzler (1971) have shown that people can even rotate three dimensional polygons. Pylyshyn (1979) and Kosslyn

(1980) did experiments on mental rotation using figures with subparts, internal patterns or overlapping figures. Clearly, people have the capability to rotate fairly complex mental images. However, all of the stimuli used in the preceeding experiments were line drawings and had a degree of inherent unity--that is, they tended to be one object, no matter how complex. It was not clear that people could or would try to rotate a spatial array of independent objects. A map differs from the previously mentioned stimuli in that it is a representation of independent objects (buildings, trees, streets, etc.) and the spatial relationships between these objects. In addition, when people try to translate between a map and what they see they must translate from a two dimensional graphical representation to a three dimensional pictorial view. One study that does deal with independent objects and differences in perspective was done by Pinker and Finke (1980). They had subjects make a mental image of four objects suspended in a three dimensional space. The subjects' task was to describe the two dimensional pattern that resulted from rotating their image of the four objects. Pinker and Finke found that their subjects were able to rotate the three dimensional image into a two dimensional image. The current experiment was designed to investigate whether people could or would mentally rotate map-like stimuli.

PRETEST

Method

Subjects. Twenty eight undergraduates from New College of the University of South Florida were paid to participate in this experiment. Thirteen of the subjects were female and fifteen were male.
Apparatus. An Apple IIe microcomputer was used to present stimuli and collect responses. The stimuli were presented on a Video 100 black and white monitor.
Stimuli. Nine different letters of the alphabet (B, C, E, G, J, K, L, P, R) were presented in six different degrees of rotation (0, 30, 60, 90, 120, 150). All of the rotations were measured from the upright going clockwise.
Procedure. Each subject started with a simple mental rotation task similar to that used by Cooper and Shepard (1973). Letters were presented one at a time and the subjects had to respond as quickly as possible whether the letters were "standard" or "reflected" (mirror image). Subjects responded by pressing keys on the computer keyboard, s for standard or m for mirror image.

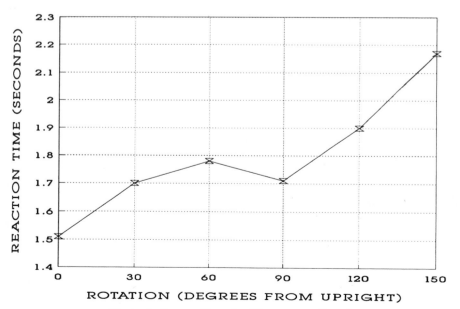

Figure 1. Pretest: Reaction Time versus Rotation

18

Results

The pretest was done to insure that all subjects were capable of doing mental rotation. Six of the subjects were dropped after the pretest. The subjects who were dropped had extreme difficulty with the task and had reaction times greater than three standard deviations above the mean of the group.

The results from the remaining 22 subjects showed an increase in reaction time with increasing degrees of rotation. These results are shown in Figure 1. The one-way repeated measures analysis of variance showed a significant difference in reaction time based on degree of rotation, $F(5,105) = 8.22$, $p<.001$. People familiar with the mental rotation literature may notice that I did not get the straight line function usually reported. Subjects in the previously published experiments had extensive practice before any data were collected. My subjects did not have any practice and therefore had a great deal more variability in their reaction times. It was sufficient for my purposes that the subjects show an increase in reaction time with increasing degrees of rotation.

MAIN EXPERIMENT

Method

Subjects. The 22 subjects who passed the pretest participated in this experiment.

Apparatus. An Apple IIe microcomputer controlled the experiment and collected the subjects' responses. The stimuli were presented using two Kodak Carousel 650 slide projectors interfaced to the microcomputer.

Stimuli. The stimuli were slides taken of three dimensional styrofoam objects on a circular surface. Both the objects and the surface were white. Each slide used five distinct objects: a ball, a sliced-off cone, a cone, a semi-circle, and a triangle. The circular surface was 90 centimeters in diameter and the objects ranged in size from 7.5 centimeters in diameter (the ball) to 18.75 centimeters (the long axis of the triangle).

There were ten different configurations of these objects. Each of the ten configurations was photographed from five different viewpoints: the bird's eye view (0 degrees), 22 degrees down from the bird's eye, 45 degrees down, 66 degrees down and 90 degrees down which brings you to the horizontal view. An additional set of slides contained the bird's eye view; however, rather than using the actual objects the name of each object was typed in the appropriate location. These last slides are equivalent to a map or diagram of the configuration.

All but the diagram stimuli were also photographed in two more ways: with two of the five objects exchanging positions and with one of the objects moved fifteen centimeters out of position. These last slides formed part of the set of "different" stimuli for the comparison task. Three types of differences were used in the comparison task. The arrangement could have been a mirror image: similar to the pretest. One of the objects could have been displaced fifteen centimeters: this encouraged the subjects to attend to the specific spatial arrangement. Two of the objects could have been interchanged: this encouraged the subjects to attend to which specific object was at each location. The three variations were used to encourage subjects to be as careful as possible about encoding the stimuli.

Procedure. The slides were projected on a white wall 2.89 meters in front of the subjects. The slides were shown in sequential pairs. The first slide in a pair was either the bird's eye view of the objects, the diagram, or the horizontal view of the objects. The second slide in the pair was any one of the five rotations of the same arrangement or one of the different versions of the arrangement. Subjects viewed thirty pairs that were the same and thirty pairs that were different. The pairs of slides were numbered one through sixty. Half the subjects saw the slides in numerical order, and half saw them in reverse numerical order.

For each trial the first slide was shown for five seconds and after a three second interval the second slide was shown. Subjects were instructed to indicate quickly and accurately whether the slides were the same or different. The subjects were given lengthy instructions about what the stimuli looked like and what kinds of differences to expect.

Results

Figure 2 shows the reaction times for the mental rotation of the objects displays. Note that the abscissa (x -axis) is degree of rotation from the first view, which would be different images

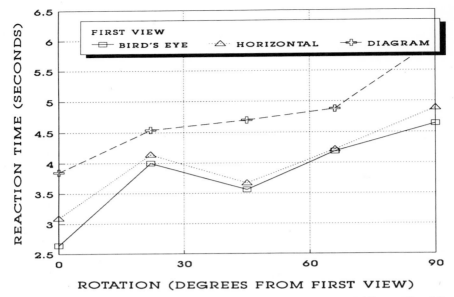

Figure 2. Main Experiment: Reaction Time versus Rotation for Three Different First Views

depending on whether subjects started with the bird's eye or the horizontal view. A two-way repeated measures analysis of variance showed a significant main effect of degree of rotation, $F(4, 84) = 53.39$, p< .001. There was an increase in reaction time with increasing degrees of rotation. There was also a significant main effect of view, $F(2,42) = 11.85$ p< .001. On the average it took the same amount of time to rotate to the horizontal view as to the bird's eye view. However, it took the subjects significantly longer to match up a given view to the map-like diagram. The interaction between the variables was not significant.

The subjects' error rates were also analyzed. There was no significant difference in number of errors for the different starting configurations. Across all subjects there were a total of 17 errors for the bird's eye view (a 4% error rate), 11 errors for the horizontal view (a 3% error rate) and 17 errors for the diagram (a 4% error rate). In fact, 57% of all the errors were accounted for by three subjects. Out of a total of 45 errors, subject #11 had 6 errors, subject # 13 had 12 errors and subject # 18 had 8 errors. No other individual subject made more than 3 errors.

CONCLUSIONS

The increase in reaction time with increasing degrees of rotation is consistent with the accepted results of Cooper and Shepard (and many others) which indicate that subjects can translate between the different views by means of mental rotation. It is interesting that subjects can rotate with equal speed to either the bird's eye or horizontal view. Intuitively, it seems more difficult to judge the spatial relationships from the horizontal viewpoint. However, neither the subjects' speed nor accuracy reflected any difficulty in dealing with the horizontal viewpoint. Subjects did take longer to translate between the slides of the actual objects and the diagram. This condition is most similar to the situation of using a map. Translating from the diagram to the horizontal view took the longest amount of time, an average of 5.97 seconds. This particular condition represents a simplified version of what someone might do when looking from a map to their surroundings.

It should be noted that the type of diagram used, simply having the names typed in the appropriate locations, would be one of the most difficult to interpret. Most maps, such as you would get of a college campus or city downtown area, provide you with outline drawings of buildings to give you a sense of their size and orientation. It would be interesting to replicate the study with diagrams that did provide outlines to see if that would reduce the translation time.

This experiment indicates that mental rotation is one way that subjects might translate between a map and their view of the surroundings. However, it does not indicate that subjects necessarily use mental rotation with maps. I was rather surprised that subjects seemed to use mental rotation for this task. I thought that with multiple independent objects to view subjects might do a more piecemeal comparison process. However, I did use only five objects. Real maps present a much more complicated array and more types of information (roads, buildings, parks, etc.) to be manipulated.

This experiment dealt with one type of mental manipulation of maps, rotations in depth. There have been other experiments done looking at other types of mental "reorientations" of maps. Shepard and Hurwitz (1984) found that subjects had to mentally rotate a map to correctly interpret left and right turns when the line they were following was not going toward the top of the map. Levine, Jankovic and Palij (1982) looked at a variety of situations in which the top of the map did not correspond to straight ahead in the environment. In these situations subjects had to mentally rotate the map in order to successfully use it for navigation. These studies provide support for the idea that subjects can mentally rotate maps. However, the rotations done in these studies are within the plane and do not change the geometric perspective. The rotations in depth required in my study are more complicated in that they introduce changes in perspective and in occlusions of the various objects.

Presumably, subjects rotate the map within the plane in order to match up the relative spatial locations of objects on the map to the corresponding objects they see in front of them. Alignment of the objects on the map with the objects in the environment may be a prerequisite to the more complicated rotation in depth. It would be interesting to do a study in which rotations both in the plane and in depth were required and to see if the reaction time for both rotations was the sum of the reactions times for each type of rotation.

In discussions about map reading a number of people have stated they do not rotate an image. These people claim to imagine themselves standing at the appropriate position and to imagine what they would see from that location. It is not clear how they derive the information to construct the image. Some sort of translation of the map information must be going on. There are probably a variety of strategies for using the information in a map. As illustrated by the pretest, not everyone can do mental rotation. These people would have to use some other method to work with a map. There is much more research to be done on the types of strategies people use to interpret maps; and on the degree to which mental imagery is an important component of map reading ability.

REFERENCES

Cooper, L. (1975). Mental rotation of random two-dimensional shapes. *Cognitive Psychology, 7*, 20-43.

Cooper, L., & Podgorny, P. (1976). Mental transformations and visual comparison processes: effects of complexity and similarity. *Journal of Experimental Psychology: Human Perception and Performance, 2*, 503-514.

Cooper, L., & Shepard, R. N. (1973). Chronometric studies of the rotation of mental images. In W. G. Chase (Ed.), *Visual information processing*. New York: Academic Press.

Dodds, A. G., Howarth, C. I., & Carter, D. C. (1982). The mental maps of the blind: The role of previous visual experience. *Journal of Visual Impairment and Blindness, 76* (1), 5-12.

Downs, R. M., & Stea, D. (1977). *Maps in mind*. New York: Harper & Row.

Evans, G. W., Marrero, D. G., & Butler, P. A. (1981). Environmental learning and cognitive mapping. *Environment and behavior, 13* (1), 83-104.

Fletcher, J. F. (1980). Spatial representation in blind children. 1:Development compared to sighted children. *Journal of Visual Impairment and Blindness, 74* (10), 381-385.

Foley, J., & Cohen, A. (1984). Working mental representations of the environment. *Environment and Behavior, 16* (6), 713-729.

Herman, J. F., Chapman, S. P., & Roth, S. F. (1983). Cognitive mapping in blind people: Acquisition of spatial relationship in a large-scale environment. *Journal of Visual Impairment and Blindness, 77* (4), 161-166.

Kosslyn, S. M. (1980). *Image and mind*. Massachusetts: HarvardUniversity Press.

Levine, M., Jankovic, I. N., & Palij, M. (1982). Principles of spatial problem solving. *Journal of Experimental Psychology: General, 111*, 157-175.

Lieblich, I., & Arbib, M. A. (1982). Multiple representations of space underlying behavior. *Behavioral and Brain Sciences, 5*, 627-659.

Millar, S. (1976). Spatial representation by blind and sighted children. *Journal of Experimental Child Psychology, 21*, 460-470.

Perkins, D. N. (1983).Why the human perceiver is a bad machine. In Beck, J., Hope, B., & Rosenfeld, A. (Eds.), *Human andmachine vision*. New York: Academic Press.

Pinker, S., & Finke, R. A. (1980). Emergent two-dimensional patterns in images rotated in depth. *Journal of Experimental Psychology: Human Perception and Performance, 6* (2), 244-264.

Presson, C. C., & Hazelrigg, M. D. (1984). Building spatial representation through primary and secondary learning. *Journal of Experimental Psychology: Learning, Memory, and Cognition, 10* (4), 716-722.

Pylyshyn, Z. W. (1979a). The rate of "mental rotation" of images: a test of a holistic analogue hypothesis. *Memory and Cognition, 7*, 19-28.

Rosencranz, D., & Suslick, R. (1976). Cognitive models for spatial representations in congenitally blind, adventitiously blind, and sighted subjects. *The New Outlook, 70* (5), 188-194.

Shepard, R. N., & Hurwitz, S. (1984). Upward direction, mental rotation, and discrimination of left and right turns in maps. *Cognition, 18*, 161-193.

Shepard R. N., & Metzler, J. (1971). Mental rotation of three dimensional objects. *Science, 171*, 701-703.

Strelow, E. R. (1985). What is needed for a theory of mobility: Direct perception and cognitive maps - Lessons from the blind. *Psychological Review, 92* (2), 226-248.

Tolman, E. C. (1948). Cognitive maps in rats and men. *Psychological Review, 55*, 189-208.

AGING, IMAGERY, AND IMAGERY VIVIDNESS IN DAYDREAMS:

CROSS-SECTIONAL AND LONGITUDINAL PERSPECTIVES

Leonard M. Giambra, Ph.D., and Alicia Grodsky, Ph.D.

Gerontology Research Center
National Institute on Aging
Baltimore, Maryland 21224

There are two salient components of mental imagery and aging: the spontaneous occurrence of images and the deliberate evocation and mental manipulation of images. Of specific interest in this study is the frequency, clarity and semblance to reality of visual and auditory images in daydreams as a function of age. When asked to use images to increase memory it has been generally shown that the elderly are capable of utilizing such a strategy (see Poon, Walsh-Sweeney, & Fozard for a review). However, Hulicka and Grossman (1967) have reported that the spontaneous use of visual imagery in memorization tasks is less likely to occur in the elderly as opposed to younger individuals. Hulicka and Grossman's results have formed the basis for the frequent claim that the elderly are less likely than the young to have spontaneous imagery--see for example, Pierce & Storandt (1988) and Poon et al (1980). There does not appear to be any independent corroboration of Hulicka and Grossman's claim. Indeed, Wood and Pratt (1987) have reported virtually the same percentage of subjects spontaneously using imagery in a memory task in both young (8%) and elderly (7%) subjects.

Pierce and Storandt (1988) looked at self-rated imagery vividness, as measured by a shortened form of the Betts Questionnaire Upon Mental Imagery, in young and elderly women. Both the young and the elderly reported equally high vividness in their visual and auditory imagery. Participants were also asked to imagine specific visual scenes using the Gordon Test of Visual Imagery Control. Young women reported more success in imagining the scenes than did the elderly women yet the difference was not significant. The elderly women were however significantly less likely to be successful in a mental rotation task, the Object Rotation test of the Schaie-Thurstone Adult Mental Abilities Test. Schaie and Labouvie-Vief (1974) have reported both cross-sectional differences and longitudinal changes, after 70 years, in mental rotation using essentially the same test. Gaylord and Marsh (1975) have also shown that the elderly produce more errors and work slower than the young on a mental rotation task.

In summary, it appears that there is no consistent evidence that the elderly are less likely to spontaneously produce imagery during verbal learning tasks like paired-associates. However, there is more consistent evidence indicating that the elderly experience more difficulty--than the young--manipulating images when requested to do so. Nonetheless, when asked to construct images linking the stimulus and response components of a paired associate the elderly seem to be as successful as the young in terms of improved memory performance.

Another source of information on age differences in frequency of the spontaneous occurrence of images comes from retrospective self-reports of imagery during daydreaming. Giambra (1977-78, 1979-80) has reported, using the Imaginal Processes Inventory (IPI), that both visual and auditory imagery in daydreams, as well as imagery vividness, had significant negative correlations with age. The largest age differences were found to occur after age 25 years and after age 70 years. Parks, Klinger, & Perlmutter (1988-89) also reported less visual imagery in daydreams in an old (60-82 years) than in a young (17-28 years) sample. These outcomes support the view that increased age results in decreased likelihood of spontaneous imagery. The present study examines likelihood and vividness of imagery in daydreams in another life span sample of men and women. Furthermore, intraindividual change is investigated by obtaining imagery and daydream vividness measures at two points separated by six to eight years.

METHOD

Subjects

There were two samples. The first or "Cross-Sectional Sample" included 908 men and 1153 women who took the IPI for the first time during a 1972-1976 period and a 1979-1984 period. Most of the Cross-Sectional Sample was drawn from participants in the Baltimore Longitudinal Study of Aging (BLSA), (Shock et al., 1984) at the Gerontology Research Center of the National Institute on Aging. The participants who were sampled during the 1972-1976 period were previously reported in Giambra (1977-78, 1979-80). The 18-23 year-old members of the sample were students recruited from Miami Univ. of Ohio, Towson State Univ. of Maryland, Community College of Baltimore, and Notre Dame College of Maryland. The sample was predominantly Caucasian, Protestant, middle- to upper-middle class, with at least some college education. For purposes of analysis, nine age groups were composed: 18-23 years (men = 337, women = 499), 24-29 (m = 53, w = 86), 30-35 (m = 83, w = 117), 36-41 (m = 65, w =103), 42-47 (m = 61, w = 79), 48-53 (m = 80, w = 65), 54-59 (m = 81, w = 80), 60-65 (m = 94, w = 72), and 66-71 (m = 54, w = 52). The second or "Longitudinal Sample" consisted of 113 women and 173 men assembled into eight age groups based upon age at the first time of testing: 20-29 years (m = 10, w = 16), 30-35 (m = 19, w = 18), 36-41 (m = 19, w = 16), 42-47 (m = 19, w = 8), 48-53 (m = 26, w = 16), 54-59 (m = 26, w = 13), 60-65 (m = 36, w = 16), and 66-71 (m = 18, w = 10). These subjects are a subsample of the Cross-Sectional Sample. The IPI was first taken between 1972-1976 and was taken for the second time 6 to 8 years later.

The majority of men were participants in the Baltimore Longitudinal Study of Aging (BLSA; Shock, Greulich, Andres et al, 1984) at the Gerontology Research Center of the National Institute on Aging in Baltimore, Maryland. Some of the women were also participants in the BLSA but most were recruited from communities in the Baltimore/Washington D.C. corridor. The vast majority of participants in the sample were Caucasian, middle- or upper-middle-class individuals with at least one year of post-high-school education. All were unpaid volunteers.

Table 1. Sample items from the Visual Imagery Scale, the Auditory Imagery Scale, and the Hallucinatory-Vividness Scale of the IPI

Sample items from the Visual Imagery in Daydreams Scale

1. I can see the people or things in my daydreams as if they were moving around.
2. The "pictures in my mind" seem as clear as photographs.

Sample items from the Auditory Imagery in Daydreams Scale

1. The sounds I hear in my daydreams are clear and distinct.
2. I can hear music with shades of softness and loudness in my daydreams.

Sample items from the Hallucinatory-Vividness of Daydreams Scale

1. My daydreams are so clear that I often believe the people in them are in the room.
2. It is hard to distinguish my daydreams from what is actually happening in real life.

The five options for each item are:

0. Definitely not true for me
1. Usually not true for me
2. Usually true for me
3. True for me
4. Very true for me.

Each scale has 12 items so that a minimum scale value is zero and a maximum is 48.

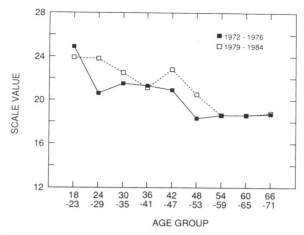

Figure 1. Mean Age Group Values for the Visual Imagery Scale
for the 1972-76 and 1979-84 Date of Testing Cohorts:
Women, Cross-Sectional Sample.

Procedure

The extent to which daydreams include visual and auditory imagery was obtained from responses to the items of Scales 7 and 8, respectively, of the Imaginal Processes Inventory (IPI; Singer & Antrobus, 1970). The vividness or clarity and semblance to reality of visual and auditory images in daydreams was measured by Scale 16 of the IPI. Each Scale value is obtained by summing responses to 12 different items of the IPI. Each of the 36 items has the same five response options which are points on a continuum indicating applicability to the individual. The options were assigned values of 0, 1, 2, 3, or 4 depending on their ordinal position on the continuum. Negatively phrased items had assigned values in the reverse order: 4, 3, 2, 1, and 0. Table 1 includes sample items from each of the three imagery IPI scales. The visual imagery scale, the auditory imagery scale, and the imagery vividness scale have both good internal consistency and test-retest reliability (Giambra, 1977-78; 1979-80).

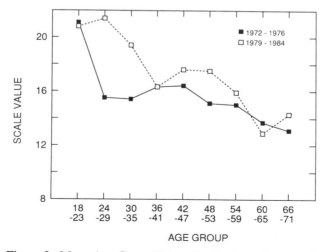

Figure 2. Mean Age Group Values for Auditory Imagery Scale
for the 1972-76 and 1979-84 Date of Testing Cohorts:
Women, Cross-Sectional Sample.

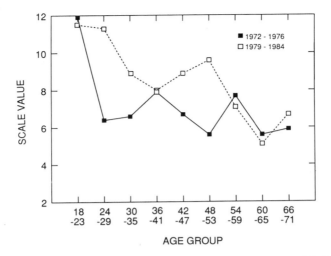

Figure 3. Mean Age Group Values For The Hallucinatory-Vividness
of Daydreaming Scale For the 1972-1976 and 1979-1984
Date of Testing Cohorts: Women, Cross-Sectional Sample.

For participants 24 years and older, the IPI was taken alone or in small groups. The 18-23 year-old college students generally completed the IPI in a classroom setting in groups of 10 to 60. Most men and some of the women completed the IPI while on a regularly scheduled visit to the Gerontology Research Center. The majority of women completed the IPI in their homes. Each participant was given a brief explanation of daydreaming and the purposes of the study. Examples of daydreaming behavior were provided and participants were advised to "make a distinction between 'thinking' about an immediate task you're performing, e.g. working, doing school work, thinking directly about it while you're doing it and 'daydreaming' which involves thought unrelated to a task you are working on or else thoughts that continue while you are getting ready for sleep or on a long bus or train ride." Instructions clarified that daydreams are spontaneous, task-unrelated images and thoughts. Longitudinal participants received identical instructions with each successive administration of the IPI.

RESULTS

Cross-Sectional Age Effects

Women. Age Group X Date of Testing analyses of variance (ANOVAs) were conducted for the three IPI scales. There were significant main effects of age for all three IPI scales, $p < .001$, i.e., Visual Imagery $(F(8,1043) = 8.53)$, Auditory Imagery $(F(8,1023) = 8.95)$, and

Table 2. Auditory Imagery and Hallucinatory-Vividness of Daydreams Scales: 1972-76 and 1979-84 Cross-Sectional Samples

Date of Testing	Sex	Visual Imagery	Auditory Imagery	Hallucinatory-Vividness
1972-76	Women	-0.23**	-0.25**	-0.24**
1979-84		-0.28**	-0.25**	-0.24**
1972-76	Men	-0.24**	-0.38**	-0.30**
1979-84		-0.24**	-0.33**	-0.13*

* p < .05, ** p < .01

26

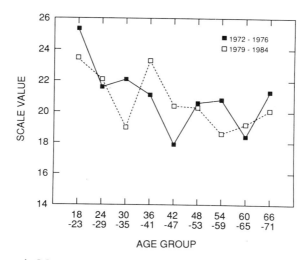

Figure 4. Mean Age Group Values for The Visual Imagery Scale
for the 1972-76 and 1979-84 Date of Testing Cohorts:
Men, Cross-Sectional Sample.

Hallucinatory-Vividness of Daydreams (H-V) ($F(8,1135) = 9.46$). All three scales showed a
general decrease with increased age, see Figures 1, 2, and 3. There were also significant Date of
Testing effects for the Auditory Imagery scale, $F(1,1023) = 5.71$, $p < .05$ and the H-V scale,
$F(1,1135) = 7.62$, $p < .01$. For both scales, the earlier mean scale values (1972-76) were greater
by 1.6 and 1.4 respectively for the Auditory Imagery and H-V scales than the later mean scale
values (1979-84). The correlation of age with each scale at each test date was calculated and is
given in Table 2. All correlations were significant, $p < .01$, and negative, $-0.28 <= r <= -0.23$.
    Men. Age Group X Date of Testing ANOVAs were conducted for the three IPI scales.
There were significant main effects of age for all three IPI scales, $p < .001$, i.e., Visual Imagery
($F(8,830) = 7.13$), Auditory Imagery ($F(8,808) = 12.71$, and H-V ($F(8,890) = 7.40$). The 18-
23 year-old group showed the largest visual imagery mean while other age groups varied
unsystematically, see Figure 4. With respect to auditory imagery, the two youngest age groups
(18-23 and 24-29 year-olds) had the largest means while again other age groups varied in an

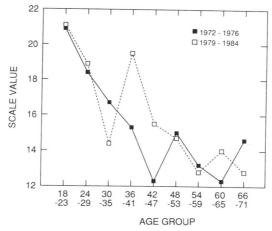

Figure 5. Mean Age Group Values for Auditory Imagery Scale
for the 1972-76 and 1979-84 Date of Testing Cohorts:
Men, Cross-Sectional Sample.

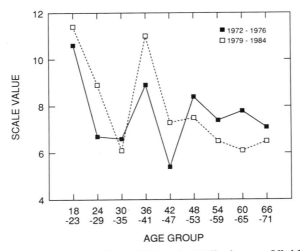

Figure 6. Mean Age Group Values for Hallucinatory-Vividness
of Daydreaming Scale for 1972-76 and 1979-84 Date
of Testing Cohorts: Men, Cross-Sectional Sample.

unsystematic manner, see Figure 5. A similar finding resulted with the H-V scale in that no general trend was noted across age groups with the exception that 18-23 year-olds displayed the greatest mean, see Figure 6. There were no significant (p > .10) Date of Testing effects for any of the three IPI scales (F < 1). The correlation of age with each scale at each time of testing is given in Table 2. All correlations were significant, p < .05, and negative, $-0.38 <= r <= -0.13$.

Longitudinal Effects

Women. An Age at First Testing X Time of Testing repeated measures ANOVA was carried out on each of the three IPI scales. Significant longitudinal changes occurred for Visual Imagery, $F(1,86) = 9.43$, p < .01; Auditory Imagery, $F(1,88) = 19.08$, p < .001; and H-V, $F(1,104) = 20.99$, p < .001. All three scales showed a decrease after a six to eight year longitudinal interval. Table 3 shows the mean change values for the three scales. Figures 7, 8, and 9 display the changes for each age group. No Age X Time of Testing interactions were significant, p > .10 (all $F(7,86-104) < 1.49$).

Table 3. Six to Eight Year Longitudinal Changes in Visual Imagery,
Auditory Imagery and the Hallucinatory-Vividness of Daydreams
Values for Men and Women: Means and Standard Deviations.

	Women		Men	
Scales	Mean	SD	Mean	SD
Visual imagery	-2.36	2.68	-0.10	1.87
Auditory imagery	-3.49	2.25	0.01	1.92
Hallucinatory-vividness	-2.17	1.61	1.08	0.77

Note. A negative change score represents a decrease after 6 to 8 years. A positive change score represents an increase after 6 to 8 years.

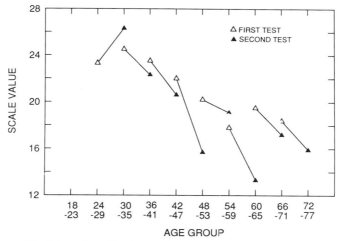

Figure 7.   Mean Age Group Values at First and Second Testing (Six
            to Eight Years Later) for Visual Imagery Scale: Women,
            Longitudinal Sample.

To increase confidence in a maturational explanation, the possibility of a non-maturational source of the Time of Testing effect was examined. As indicated in the Cross-Sectional results for women, Date of Testing effects were found for both the Auditory Imagery and the H-V Scales. The mean of the Auditory Imagery Scale values for the 1972-76 period was greater by 1.60 points than the mean for the 1979-84 period. Thus, the Auditory Imagery Scale values for the 1979-84 period for all longitudinal sample women were "adjusted" to take into account the non-maturational 1979-84 downward influence. For all women in the longitudinal sample, 1.60 scale points were added to the Auditory Imagery Scale score obtained at the second time of testing. An Age at First Testing X Time of Testing repeated measures ANOVA yielded a significant effect for longitudinal change over time, $F(1,88) = 5.60$, $p < .05$. Again, there was no significant interaction of age with time of testing ($p > .10$) in this adjusted sample.

The cross-sectional mean of the H-V Scale values for the 1972-76 period was greater by 1.44 points than the mean for the 1979-84 period. Thus the H-V Scale values for the 1979-84

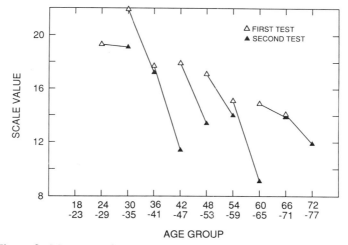

Figure 8. Mean Age Group Values at First and Second Testing (Six
           to Eight Years Later) for Auditory Imagery Scale: Women,
           Longitudinal Sample.

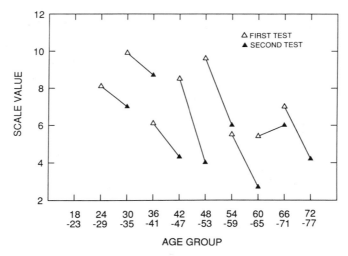

Figure 9. Mean Age Group Values at First and Second Testing (Six
to Eight Years Later) for The Hallucinatory-Vividness of
Daydreaming Scale: Women, Longitudinal Sample.

period for all longitudinal sample women were "adjusted" to account for the non-maturational 1979-84 downward influence. Therefore, for all women in the longitudinal sample, 1.44 scale points were added to the H-V Scale score obtained at the second time of testing. An Age at First Testing X Time of Testing repeated measures ANOVA indicated no significant longitudinal change over time, nor age interaction with time of testing after adjustment (p > .10). The significant longitudinal change in H-V reported in a previous paragraph became nonsignificant with the adjustment for possible non-maturational influences $(F(1,104) = 2.40, p > .10$.

Men. An Age at First Testing X Time of Testing repeated measures ANOVA was completed for all three IPI scales. Significant longitudinal changes occurred for H-V, $F(1,161) = 4.46$, p < .05, but not for Visual Imagery, $F(1,144) < 1$, or Auditory Imagery, $F(1,136) < 1$, both p > .05. There was a general increase over time in the Hallucinatory-Vividness of Daydreams for men.

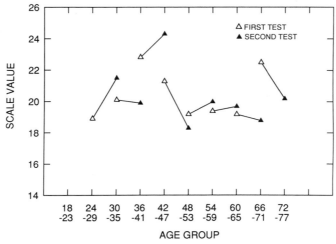

Figure 10. Mean Age Group Values at First and Second Testing
(Six to Eight Years Later) for Visual Imagery Scale:
Men, Longitudinal Sample.

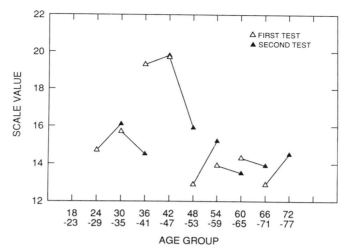

Figure 11. Mean Age Group Values at First and Second Testing
(Six to Eight Years Later) for Auditory Imagery Scale:
Men, Longitudinal Sample.

See Table 3 for mean values and Figures 10, 11, and 12 for age group means. There were no significant Age X Time of Testing interaction effects, p > .10 (all F(7,136-161) < 1.30).

DISCUSSION

The six to eight year longitudinal results concerning visual and auditory imagery in daydreams and the vividness of such images in daydreams are partially congruent with the cross-sectional results and with Giambra (1977-78, 1979-80). For women, all outcomes were the same: interindividual and intraindividual decreases occurred with age in the likelihood of visual and auditory images and in the vividness of those daydreams. However the results were less

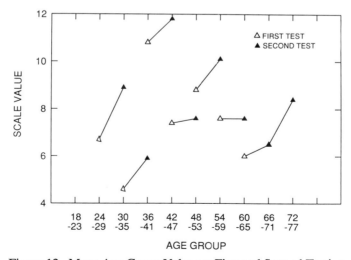

Figure 12. Mean Age Group Values at First and Second Testing
(Six to Eight Years Later) for Hallucinatory-Vividness
of Daydreaming Scale: Men, Longitudinal Sample.

Table 4. Summary of Significant Cross-Sectional Age Differences and Six to Eight Year Longitudinal Changes for the Visual Men and Women

| | Sample | | | |
| | Women | | Men | |
Scale	Cross-sectional	Longi-tudinal	Cross-sectional	Longi-tudinal
Visual imagery	yes - d	yes - d	yes - y	no - ?
Auditory imagery	yes - d	yes - d	yes - y	no - ?
Hallucinatory-vividness	yes - d	yes - d	yes - y	yes - i

Note. d -indicates decrease with increased age. However, all scales correlate negatively with age in the cross-sectional samples.
   i -indicates increase with increased age.
   y -indicates young group(s) greater than other groups which show little systematic pattern of increases or decreases with age.
   ? -indicates no systematic pattern of increases or decreases after six to eight years.

clear for the men. The youngest cross-sectional age groups had higher likelihoods of visual and auditory imagery and greater vividness than the oldest age groups. Longitudinal findings for the men demonstrated no consistent pattern or significant time effect for either auditory or visual imagery occurrence. For the hallucinatory-vividness of daydreams however, the men showed a significant increase with age over the six to eight year time period. In other words, the men reported that images in daydreams became more vivid with age. See Table 4 for a summary description of all significant and nonsignificant effects.

These results are, on the whole, consistent with the conclusion that the spontaneous occurrence of visual and auditory imagery is less likely with increased age. Together, this outcome and the reports of the reduced spontaneous use of imagery in paired-associates learning (Hulicka & Grossman, 1967; but see Wood & Pratt, 1987), the apparent success of mnemonic memory/learning training using imagery (Poon, Walsh-Sweeney, & Fozard, 1980; but see Mason & Smith, 1977) and the poorer ability of older adults in manipulating mental images (Gaylord & Marsh, 1975; Schaie & Labouvie-Vief, 1974; Pierce & Storandt, 1988) form a puzzling pattern. One can only speculate about the underlying basis of this pattern. One possibility is that image production may be extremely effortful and the older adults produce fewer spontaneous images because it requires a level of mental effort which is avoided in the interests of optimal energy expenditure. However, when required, a deliberate and successful mental effort can be made to produce images, for example, in the production of mental images to aid in simple learning tasks such as paired-associates. However,when mental manipulation of an image is required, as in mental rotation, too much effort is required and older adults do more poorly than younger adults.

SUMMARY

The frequency, clarity and semblance to reality of visual and auditory images in daydreams were investigated as a function of age. In the present study, six to eight year longitudinal changes were examined as were cross-sectional age effects. The Cross-Sectional Sample included 908 men and 1153 women partitioned into eight age groups ranging from 18 to 71 years. The Longitudinal Sample consisted of 113 women and 173 men ranging in age from 20 to 71 years. The extent to which daydreams include visual and auditory imagery and the vividness of daydreaming imagery were measured by 3 scales of the Imaginal Processes Inventory.

Analyses of variance revealed significant age effects for all three IPI scales for both the men and the women in the Cross-Sectional Sample. The women decreased in visual and auditory imagery as well as vividness imagery with age while the men showed no systematic pattern with age. Longitudinal results indicated similar findings for the women in that significant decreases over time occurred for the three IPI scales. In contrast, the men showed only significant longitudinal change for the vividness of daydreams which resulted in an increase over the six to eight year period. However, vividness was generally low for all ages and times of testing.

REFERENCES

Gaylord, S. A., & Marsh, G. R. (1975). Age differences in the speed of spatial cognitive process. *Journal of Gerontology, 30*, 674-678.

Giambra, L. M. (1977-78). Adult male daydreaming across the life span: A replication, further analyses, and tentative norms based upon retrospective reports. *International Journal of Aging and Human Development, 8*, 197-228.

Giambra, L. M. (1979-80). Sex differences in daydreaming and related mental activity from the late teens to the early nineties. *International Journal of Aging and Human Development, 10*, 1-34.

Hulicka, I. M., & Grossman, J. L. (1967). Age-group comparisons for the use of mediators in paired-associate learning. *Journal of Gerontology, 22*, 46-51.

Mason, S. E., & Smith, A. D. (1977). Imagery in the aged. *Experimental Aging Research, 3*, 17-32.

Parks, C. W., Jr., Klinger, E., & Perlmutter, M. (1988-89). Dimensions of thought as a function of age, gender, and task difficulty. *Imagination, Cognition, and Personality, 8*, 49-62.

Pierce, K., & Storandt, M. (1988). Similarities in visual imagery ability in young and old women. *Experimental Aging Research, 13*, 209-211.

Poon, L. W., Walsh-Sweeney, L., & Fozard, J. L. (1980). Memory skill training in the elderly: Salient issues on the use of imagery mnemonics. In L. W. Poon, J. L. Fozard, L. S. Cermak, D. Arenberg, & L. Thompson (Editors) *New directions in memory and aging* (pp. 461-484). Hillsdale, NJ: Lawrence Erlbaum.

Schaie, K. W., & Labouvie-Vief, G. (1974). Generational versus ontogenetic components of change in adult cognitive behavior: A fourteen year cross-sectional sequence. *Developmental Psychology, 10*, 305-320.

Winograd, E., & Simon, E. W. (1980). Visual memory and imagery in the aged. In L. W. Poon, J. L. Fozard, L. S. Cermak, D. Arenberg, & L. W. Thompson (Editors), *New directions in memory and aging* (pp.485-506). Hillsdale, NJ: Lawrence Erlbaum.

Wood, L. W., & Pratt, J. D. (1987). Pegword mnemonic as an aid to memory in the elderly: A comparison of four age groups. *Educational Gerontology, 13*, 325-339.

LEVELS OF IMAGERY AND VISUAL EXPRESSION

Vija B. Lusebrink, Ph.D.

Expressive Therapies Department
University of Louisville
Louisville, KY 40292

Images are defined as "transient, perceptlike representations that exist in short term memory" (Kosslyn, 1988, p. 319). Visual expression is imagelike representation created in an external medium with its own qualities influencing these representations. Both imagery and visual expression are multileveled and constructed over a period of time, although means of construction differ and so does time required.

Ahsen's (1982, 1984) ISM model defines the three components of imagery as image, sensation, and meaning. Different aspects and levels of imagery have been investigated from the different viewpoints, i.e. developmental (Piaget, 1962; Piaget & Inhelder, 1971), psychophysiological (Barrett & Ehrlichman, 1982; Ehrlichman & Barrett, 1983; Jacobson, 1932; Lusebrink, 1987; Lusebrink & McGuigan, 1989; Lang, 1979), cognitive (Paivio, 1971), and states of consciousness viewpoints (Groff 1976; Kluver, 1966; Masters & Houston, 1968).

Visual expression and media applications in art therapy can be placed on different hierarchically organized levels of the conceptual model of the Expressive Therapies Continuum (ETC) (Kagin & Lusebrink, 1978; Lusebrink, 1990). Consisting of four levels of increasing complexity based on the developmental sequence of mental imagery and graphic expression, the model draws its information predominantly from clinical observations. The ordering of imagery on different levels and the different studies supporting it contribute to the understanding and validity of the ETC.

The following is a brief overview of the different levels of imagery, and an introduction to the different levels of visual expression and information processing in the framework of the ETC. It also presents the commonalities and differences between imagery and visual expression as used in art therapy.

LEVELS OF IMAGERY

Developmental Levels

The developmental levels of mental imagery can be organized along the stages of development of the intellect (Piaget, 1962; Piaget & Inhelder, 1971). A stable mental image, which is a prerequisite for internal experiences using imagery, is achieved by the end of the sensory-motor period. The formation of mental images is based on deferred imitation through sensory-motor activities using objects and self-body and the internalization of these activities.

During the preconceptual stage, the next developmental level, the mental images have a static quality and require concrete objects as their external counterparts. Symbolic play facilites differentiation of the images. The static quality of images continues throughout the preoperational stage. Images achieve a dynamic and anticipatory quality in the stage of concrete operations during which the child learns to manipulate the images internally. This ability

Mental Imagery, Edited by R.G. Kunzendorf
Plenum Press, New York, 1990

blossoms with the advent of formal operations and adolescence when daydreaming is at its peak (Singer, 1975; Starker, 1982).

The developmental sequence of imagery is important in art therapy. Children's graphic development and visual expressions differ in different developmental stages and reflect their intellectual and visuo-motor development and their understanding and reference point of the world around them (Lowenfeld & Brittain, 1970). Adults may regress in their visual expression to earlier stages of graphic development because of anxiety and psychopathology; regression also can occur in creative spontaneity.

Psychophysiological Components of Imagery

The psychophysiological components of imagery present a complex pattern and do not lend themselves to easy classification on different levels. The most common approach to classifying psychophysiological components associated with imagery is along the different modalities: kinesthetic (Jacobson, 1930), visual and verbal and/or auditory reflecting the peripheral activities (Ehrlichman & Barrett, 1983), and brain wave or central activities (Ehrlichman & Wiener, 1980).

The complexity of the psychophysiological components of visual imagery is results from the different patterns of these components associated with different imagery (McGuigan, 1978). For example, the pattern of eye movement and covert arm and lip activity differentiated between the images of the letter *P, pencil,* and *pasture* in studies by Lusebrink (1987) and Lusebrink and McGuigan (1989). Different patterns of psychophysiological components also are associated with different emotions: for example the pattern of heart rate and blood pressure components have been shown to differentiate between anger and fear imagery scenes (Lang, Levin, Miller, & Kozak, 1983; Schwartz, Weinberger, & Singer, 1981).

Cognitive Levels of Imagery

Even though images can represent concrete objects, they are not "concrete pictures in our heads" in that they are constructed from parts that involve the activity in different parts of the visual cortex and temporal inferior and parietal areas of the brain (Kosslyn, 1987; Kosslyn, Cake, & Provost, 1988; Roth & Kosslyn, 1988). Thus images have a dynamic and emergent quality (Bugelski, 1983; Kosslyn, 1980, 1987).

The cognitive levels of imagery can be conceptualized as ranging from simple visual sensory components and concrete images to abstract concepts. On the *sensory level,* low level sensory visual processing reactivates sensory traces representing such features as lines, angles, lattice, and so forth (Paivio, 1971) that may be experienced as visual sensory configurations without any cognitive meaning. If not further elaborated, images on this level are experienced as transitory.

Low level visual processing provides input for the more centrally located high level processing. Imagery, for the large part parallels vision more centrally removed from the peripheral levels and assumes a functional equivalence with it (Kosslyn, 1987). Kosslyn proposes two cortical visual processing subsystems, one that analyzes what the object is, the other where the object is. The first subsystem generates images in their global shape; the other elaborates an image by constructing its parts. These two subsystems also are functional in determining the relationship between different images: the first determines coordinate location encoding; the other determines categorical relationships between between parts of the image such as up/down and left/right. The two subsystems are involved in the next level of imagery formation, *concrete representational images.* Images fade over periods of time and have to be reinstated in the visual medium (Kosslyn, 1980).

The subsequent *referential level* of imagery involves images with referential meaning formed in response to concrete words (Paivio, 1971). On this level images also are anticipatory. The anticipatory function may involve (a) rotation of images in space (Shepard & Cooper, 1982), or (b) images that anticipate or rehearse an individual's future actions. The referential level and the subsequent level of *associative meaning* may involve modalities other than the visual, such as kinesthetic, tactile, auditory, and olfactory. On the associative level, images provide the imaginal counterpart to abstract words and concepts (Paivio, 1971). Images on this level also may represent figurative aspects of a symbol (Piaget, 1962); input from other modalities elaborates on symbolic meaning.

Ultimately, from the cognitive viewpoint, knowledge is assumed to be propositional in nature: abstract, nonverbal, and nonimaginal. This assumption is based on the interaction of the two representational processes, i.e. visual and verbal, which require a common propositional basis. Such propositions have a truth value and are abstract representations of the essential features and underlying structures of knowledge (Anderson, 1978).

The level on which an image is experienced depends not only on the information it represents, but also on the awareness and attention directed towards it. A focal awareness may elaborate on the differential and detailed aspects on an image through an "attention window" that selects a region at a lower level processing of the visual system for further processing (Kosslyn, 1987). A more general view coupled with associative awareness may elaborate on the context of the image and its meaning. An emphasis on the categorical and cognitive aspects may bring out the abstract aspects of images representing the underlying structures.

Levels of Imagery Associated with Altered States of Consciousness

Images can be ordered on the different levels of consciousness in which they are experienced, from hypo-arousal to hyper-arousal. Hyper-arousal is characterized by a high rate of information processing, which can be present in acute emotional stress and acute psychosis. In mescaline and LSD intoxication this arousal is limited predominantly to the visual system (Ey, 1973). Altered states of consciousness also are associated with hypo-arousal, such as meditation and sensory deprivation. Dreams in REM state are produced in a combined state of hypo- and hyper-arousal; during REM state gross motor movement is inhibited yet the activity of the autonomic nervous system, eye movement, and brain activity is increased.

Images experienced in states of consciousness altered by drug use range from entoptic phenomena and simple perceptual distortions to the fantastic complex images present with a larger amount of drugs and later in the "trip." The imagery present under the influence of drugs or pseudo-hallucinations can be placed on three to four levels (Grof, 1976; Kluver, 1966; Masters & Houston, 1968). At the beginning of intoxication, sensory experiences are enhanced. On this *sensory level* images have a simple ornamental or geometric pattern that undergoes constant changes and lacks continuity. Such images are described as "form constants," such as grating, lattice, honeycomb, tunnel, funnel, spiral (Kluver, 1966; Siegel & Jarvick, 1975). These sensory images result from the chemical stimulation of the perceptive visual analyzers on a very basic level (Ey, 1973; Grof, 1976).

The images on the next deeper, or "Freudian," level are *recollective* and reflect, symbolically, emotionally charged personal experiences. These images are based on the release of stored traumatic tensions present in the different parts of the body, such as muscles, the cardiovascular and urogenital systems, and bowels (Grof, 1976).

The subsequent *symbolic* (Masters & Houston, 1968), or "perinatal" (Grof, 1976), level may involve images of birth and death and dying; evolutionary and historical themes; and archetypal images of galaxies and solar systems, sacrificial ceremonies, devils, and wrathful deities. On this level individuals experience participation in the dreamlike imagery with all their senses and profound emotions. These images are most likely communicated through graphic means, such as painting (Masters & Houston, 1968).

The deepest level, or *transpersonal* level, is experienced basically as uncommunicable. It may involve religious and mystical experiences of the dissolution of ego boundaries beyond space and time, and it is often associated with self-integration.

The images present on the first and third level also are experienced in psychosis and schizophrenia, depending on the type and depth of psychosis. The transpersonal level may be experienced as "being in heaven." The more personal, or "Freudian", images may appear in the later stages of reconstitution.

According to Kunzendorf (1985-86, 1986-87, 1987-88), subconscious percepts consist of unmonitored sensations and repressed memories composed of conscious sensory qualities, but they are prevented from becoming sensory images during everyday experiences. Images experienced on the different levels of consciousness depend on the individual differences in openness to these experiences, or on the depth of psychosis or drug intoxication.

Imagery and Emotional Components

In addition to the structural aspect, imagery--especially imagery with personal references-- incorporates an emotional aspect. According to Lang's bio-informational theory of emotional imagery, an emotional image is defined as "a conceptual network in the brain, integrating perceptual, meaning, and somatovisceral propositions" (Lang, Levin, Miller, & Kozak, 1983, p. 279). The pattern of the psychophysiological components is a significant part of the emotional image. For example, the pattern of heart rate and blood pressure responses differentiates between anger and fear imagery scenes (Lang, 1979; Schwartz, Weinberger, & Singer, 1981). Emphasis on the different components of the emotional imagery differentially influences its physiological components: Descriptions of bodily sensations increase the activity of the physiological components; this increase is not present when the descriptions of the stimulus emphasize the structural aspects of form and color (Lang, 1979).

Leventhal's perceptual-motor theory of emotions (Leventhal & Mosbach, 1983; Leventhal & Tomarken, 1986) proposes that emotional experiences are constructed within the central nervous system by a hierarchical system consisting of three levels: sensory motor level, schematic encoding level, and conceptual level.

Opinions differ as to whether emotions are based on separate systems (Zajonc & Markus, 1984) or on a fused, reciprocally interactive system (Lazarus, 1982; Mahoney, 1984). Regardless to which hypothesis one adheres, the conceptual differentiation of emotions into sensory-motor, perceptive, and cognitive subsystems provides different avenues for dealing with emotions in everyday life and therapy. Greenberg and Safran (1984) propose that the conceptualization of emotions on different levels facilitates therapeutic decisions about the level of the process of emotional synthesis on which to intervene. Rachman (1984) suggests to use nonverbal means, such as music, to modify affective reactions, because the nonverbal procedures are more compatable with the nonverbal nature of emotions.

LEVELS OF EXPRESSION IN ART THERAPY:
THE EXPRESSIVE THERAPIES CONTINUUM

All the above dimensions and levels of imagery can be applied to elaborate on the multileveled nature of visual expression. The conceptual framework of the ETC (Kagin & Lusebrink, 1978; Lusebrink, 1990) incorporates these levels in a hierarchical, developmentally based sequence.

The ETC consists of three levels of increasing complexity of expression and interaction with media: kinesthetic/sensory (K/S), perceptual/affective (P/A), and cognitive/symbolic (C/SY). The progression of the levels reflects the developmental sequence of imagery formation and also the modes of representation of thought as proposed by Bruner (1964) and Horowitz (1970, 1978, 1983).

A fourth or creative (CR) level of the ETC can be present on any of the other three levels, incorporating their emergent functions (Lusebrink, 1990). The two poles of each level can interact in a complementary manner, thus giving rise to the emergent functions. The two poles of each level also can be exclusive of each other in that the focus of the expression can be on one polarity at the exclusion of the other.

The Kinesthetic/Sensory Level

The *kinesthetic* component of the K/S level focuses primarily on the release of energy and expression of it through bodily action and movement. The *sensory* component emphasizes the tactile, haptic and other sensations experienced and expressed by interaction with art media. Art media on this level act as facilitators for kinesthetic actions or the awareness of sensations. The pounding of clay is an example of kinesthetic use of the media. Explorations with fingerpaints amplify the tactile as well as visual sensations through texture and color. Sensory activities require that individuals let go of conscious control, and "immerse themselves in unpredictable sensory activities" (McNiff, 1981, p.51). Sensations are amplified through relaxation and withdrawal from external stimuli; they also can be amplified through verbal descriptions of sensory images. On the K/S level the reflective distance between the stimulus and action or sensation is minimal. The K/S level of expression deals with kinesthetic, tactile, or visual peripheral stimulation and has a minimal equivalence with images which are based on more centrally located brain structures (Kosslyn, 1987).

From the imagery viewpoint, though, an early aspect of imagery formation is deferred imitation through depicted action and its internalization (Piaget, 1962). The same applies for the internalization of images of objects: the latter have to be explored through the senses before they can be internalized as images. Images depicting action or action-related subjects have a covert kinesthetic component (Jacobson, 1930; Lusebrink, 1987; Lusebrink & McGuigan, 1989). Sensations and sensory images can be below the level of awareness (Kunzendorf, 1987-88). Through kinesthetic and sensory activities the covert components and images may be brought to awareness.

Each level of the ETC also has a healing or emergent dimension that leads to a developmentally higher level of information processing and more integrated sense of self. The kinesthetic action may lead to a rhythmic expression and perception of form. Exploration of media through kinesthetic and sensory involvement is especially valuable for young children (Kramer, 1971) because they need to handle objects and materials physically to internalize images. Kinesthetic actions, such as pounding clay, can be an expression of negative feelings, which can be transformed by subsequently using the clay to make forms (Betensky, 1973).

Sensory images--visceral, tactile, or visual--can become building components for emotions, images, and verbal expressions. The importance of the sensory component has been pointed out by Ahsen (1982, 1984) as one of the tripartite constituents of imagery. The emergent dimension of the sensory level contributes to the expression of emotions and formation of emotional images on the affective level.

The Perceptual/Affective Level

The *perceptual* pole of the P/A level focuses on the formation of representational images through form, color, and pattern. This level emphasizes the structural qualities of images and utilizes the structural qualities of media. The creation of regular configurations, either representational or patterned, also helps children to develop schemas that can be used to describe the real world (Kramer, 1979). One of the first goals in therapy with the mentally retarded is expansion of their motor, sensory, and perceptual capacities because their symbol formation is impaired. The transition to a level involving organized imagery can be enhanced by the therapist's modeling the drawing of circles and vertical lines (Wilson, 1977, 1985a, 1985b).

The dialogue between the medium and the individual depicting images creates an isomorphic interaction (Arnheim, 1972) between the two. The *affective* pole of the P/A level emphasizes the expression of emotions and affective images. Fluid media, such as paints, and their sensory components facilitate expressions on the affective level. The perceptual and affective aspects of the P/A level interact in that the perceptual aspect gives form to emotions, i.e. this aspect emphasizes the schematic component of emotions. The affective component, in turn, gives the form a dynamic quality through emphasis on certain aspects of the structure or form. The pattern of lines and forms constitutes a differential pattern expressive of the different emotions represented (Rhyne, 1979a).

Expression can manifest in the extreme of either the perceptual or affective pole. Elaboration and accentuation of the form and structure become means to control emotions. An emphasis on the emotional qualities of the expression distorts or defies the restrictions of structure and form.

In relation to imagery, the perceptual aspects of the P/A level deal with concrete representational imagery and patterns constructed through the combination of simple visual sensory elements--lines, angles, and areas formed through their interaction. On the affective level different patterns of imagery are associated with different emotions (Lyman & Waters, 1989). For example, in this study, man-made objects, places, and events were associated with four negative emotions--anxiety, boredom, envy, and loneliness--but not with positive emotions. Contentment and happiness, on the other hand, were associated with images of nature places, objects, events, and activities.

The intensity of affect associated with specific images may mark them for recall or repression. The intensity of emotions in memory activate other mood and intensity associated areas. The lack or inability to experience affect, such as in alexithymia, may go hand in hand with the inability to experience images. Overwhelming affect associated with images may lead to repression of the images or their affective component and eventually to regression in observable behavior, including visual expression (Rubin, 1978). On the P/A level, reflective distance varies from minimal distance in an overwhelming experience of affect to considerable affective distance when the perceptual aspects of the expression are overemphasized.

Interaction between the affective and perceptual components may lead to a creative expression and emergent components of cognition and symbolism. The transition to spatial integration can be elucidated in comparing the mechanisms involved in Kosslyn's (1987) proposed subsystems of imagery formation to the stages of graphic development. The two subsystems of imagery formation are involved in pattern recognition and location recognition. The visual expressions of young children and regressed schizophrenics reveal two separate stages of organizing form. In the first, developmentally-based, preschematic stage (Lowenfeld & Brittain, 1970), the child portrays isolated objects or parts of objects. The regressed schizophrenic visually represents isolated objects or objects with incongruously fused parts.

Spatial organization emerges in children's drawing in the subsequent schematic stage; early phases of this stage involve x-pictures and fold-over space (Lowenfeld & Brittain, 1970). The schizophrenics' representation of space displays similar elements (Plokker, 1965). In deep regression, spatial concepts become incohesive and space may be experienced as limitless. Billig (Billig, 1968; Billig & Burton-Bradlley, 1978) compares the change of spatial representations in schizophrenic regression as inversely to related to the stages of development of spatial integration in primitive art.

When the stages of graphic development and the subsystems involved in imagery construction are compared, it appears that the subsystem active in pattern recognition is predominant in the preschematic stage, and the location recognition subsystem is increasingly active in the schematic stage. In applying Kosslyn's (1987) concept of the "attention window" to the regressed schizophrenic drawings, it appears that here the "window" does not function in a stable, object directed manner, but that, through shifting, leads to synthesis of objects with incongruous parts.

The Cognitive/Symbolic Level

Emphasis on the categorical and spatial relations between individual images and representational depiction of objects leads to the cognitive/symbolic aspects of the ETC. The C/SY level is qualitatively different from the previous levels in that it encompasses conceptual and anticipatory operations with images. The cognitive component of this level focuses on analytical, sequential operations, logical thought, and problem solving. For example, by representing different aspects of a problem through abstract shapes, a visual expression can be used in problem solving (Rhyne, 1979b). Alternative solutions to a problem can be arrived at through defining the constructs associated with the images (Rhyne, 1979a). Construction of a topic-directed collage with inserted word is another expression on the cognitive level (Landgarten, 1981). In art therapy involvement with concrete objects leads to abstraction and systematic elaboration of concepts (Roth, 1978, 1987). Abstractions and concept representation through visual forms are part of operations on the cognitive level.

The exploration of media properties and their internalization at the lower levels of the ETC contributes to the understanding of actions necessary to execute complex oerations. Differentiation of spatial relationships can be improved through warm-up exercises that observe and depict relationships among objects in external world--left/right or front/back (Silver, 1978). Compared to the previous levels, increased reflective distance contributes to the ability to plan actions on the cognitive level. This level encompasses images with referential and associative meaning denoting general categories and categorical operations.

The *symbolic* component of the ETC at this level focuses on intuitive concept formation, realization and actualization of symbols, and the symbolic expression of meaning. Images can represent objects, feelings and ideas (Levick, 1984). A symbolic image is defined here predominantly in psychodynamic terms in that an aspect of the symbol refers to a consciously not known quality, either repressed or not yet formulated in conscious terms. Symbols are multileveled and multidimensional and encompass kinesthetic, affective, and structural components. Part of the meaning of symbolic images is implied through the structure of the images. The affective component endows symbolic images with a special personal meaning for the individual. Symbols on this level can be either regressive or progressive. As defense mechanisms they are manifested in drawings through subjective graphic representation or omission of specific objects or thoughts (Levick, 1983). In regression, the referential aspect of symbolic images can become self-referential or as a result in a shift of consciousness the external reality can be perceived on symbolic terms. Progressive symbols refer to future occurences and anticipations. The use of fluid media influence symbol formation incorporating affective aspects. The concretization of symbols and their resolution on personal terms is enhanced through the use of resistive media.

Images with symbolic meaning can be experienced and expressed on different levels of consciousness that parallel the levels described by Groff (1976) and Masters and Houston (1968). The basic level, with its emphasis on simple perceptual elements, can be used as a means to avoid the further development of threatening symbolic images. The mechanisms of suppression or repression of sensory images have been elucidated by Kunzendorf (1985-86, 1986-87, 1987-88) as discussed before.

The next level of consciousness deals with personal symbolic images, followed by a deeper level of consciousness that involves universal symbolic images. This latter level is accessed mainly in dreams, during periods of stress, and also in psychosis. At times symbolic visual expressions reflect the different levels of consciousness distinctly; at other times a combination of levels two and three. Interaction between the cognitive and symbolic aspects leads to a goal directed creative expression, self-actualization, and transformation of the environment.

The Creative Level

On the *creative level* images, along with verbal processing, provide an alternate view and thus enhance creative synthesis. Similarly, the interaction of the cognitive and intuitive symbolic aspects of knowledge contributes to the creative product. The creative synthesis incorporates the contribution of the component parts of imagery, be they kinesthetic or sensory, perceptual or affective, cognitive or symbolic.

In visual expression creativity is manifested through the ability to create order out of unstructured media, especially if the product has an emotional impact (Rubin, 1978). According to Kramer (1979), "the creative art expression is characterized by economy of means, inner consistency, and evocative power" (p.50). In the creative act, the reflective distance alternates between minimal (the creator involved in the work), and considerable (the creator examining the work) (Kagin & Lusebrink, 1978). Creative interactions between the polarities on each level of the ETC (Kagin & Lusebrink, 1978) were highlighted before in connection with particular levels.

THERAPEUTIC ASPECTS INTRINSIC TO IMAGERY AND VISUAL EXPRESSION

Imagery approaches to therapy differ from other modes of therapy in that free and guided imagery can produce change without the mediating aspects of interpretation (Sheikh & Jordan, 1983). Similarly, awareness in art therapy does not need to be translated into words in that the awareness gained through the expression can be effective by remaining on the perceptual/emotional level in that the individual gives form to feeling (Rhyne, 1973).

In art therapy the creative aspects of visual expression can be healing through the realization of aesthetic form and balance (Kramer, 1971; McNiff, 1978; Rubin, 1978; Ulman, 1975), and synthesis of form and content (Kramer, 1971, 1979). Such qualities of the visual expression represent one aspect which differentiates the therapeutic characteristics of imagery and art therapy (Lusebrink, 1989).

Imagery spans the continuum between consciousness and the unconscious through its physiological and emotional components (Sheikh and Jordan 1983). In therapy the conceptualization and elaboration of different levels of imagery and visual expression takes advantage of their multileveled nature. Different levels of imagery reflect the development and the process of construction of imagery. The concept of levels also clarifies the understanding of the structures involved in this constructive process. The multileveled characteristics of imagery contribute to the understanding of the multileveled application of visual expression in therapy. Elaboration of the different levels facilitates differential interventions through verbal directions and media applications, which, in turn, influence both the structures and processes involved.

REFERENCES

Ahsen, A. (1982). Imagery in perceptual learning and clinical application. *Journal of Mental Imagery, 6,* 157-186.

Ahsen, A. (1984). ISM: The triple code model for imagery and psychophysiology. *Journal of Mental Imagery, 8* (4), 15-42.

Anderson, J.R. (1978). Arguments concerning representations for mental imagery. *Psychological Review, 85* (4), 249-277.

Arnheim, R. (1972). *Toward a psychology of art.* Berkeley: University of California Press.

Barrett, J. & Ehrlichman, H. (1982). Bilateral hemispheric alpha activity during visual imagery. *Neuropsychologia, 20* (6), 703-708.

Betensky, M. (1973b). *Self-discovery through self-expression.* Springfield, Ill: Charles C. Thomas.

Billig, O. (1968). Spatial structure in schizophrenic art. In I. Jakob (Ed.), *Psychiatry and art* (pp. 1-16). Basel: Karger.

Billig, O., & Burton-Bradley, B.G. (1978). *The painted message.* New York: John Wiley.

Bruner, J.S. (1964). The course of cognitive growth. *American Psychologist, 19,* 1-15.

Bugelski, B.R. (1983). Imagery and thought processes. In A.A. Sheikh, (Ed.). *Imagery: Current theory, research and applications* (pp. 72-95). New York: John Wiley & Sons.

Ehrlichman, H. & Barrett, J. (1983). 'Random'saccadic eye movements during verbal-linguistic and visual-imaginal tasks. *Acta Psychologica, 53*, 9-26.

Ehrlichman, H. & Wiener, M.S. (1980). EEG asymmetry during covert mental activity. *Psychophysiology, 17* (3), 228-235.

Ey, H. (1973). *Traite des hallucinations* (Tome 1 et 2). Paris: Masson et Ci, Editeurs.

Greenberg, L.S. & Safran, J.D. (1984). Integrating affect and cognition: A perspective on the process of therapeutic change. *Cognitive Therapy and Research ,8* (6), 559-578.

Grof, S. (1976). *Realms of the human unconscious. Observations from LSD Research.* New York: E.P. Dutton.

Horowitz, M.J. (1970). *Image formation and cognition.* New York: Appleton-Century-Crofts.

Horowitz, M.J. (1978). Controls of visual imagery and therapist   intervention. In J. Singer & K.S. Pope (Eds.), *The power of human imagination* (pp. 37-49). New York: Plenum.

Horowitz, M.J. (1983). *Image formation and psychotherapy* (rev. ed., *Image formation and cognition*). New York: Jason Aronson.

Jacobson, E. (1930). Electrical measurements of neuromuscular states during mental activities: II. Imagination and recollection of various muscular acts. *American Journal of Physiology, 94*, 22-34.

Jacobson, E. (1932). Electrophysiology of mental activities. *American Journal of Physiology, 44*, 677-694.

Kagin, S.L. & Lusebrink, V.B. (1978). The Expressive Therapies Continuum. *Art Psychotherapy, 5* (4), 171-179.

Kluver, H. (1966). *Mescal and mechanisms of hallucinations.* Chicago: The University of Chicago Press.

Kosslyn, S.M. (1980). *Image and mind.* Cambridge, Mass.: Harvard Univ. Press.

Kosslyn, S.M. (1987). Seeing and imagining in the cerebral hemispheres: A computational approach. *Psychological Review, 94* (2), 148-75.

Kosslyn, S.M. Cake, C.B., & Provost, D.A. (1988). Sequential processes in image generation. *Cognitive Psychology, 20*, 319-343.

Kramer, E. (1971). *Art as therapy with children.* New York: Schocken.

Kramer, E. (1979). *Childhood and art therapy.* New York: Schocken.

Kreitler, H., & Kreitler, S. (1972). *Psychology of the arts.* Durham, NC: Duke University Press.

Kunzendorf, R.G. (1984-85). Subconscious percepts as "unmonitored" percepts.: An empirical study. *Imagination, Cognition, and Personality, 4* (4), 365-373.

Kunzendorf, R.G. (1985-86). Repression as the monitoring and censoring   of images: An empirical study. *Imagination, Cognition, and Personality, 5* (1), 31-39.

Kunzendorf, R.G (1987-1988). Self-consciousness as the monitoring of   cognitive states: A theoretical perspective. *Imagination, Cognition, and Personality, 7* (1), 1987-88.

Landgarten, H.B. (1981). *Clinical art therapy.* New York: Brunner/Mazel.

Lang, P.J (1979). Presidential address, 1978: a bioinformational theory of emotional imagery, *Psychophysiology, 16* (6), 495-512.

Lang, P.J., Levin, D.N., Miller, G.A., & Kozak, M.J. (1983). Fear behavior, fear imagery and the psychophysiology of emotion: The problem of affective response integration. *Journal of Abnormal Psychology, 92* (3), 276-306.

Lazarus, R.S. (1982). Thought on the relations between emotion and cognition. *American Psychologist, 37* (9), 1019-1024.

Leventhal, H. & Mosbach, P.A. (1983). The perceptual-motor theory of emotion. In J.T. Cacioppo & R.E. Petty (Eds), *Social psychophysiology* (pp. 353-388). New York: Guilford.

Leventhal, H. & Tomarken, A.J. (1986). Emotion: Today's problem. *Annual Reviews of Psychology, 37*, 565-610.

Levick, M.F. (1983). *They could not talk and so they drew: Children's styles of coping and thinking.* Springfield, Ill: Charles C. Thomas.

Levick, M.F. (1984). Imagery as a style of thinking. *Art Therapy, 1* (3), 119-124.

Lowenfeld, V. & Brittain, W.L. (1970). *Creative and mental growth* (5th ed.). New York: Macmillan.

Lusebrink, V.B. (1986-87). Visual imagery: Its psychophysiological components and levels of information processing. *Imagination, Cognition, and Personaltiy, 6* (3), 205-218.

Lusebrink, V.B. (1989). Art therapy and imagery in verbal therapy: A comparison of therapeutic characteristics. *The American Journal of Art Therapy, 28* (1), 2-3.

Lusebrink, V.B. (1990). *Imagery and visual expression in therapy.* New York: Plenum Press.

Lusebrink, V.B. & McGuigan, F.J. (1989). Psychophysiological components of imagery. *Pavlovian Journal of Biological Sciences, 24* (2), 58-62.

Lyman, B. & Waters, J.C.E. (1989). Pattern of imagery in various emotions. *Journal of Mental Imagery, 13* (1), 63-74.

Masters, R.E.L., & Houston, J. (1968). *Psychedelic art.* New York: Blanche House.

Mahoney, M.J. (1984). Integrating cognition, affect, and action: A comment. *Cognitive Therapy and Research, 8* (6), 585-589.

McGuigan, F.J. (1978). *Cognitive psychophysiology: Principles of covert behavior.* Englewood Cliffs, NJ: Prentice-Hall.

McNiff, S.A. (1981). *The arts and psychotherapy.* Springfield, Ill: Charles C. Thomas.

Paivio, A. (1971). *Imagery and verbal processes.* New York: Holt, Rinehart & Winston.

Piaget, J. (1962). *Play dreams, and imitation in childhood.* New York: Norton.

Piaget, J. & Inhelder, B. (1971). *Mental imagery in the child.* New York: Basic Books.

Plokker, J.H. (1965). *Art from the mentally disturbed.* Boston: Little, Brown.

Rachman, S. (1984). A reassessment of the "primacy of affect". *Cognitive Therapy and Research, 8* (6), 579-584.

Rhyne, J. (1973). *The gestalt art experience.* Monterey, Calif.: Brooks/Cole.

Rhyne, J. (1979a). Drawings as personal constructs: A study in visual dynamics. *Dissertation Abstracts International, 40* , 2411B. (University Microfilms International No. Tx 375-487).

Rhyne, J. (1979b). Gestalt art experience. In L. Gantt, G. Forrest, D. Silverman, R.J. H. Shoemaker (Eds), *Art Therapy: Expanding horizons. Proceedings of the 9th Annual Conference of the American Art Therapy Association.* (pp. 125-126).

Roth, E.A. (1978). Art therapy with emotionally disturbed--mentally retarded children: A technique of reality sharing. In B.K. Mandel, R.H. Shoemaker, & R.E. Hays (Eds), *The dynamics of creativity. Proceedings of the 8th Annual Art Therapy Association Conference.*

Roth, E.A. (1987). A behavioral approach to art therapy. In J.A. Rubin (Ed.), *Approaches to art therapy: Theory and technique.* New York: Brunner/Mazel.

Roth, J.D. & Kosslyn, S.M. (1988). Construction of the third dimension in mental imagery. *Cognitive Psychology, 20*, 344-361.

Rubin, J.A. (1978). *Child art therapy: Understanding and helping children grow through art.* New York: Van Nostrand Reinhold.

Schwartz, G.E., Winberger, D.A. & Singer, J.A. (1981). Cardiovascular differentiation of happiness, sadness, anger and fear following imagery and exercise. *Psychosomatic Medicine, 43* (4), 343-364.

Shepard, R.N. & Cooper, L.A. (1982). *Mental images and their transformations.* Cambridge, MA: The MIT Press/Bradford Books.

Siegel, R.K. & Jarvik, M.E. (1975). Drug induced hallucinations in animals and man. In R.K. Siegel & L.J. West (Eds.), *Hallucinations: Behavior, experience and theory* (pp. 81-161). New York: Wiley.

Silver, R. (1978). *Developing cognitive and creative skills through art.* Baltimore, Md.: University Park Press.

Singer, J.L. (1975). *The inner world of daydreaming.* New York: Harper & Row.

Starker, S. (1982). *Fantastic thoughts: All about dreams, daydreams, hallucinations and hypnosis.* Englewood Cliffs, N.J.: Prentice-Hall.

Wilson, L. (1977). Art therapy with the mentally retarded. *American Journal of Art Therapy, 16* (3), 87-97.

Wilson, L. (1985a). Symbolism and art therapy: I. Symbolism's role in the development of ego functions. *American Journal of Art Therapy, 23* (3), 79-88.

Wilson, L. (1985b). Symbolism and art therapy: I. Symbolism's relationship to the basic psychic functioning. *American Journal of Art Therapy, 23* (4), 129-133.

Zajonc, R.B., & Markus, H. (1984). Affect and cognition: The Hard interface. In C.E. Izard, J. Kagan, & R.B. Zajonc (Eds.), *Emotions, cognition, and behavior* (pp. 73-102). Cambridge, England: Cambridge University Press.

TRANSFORMING IMAGERY INTO ART: A STUDY OF THE LIFE AND WORK OF GEORGIA O'KEEFFE

Selina Kassels, Ph.D.

Clinical Supervisor
Newton-Wellesley Hospital
Newton, MA 02162

Rosemary Gordon (1970) noted that art serves as a means of communicating private imagery and stated that art is "the most adequate way of giving substance to images" (p. 78). This paper traces the role that imagery processes played in the life and work of Georgia O'Keeffe demonstrating that the artist's drawings and paintings did give "substance" to her images.

Visual artists frequently use the word image interchangeably refering both to the picture in the mind's eye of the artist and to the outward expression of that picture on a completed canvas. This study explores the continuum between the inner imagery and the outward expression by identifying five phases of the artist's career that illustrate varying processes by which imagery was transformed into art. The study applies Rosenberg's (1987) model for studying processes by which visual artists use imagery in their art-making. It is also consistent with a case-study method developed by Wallace (1989) and Gruber (1989) that seeks links between the life and work of creative artists. The evolving imagery and phases of Georgia O'Keeffe's career mark significant transitions and emotional crises during her adult life. The artist's oeuvre can be viewed as an expression of her inner world and of the ways she used her work to communicate and transform her private world of imagery into artistic expressions.

IMAGERY, ART AND CREATIVITY

Georgia O'Keeffe experienced exceptionally vivid mental imagery, not only in the visual modality but also in other modalities, especially auditory and kinesthetic imagery. Her capacity for imagery and her propensity to experience a rich variety of imagery is documented in the artist's personal correspondence and letters (1988) as well as in the memoirs of her close friend, Anita Pollitzer (1988). Although Georgia O'Keeffe thought of herself as relatively inarticulate, she frequently wrote letters that contained poetic descriptions replete with vivid imagery. For example, in a letter written to Anita Pollitzer in 1915, Georgia was struggling to articulate her own definition of art. She could not find an answer to that abstract question, but she wrote instead in another letter:

> It's a wonderful night. I'm going to try to tell you about tonight...I'm going to try to tell you about the music of it with charcoal--a miserable medium for things that seem alive and sing...(Pollitzer, 1988, p.39).

Art for Georgia O'Keeffe was the act of expressing herself in a visual language; it was a way of communicating her passion for nature and a way of translating inner imagery into shapes and colors on canvas.

Subsequent sections of this paper will delineate both the role that imagery played in inspiring the artist's subjects and her flexibility in manipulating and transforming imagery into a range of representational and abstract styles.

Mental Imagery, Edited by R.G. Kunzendorf
Plenum Press, New York, 1990

This case study of the work of a successful artist substantiates other investigations which explore relationships between imagery abilities and artistic accomplishments. Empirical and experimental investigations of the relationships between imagery and creativity have proved inconclusive (Forisha, 1978) despite anecdotal evidence describing the role images play in illumination of creative ideas (Ghiselin, 1952; Gowan, 1978). Methodological limitations, individual differences in imagery abilities (in respect to vividness, modality, autonomy) and the importance of moderating variables, such as mastery of aesthetic principles, are all possible explanations for the difficulties in empirically demonstrating relationships between creative abilities and imagery abilities (Kunzendorf, 1982). Interviews and phenomenological research strategies have been the most successful approaches in exploring the relationship between imagery abilities and artistic creativity (Lindauer, 1983; Rosenberg 1987b). Rosenberg (1987b) studied 13 professional artists and through a content analysis of intensive interviews confirmed the existence of imagery in their procedures and demonstrated the value of applying her theoretical model (1987a) to understand how visual artists use imagery in their art-making. Rosenberg's (1987b) model identifies the processes involved in transforming internal aspects of mental images into external artistic products. Transformational processes include "viewing the world as material for art" (p. 80) experimenting with forms, and processes of simultaneously painting and monitoring the production of the completed product. Rosenberg found many artists in her study developed a rich storehouse of mental images and facilitated their work by placing themselves in a receptive frame of mind to conjure up their images.

Our examination of Georgia O'Keeffe's life will illustrate several processes that were involved in her connecting and transforming her inner emotions, sensations, and imagery experiences into works of art. Her devotion to art was the primary passion of her life and at the point where personal relationships and intimacy threatened her work, she chose to arrange a lifestyle that gave priority to her needs for viewing the world as material for art, and living a life that kept her close to nature and to what she described as the "wideness and wonder of the world" (O'Keeffe, 1976, p. 71).

Solitude and Risk-taking

Georgia O'Keeffe was born on a farm in Wisconsin in 1887 and died in New Mexico in 1986. She was an original, innovative painter who achieved both creative and commercial success in an era when women could aspire to be art teachers but not artists (Munroe, 1979). Her willingness to take risks and her need for solitude are key themes that characterize her life and work. Risk-taking was essential in enabling her to transform private, personal imagery into artistic productions; it was also essential in enabling her to design a life-style that deviated from social mores and supported her desire to make painting a priority. Her drive for autonomy conflicted with wishes for intimacy, and these conflicts were initially resolved through her relationship with Alfred Stieglitz and then surfaced as their relationship matured, contributing to crises in the marriage.

This paper interprets Georgia O'Keeffe's life as a spiritual and psychological journey in which the artist sought and found relationships and places she needed to nourish and liberate her spirit and fulfill her sense of mission as an artist. The story of O'Keeffe's life, especially her relationship with Alfred Stieglitz, provides a role model for understanding the challenges and opportunities that face creative women as they struggle to take career risks and to combine marriage and career.

Georgia O'Keeffe's life is consistent with Storr's (1988) analysis that creative people often need solitude as a prerequisite for creative work. Long periods of solitude often preceded bursts of creative activity in her life. Georgia O'Keeffe's life and work also is consistent with other formulations presented in Storr's (1988) description of dynamics that influence creative work.

The evolving imagery of Georgia O'Keeffe's art suggests that the artist's work served as a means of self-fulfillment, self-actualization, and possibly served to restore psychological equilibrium at times of crisis in personal relationships. Georgia O'Keeffe's attachment to nature and to the land she loved was as deep and rewarding as her most intimate relationship. She was gifted in her ability to translate her imagery and her spirit onto canvas.

John Sloan (1977) in *Gist of Art* has offered a description of an artist's function: "The artist...crystallizes the prose of nature into poetic images" (p. 18). This quote is an apt description of Georgia O'Keeffe's use of art to communicate, to transform, and to depict her view of the world.

A CASE STUDY: TRANSFORMING IMAGERY INTO ART

In this section of the presentation, the varying impact of imagery is traced throughout five phases of the artist's career.

Role of Imagery in the Birth of an Artist: The Early Drawings

The role that mental imagery played in Georgia O'Keeffe's development as an artist is most evident in her early charcoal drawings.

Vera John-Stiener (1985) in describing the power of visual thinking suggests that images are essential in the development of an artist's career. The development of an artist's career hinges on her capacity to discover and express "an image that signifies the self" (p. 97). The "image that signifies the self" is described as a strong, original, and creative view of the world or synthesis of the artist's experience which introduces a composition that is exciting and memorable. The work of the artist "is constructed from varied flights of the artist's thought...Once completed a painting becomes...a framed moment in the shared visual culture of the time" (p. 102).

Georgia O'Keeffe's early drawings depict the spiritual and aesthetic birth of the artist as a young woman To appreciate the originality of these drawings, we need to recall that the artist drew these in 1915 when she was 27 years old. She had assumed a position teaching art at a women's college in South Carolina and found this environment stifling because of the emphasis on conforming and convention. In her letters to her friend Anita Pollitzer, O'Keeffe described her experiences and thoughts at the time she produced the drawings - her excitement and joy, as well as her self-doubts:

> Did you ever have something to say and feel as if the whole side of the wall wouldn't be big enough to say it in and then sit down on the floor and try to get it onto a sheet of charcoal paper...I wasn't even sure I had anything worth expressing--There are things we want to say but saying them is pretty nervy...(Cowart, Hamilton, and Greenough, 1987, pp. 146-147).

The letters indicate that Georgia experienced a sense of being flooded with images, driven to express these on paper, and felt that the forms she produced were the "purest" expression of original images and a way to break with past influences in her artistic training. She also wrote to Anita that it was emotionally safer for her to pour her feelings into charcoal drawings than risk losing herself in romantic relationships. Many years later when encouraged to write her memoirs, the artist (O'Keeffe, 1976, p.1) described the boldness involved in risking using her own mental imagery as the source of a unique, individual style. She wrote that while she had been taught to paint by copying the masters, she had decided ignore those lessons and be innovative, using her own personal imagery as a source of inspiration. She discovered that forms that arose from her own imagination were completely original and realized that these forms and images could be subjects for her art.

She made a fresh start by relinquishing all colors, using only charcoal on paper to express herself. This technique left her feeling "alone and free, working into my own unknown." (O'Keeffe, 1976, p. 1). In later letters, O'Keeffe described her process of risk-taking as "working into my unknown."

Although the artist attributed the inspiration for her early charcoal drawings solely to her imagination, these abstract drawings contain many of the basic forms of nature which inspired the artist's later works (Messinger, 1988). Note especially the components of *Drawing #13*: jagged edges which will represent bolts of lightening in later paintings; meandering flowing lines and elliptical bud shapes that could suggest female forms and are evocative of the hills that dominate the later paintings of New Mexico landscapes. Georgia O'Keeffe playfully associates "maybe a kiss" (Bry, 1988, p.9) to *Drawing #12* that exudes sensuousness. She attributes *Abstraction IX* (1917) to a stored memory image of a woman's face (Bry, 1988). Many years later similar forms and lines were used to represent a painting of roads in the New Mexico desert (*Road Past the View*).

These early drawings of Georgia O'Keeffe became legendary in the world of art. Georgia had sent a roll of these drawings to her friend Anita Pollitzer. Ignoring Georgia's instructions not to show them to anyone, Anita took the drawings to Alfred Stieglitz who owned a gallery in New York called 291. Stieglitz was a pioneer in introducing contemporary and modern art to America. When he saw the early drawings of Georgia O'Keeffe he is rumoured as having exclaimed "Finally a woman on paper!" (Pollitzer, 1988, p. 48). Recognizing the original quality of the drawings, he included them in a show in his gallery in the Spring of 1916. Georgia returned to New York for a semester of studying art, and when she left, she also began to correspond with Stieglitz. Their letters also trace the artist's imagery as she continued to develop a distinctive style in her work.

In 1917 and 1918, the artist began to add color, using water colors to continue her explorations in abstraction. *Blue Lines* in 1916 is a famous early drawing often thought to symbolize a male and female image. Several other early watercolors reveal the influence of nature on the artist's work and her propensity to transform images drawn from nature into abstract compositions. For example, the 1917 watercolors entitled *Light Coming from the Plains* and *Starlight Night* are abstractions distilled from how the artist visualized and experienced the sky in the country. Georgia had moved to the deserted plains of a town called Canyon in Texas where she also taught art in a small college. She filled her letters with descriptions of the evening sky and a nearby canyon which were exhilarating to her. She delighted not only in visual images but in the sounds of the Texas plains and their capacity to evoke kinesthetic imagery which was transformed into her watercolors.

Tonight I walked into the sunset to mail some letters--the whole sky, and there is so much of it out here, was just blazing and the blue grey clouds were rioting all through the hotness of it...

The Eastern sky was all grey blue--different kinds of clouds...there was nothing but sky and flat prairie land...land that seems more like the ocean than anything else I know...(Cowart et al., 1987, pp. 156-157).

Georgia spent much of her time in long solitary walks, soaking up the sounds, sights, and feel of the land, or in the model suggested by Rosenberg (1987b), viewing the world as material for art and storing images which are later retrieved and transformed. Her famous *Evening Star* was a series of 10 watercolors which evolved over the course of the year of 1917. It is the design which represented Georgia's image of the evening sky on the plains. The artist (O'Keeffe, 1976, p.6) reminisced that she frequently walked in the late afternoon away from town looking at the horizon which stretched wide "like the ocean". She was fascinated with the scene of the evening star rising up high while the sun was still setting.

Years later Georgia O'Keeffe wrote of the importance of transforming her perceptions of landscapes into imaginative images:

The memory or dream thing that I do for me comes nearer reality than my objective kind of work. (Cowart et al., 1987, p. 206)

Imagery that Merges Art and Love

Stieglitz's letters to Georgia O'Keeffe during her year of teaching in Canyon Texas drew them closer together. This was the first time O'Keeffe had found a man she could completely trust, a soulmate. It is interesting to note O'Keeffe's capacity for expressing herself in images extending to her verbal communication. For example, she wrote Anita describing the way Stieglitz's letters fulfilled her needs:

his letters...have been like fine cold water when you are terribly thirsty...I think letters with so much humanness in them have never come to me before...they seem to give me a great big quietness. (Pollitzer, 1988, pp. 141-142)

Worried about her health, Stieglitz sent for Georgia to join him in New York in 1918, and they became lovers shortly afterwards. Stieglitz was 54 years old; Georgia 31. They were united by their love for art, and defiance of convention. She provided him with the courage and excuse to leave a stultifying marriage. O'Keeffe and Stieglitz began a passionate love affair, living during the winters in the New York studio of Alfred's niece and during the summers at the Stieglitz family home at Lake George. He took the role of her mentor, freeing her from the responsibility of teaching to support herself, and encouraging her to put all her energy into her painting.

For both Stieglitz and O'Keeffe, the early years of their relationship were years of heightened emotionality and intimacy in which their art and their love was fused. It was during these years that Stieglitz photographed his lover in one of the most remarkable series of nude photographs of a woman's body that had ever been made. O'Keeffe began painting in oils and

48

her paintings, especially her abstractions, became infused with a heightened sensuality that seemed to vibrate with passionate imagery. *Music, Pink and Blue,* 1919, was a personal favorite of O'Keeffe's and remained in her personal collection for 50 years. Its warm colors and sensuous fluid lines seem to evoke inner and outer harmony and the whole canvas communicates a celebration of joy. The artist herself (O'Keeffe, 1976) ascribed the source of this imagery to exercises in which she translated sound into color. In 1914, while Georgia was taking courses at Teachers College, Columbia University to meet requirements for teaching art, she overheard music coming from a classroom. She entered and joined in exercises that were taught by an innovative instructor, Alan Bemet. He played records, instructing his students first to paint while listening to soft low tones and then to paint while listening to notes from much higher octaves. Georgia, who was very sensitive to sounds in nature, was thus formally exposed to an idea she later incorporated in her paintings - "the idea that music could be translated as something for the eye" (O'Keeffe, 1976, p.14).

As O'Keeffe continued to work in oils, her subject matter broadened, ranging from abstractions to representational paintings. She began a pattern of exploring the same subject in styles that ranged along a continuum from abstract to representational, or vice versa. Her paintings, therefore, began to reflect her capacity to take an image, to manipulate it, and to play with it, and then to express many variations on her canvasses. While there is a lack of empirical research on how artists use imagery in their work, psychologists and scholars interested in how artists use imagery in their work, speculate that many artists may have unusual abilities to manipulate and transform the inner world of mental images (Gordon, 1972; Lindauer, 1977; Mandelbrojt, 1970). There are several subjects that can illustrate how Georgia O'Keeffe transformed and painted what she saw in her mind's eye, turning her perceptions into imaginative compositions. Two compositions, for example, were inspired by the artist's impressions of her summer home at Lake George. First, the more representational view entitled, *Lake George* (1924) and then the more abstract, *From The Lake, No. 1* (1924). There are also two canvasses which depict different renditions of a view of a stormy sky over the ocean. The first is entitled *A Storm* (1922) and the second is *Lightening At Sea* also painted in 1922. Note that both paintings feature the jagged line depicting lightening and that this image originally appeared in O'Keeffe's abstract drawings and was most likely inspired by the wild quality of the lightening that she observed in the storms over the Texas plains. These canvasses illustrate how memory images, perceptions, and imagination images can also become threaded into the final composition of the artist. The process of interweaving memory and imagination is a key function that imagery plays in the process of transforming experience into art (Arieti, 1976).

Flowers: The Images that Became Symbols

Georgia O'Keeffe is best known for her paintings of flowers. A recent centennial publication *Georgia O'Keeffe: One Hundred Flowers* featured over a hundred of these paintings and documented that she painted over 200 flowers between 1918 and 1930, painting lillies, poppies, hollyhocks, irises, pansies and many other flowers. The images are striking because of their vivid colors, and because of the distinctive style of projecting the blossom right at the viewer so that it fills the whole canvas and seems to pull the viewer right into the center of the flower. In the Exhibition Catalogue of 1939, Georgia O'Keeffe described her own intention to coax her audience into looking closely at enlarged flowers, and to shock them into seeing flowers as she saw them.

The artist began her flower series in part as a reaction to what she felt was excessive interpretation of her abstract paintings as female sexual symbols. Ironically, the flowers were her attempt to disclose less of her private self in her imagery and to find subjects that she considered representational. The flowers serve to illustrate the processes by which images are transformed into symbols, since O'Keeffe's flowers have become among the most famous of erotic symbols in American 20th century painting. Images have been described as becoming symbols by virtue of the abstract ideas and associations that become attached to a tangible visible object (Gordon, 1972). O'Keeffe (1976) resented this treatment of her flowers. She chided her audience for hanging their sexual "associations" on her flowers.

The joy and brilliance of the early flower paintings lends to their being interpreted as a symbol and self-portrait of the flowering of O'Keeffe's career and her love (Schaire, 1987). O'Keeffe and Stieglitz were married in 1924 and by the mid 1920's the flower paintings were creating a sensation in New York exhibitions. It is also interesting to speculate that O'Keeffe's flowers are an example of Arnheim's (1971) concept that "all art is symbolic" (p. 440-442). Artistic objects, according to Arnheim, are not symbolic by virtue of representing other objects (which is the psychoanalytic interpretation of flowers as symbols of genitalia). The symbolism is inherent in the perceptual characteristics of a composition since those characteristics illustrate universal truths of nature. In this respect, Georgia O'Keeffe's flowers symbolize the blossoming that exists both in the physical world of nature and in our human consciousness when we experience our enterprises or our love realizing their potential.

Images that Express the Darker Side of Life

Throughout Georgia O'Keeffe's career, the source of most of her imagery was some object of her passion--either the passion for landscapes, for nature, or other objects and experiences that represent a strong attachment for her. O'Keeffe (1976) explained that she had painted flowers, sea shells, and rocks because they were objects that she had found fascinating. Similarly, she described "beautiful white bones on the desert" as objects that she had admired, collected, and later painted. All these objects were ways she expressed on canvass "the wideness and wonder of the world as I live in it" (p. 71).

Biographical studies indicate that the artist did sustain at least one and more likely two episodes of depression that did threaten to halt her career in mid-life. It is interesting to try to trace the impact of these emotional crises on her imagery and paintings.

Although limited mention is made of these episodes in available biographies (Castro, 1985; Lisle, 1980; Robinson, 1989), sources indicate the artist suffered from an ambiguous illness called "nervous exhaustion" in 1928. She also experienced an episode of depression and panic in the winter of 1932 and 1933 which finally resulted in a hospitalization for treatment (Lisle, 1980, p. 261).

Her emotional crisis coincided with changes and tension in her relationship to Stieglitz and her sense that the relationship threatened her sense of autonomy, and threatened the development of her career. By 1927, there had been a shift in the balance of power in their relationship. Georgia had become the successful artist who was supporting the household. Alfred was aging, had been strickened with a heart attack, and made demands that drained Georgia's time and attention. Their lifestyles clashed. She needed and valued a solitary existence in the country which nourished her painting. He craved the conversation and audiences of New York City.

It is possible that the artist's sense of an impending emotional crisis in her life and marriage is represented in the painting *Black Abstraction* (1927). It is a unique work for her, one of her most abstract statements with paint and lines as the only compositional element and presenting an image of darkness closing in on a center core of light. In her later memoirs, O'Keeffe (1976) herself ascribed this image to a memory that dominated her consciousness just before she succumbed to the effects of anaesthesia when undergoing surgery for a benign tumour on her breast. We may also speculate that she was representing her sense of loss of control and the fear of other losses. The picture creates a tense ominous mood and a sense of being lost in space. One of Georgia O'Keeffe's most famous flowers, *The Black Iris*, was also painted in 1927 and its dark beauty may also portend the artist's sense that she is beginning to be enveloped in darker emotions.

Images that Revitalized the Artist

Georgia decided that a change of scenery would help her recover from her "illness" and she reasserted her courage and boldness in 1929 by defying Stieglitz's wishes and taking her first separate vacation from him. During the summer, she traveled to Taos and spent the summer months there. This trip marked a turning point in her life and career. Her enthusiastic letters home to Stieglitz and to friends describe her feeling that she had found herself again. A letter written to Henry McBride, a New York art critic, communicates a passion for the New Mexico landscape that resembled the artist's sense of excitement in experiencing the vast Texas plains when she was a young art teacher:

> I never feel at home in the East as I do out here--and finally feeling in the right place again, I feel like myself--and I like it...Yours till the mountain out Yonder sinks (Cowart, et al., 1987, pp. 189-190).

New images inspired by New Mexico started appearing in Georgia O'Keeffe's paintings in 1929 (*Ranchos Church*, 1929 and *Black Cross, New Mexico*, 1929). She wrote of her conflict between the love she felt for this land and the loyalty and attachment she felt to Stieglitz which drew her back East. Eventually she resolved this conflict by spending part of each year in New

Mexico, buying a small adobe house at Ghost Ranch which had a sweeping vista of the Pedernal mesa and Jamez mountains, and eventually another home in the village of Abiquiu which overlooked a green river valley. She moved permanently to New Mexico after Stieglitz's death in 1946. Her art has come to be almost as much identified with the images of the desert as it has with flowers and abstractions. Red hills, pelvis bones, and skulls--these were the objects and vistas from the land she called the "Faraway" (*From the Faraway Nearby*, 1937) and this imagery represented her new passions and the revitalized sense of self that she derived from the land (*The Pedernal and Red Hills; The Grey Hills*, 1942).

There are fewer letters describing O'Keeffe's imagery processes in her later years. The paintings, themselves, give the visual record of landscapes and objects she studied--many of them closely connected to her homes. She lived a solitary life, devoted much time to paintings and while she traveled widely in her later years, she returned to her New Mexico homes describing them as the most wonderful place in the world.

In an Exhibition Catalogue, she explained that her landscapes represented the expression of her passionate attachment to the vistas she loved. She acknowledged that her connection to these images paralleled the earlier attachment to flowers although she realized that her audience would not necessarily appreciate her degree of passion.

Her friend Anita Pollitzer visited Georgia in 1951 and in her book (1988) described the early morning ritual in which the artist would rise to view panoramic sunrise from her Abiquiu patio. The artist had constructed her daily life in New Mexico to witness the visual drama of the sky, and the space--images which found their way into many of her later paintings. One of the most striking images that Georgia O'Keeffe painted in later years was a dream-like picture entitled *Ladder to the Moon* (1958).

The object of this painting was the ladder that led to the roof of the artist's home at Ghost Ranch. O'Keeffe (1976) wrote about climbing this ladder several times daily to view the surrounding panoramic view, especially the image of the Pedernal mesa and the surrounding mountain range. Her inspiration for the painting arose from a spontaneous insight she had one evening while observing a high, white moon: "Painting the ladder had been in my mind for a long time and there it was--with the dark Pedernal and high white moon--all ready to be put down" (O'Keeffe, 1976, p. 102).

In her words Georgia O'Keeffe has illustrated how imagery processes were transformed into memorable and exciting canvasses, and how the spiritual home she found in the desert inspired a long and creative career. In another Exhibition Catalogue, Georgia O'Keeffe wrote that her drive for autonomy had led her into expressing original images on canvass. She wrote about the start of her career at age 27. She wrote that she had a typical upbringing but that, by age 20, her life was constricted by convention. She had felt that she could neither live where she wanted to, nor express her ideas freely. This carried over to her painting. She felt her formal training in art institutes had stifled her originality. It was through her art that she chose to assert her wish for autonomy. She decided that her painting was her private concern and that she could at least express herself freely in her art. She found she could "say things with colors and shapes" and use her images to express "things I had no words for" (O'Keeffe, 1976, p. 13).

By the time Georgia O'Keeffe died in 1986 she had lived almost 100 years. She had in fact not only painted what she wanted, but she had lived where she wanted and gone where she wanted. And in the process she had transformed her life and experiences into canvasses that expand our own view of the possibilities in our lives.

ACKNOWLEDGMENT

The author wishes to express appreciation to the National Gallery of Art which has given permission to quote from *Georgia O'Keeffe, Art and Letters* . 1988.

REFERENCES

An American Place. (1939). *Exhibition Catalogue* .
Anderson Galleries. (1923). *Exhibition Catalogue* .
Arieti, S. (1976). *Creativity: The Magic Synthesis*. New York: Basic Books.
Arnheim, R. (1971). *Art and Visual Perception*. Berkeley: University of California Press.
Bry, D. (Ed.). (1988). *Georgia O'Keeffe: Some Memories of Drawings*. Albuquerque: University of New Mexico Press.

Castro, J. (1985). *The Art and Life of Georgia O'Keeffe*. New York: Crown Publishers.

Cowart, J., Hamilton, J., and Greenough, S. (1988). *Georgia O'Keeffe: Art and Letters*. Washington and New York: New York Graphic Society Books.

Forisha, B. (1978). Mental Imagery and Creativity: Review and Speculations. *Journal of Mental Imagery, 2,* 23-32.

Ghiselin, B. (Ed.). (1952). *The Creative Process*. New York: Mentor.

Gordon, R.A. (1972). A Very Private World. In P.W. Sheehan (Ed.), *The Function and Nature of Imagery* (pp. 63-80). New York: Academic Press.

Gowan, J.C. (1978). Incubation, Imagery, and Creativity. *Journal of Mental Imagery, 2,* 23-32.

Gruber, H. (1989). The evolving systems approach to creative work. In D.B. Wallace and H.E. Gruber (Eds.) *Creative People at Work* (pp. 3-24). New York: Oxford University Press.

John-Steiner, V. (1985). *Notebooks of the Mind*. Albuquerque: University of New Mexico Press.

Kuzendorf, R. (1982). Mental Images, Appreciation of Grammatical Patterns, and Creativity. *Journal of Mental Imagery, 6,* 183-202.

Lindauer, M. (1983). Imagery and the Arts. In A.A. Sheikh (Ed.), *Imagery: Current Theory, Research, and Applications* (pp. 468-506). New York: John Wiley and Sons.

Lisle, L. (1980). *Portrait of an Artist*. New York: Washington Square Press.

Mandelbrojt, J. (1970). On Mental Images and Their Pictorial Representation. *Leonardo, 3,* 19-26.

Messinger, L. (1988). *Georgia O'Keeffe*. New York: Thames and Hudson.

Munroe, E. (1979). *Originals: American Women Artists*. New York: Simon and Schuster.

O'Keeffe, G. (1976). *Georgia O'Keeffe*. New York, The Viking Press.

O'Keeffe, G. (1985). *Works on Paper*. Albuquerque: University of New Mexico Press.

Pollitzer, A. (1988). *A Women on Paper*. New York: Touchstone.

Robinson, R. (1989). *Georgia O'Keeffe*. New York: Harper and Row.

Rosenberg, H. (1987a). *Creative Drama and Imagination*. New York: Holt Rinehart, and Winston.

Rosenberg, H. (1987b). Visual Artists and Imagery. *Imagination, Cognition, and Personality, 7,* 77-93.

Schaire, J. (1987). Georgia O'Keeffe in love. *Arts and Antiques,* 61-72.

Sloan, J. (1977). *Gist of Art*. New York: Dover Publications.

Storr, A. (1988). *Solitude: A Return to the Self*. New York: Ballantine Books.

Wallace, D. (1989). Studying the Individual: The Case Study Method and Other Genres. In D.B. Wallace and H.E. Gruber (Eds.), *Creative People at Work* (pp. 25-41). New York: Oxford University Press.

THE NATURE OF THE THEATRICAL IMAGINATION:
HOW THEATRE GOING AFFECTS CHILDREN'S IMAGINATION,
AND WHAT CHILDREN SAY ABOUT THEIR THEATRE EXPERIENCES

Helane S. Rosenberg, Ph.D.,   and   Yakov M. Epstein, Ph.D.

Graduate School of Education   Department of Psychology
Rutgers University   Rutgers University
New Brunswick, NJ 08903   New Brunswick, NJ 08903

In 1986, the state of Massachusetts passed legislation called the Performing Arts Student Series (PASS) which provided funding to allow school children to see selected performing arts events for a small fee. The following investigations are part of the evaluation study of this program. One of the key questions of this three-year investigation focused on the effect of theatre attendance on mental imagery abilities.

THE QUANTITATIVE INVESTIGATION

The Method

The purpose of this study was to investigate the effects of theatre attendance on the mental imagery abilities of selected Massachusetts children participating in the PASS Program. The sample consisted of 990 children (in grades three to five), 46 of whom were in a control group that did not attend the theatre, and 944 children in an experimental group who attended the theatre under funding provided by this arts program. In November 1986, we administered the Cognitive Visual Mental Imagery Test (CVMI) (Smith, 1986) as part of a pre-test package.

The Cognitive Visual Mental Imagery Test consists of two stories read aloud to the children, to which they make written responses. Just as in responding to a theatrical story, the children are asked to recall, conjecture, provide their own detail, and draw conclusions to this narrative story. Their responses are scored for fluency, flexibility, elaboration, and accuracy, as well given a total score. (For this study, we only looked at total scores.) From November 1986 through May 1987, the children were taken to at least one (several groups of children did attend two performing arts events) professional theatre performance. They saw such performing arts events as *Christmas Carol, Mary Poppins, Pinocchio,* and *Most Valuable Player.* We then returned again to their classrooms and administered as part of our posttest package the posttest version of the Cognitive Visual Mental Imagery Test.

The Analysis

Total scores for each of the two stories were summed, once for the pre-test and once for the post-test. Pretest scores ranged 1 to 64 and post-test scores ranged from 1 to 72. A 2 X 2 General Linear Model Analysis of Variance (ANOVA) for unequal numbers of observations was performed on these summed scores. The ANOVA model consisted of one between groups factor (Experimental vs: Control groups) and one within groups repeated measures factor (pre vs: post-test scores).

Mental Imagery, Edited by R.G. Kunzendorf
Plenum Press, New York, 1990

Table 1. Mean Imagery Scores: Total Sample

	Story Pre	Story Post
Experimental	32.85	37.50
Control	36.07	38.33

The Results

Table 1 shows the pre-test and post-test means for children in the Experimental and in the Control groups. The data reveal that the control group of students had significantly higher imagery scores at the outset than the experimental group ($Mean_{con}$=36.06; $Mean_{exp}$=32.85). In contrast, post-test scores for the two groups were not significantly different ($Mean_{con}$=38.33; $Mean_{exp}$=37.50). The F statistics indicate that there was a significant Pre/Post effect (F (1,988) = 32.70; p <.0001) and a significant Pre/Post by Experimental/Control group effect (F (1,988) = 3.91; p < .05). The highly significant Pre/Post effect is the result of the lower pre-test score contributed by the experimental group. The most meaningful pattern revealed by these data is the greater increase in imagery scores for the experimental group than for the control group.

It is difficult to know why the experimental group had lower pre-test imagery scores than the control group. The sizes of the two groups were very disproportionate (N_{con}=46; N_{exp}=944). The greater increase in pre/post imagery scores for the experimental group may indicate that theatre attendance has a stimulating effect on the imagination of children. However, this conclusion cannot be defended easily from these data.

Fortunately, another data analytic strategy was possible - one which could potentially reveal a clearer pattern of results. In an effort to find such a pattern, we used a stratified random sampling procedure for our experimental group. For each of the control group scores on the pretest, we found the corresponding subset of experimental group pre-test scores. From this subset we randomly selected one subject. Using this procedure, we obtained a small random experimental sample, equal in size to the control group sample, whose pre-test scores were comparable to the pre-test scores of the control group. We then performed the analysis of variance that we had done with the total sample. Table 2 shows the means for both groups.

As expected, the stratified random sampling procedure resulted in extremely similar pre-test scores ($Mean_{con}$ = 36.06; $Mean_{exp}$ = 36.15). However, post-test scores for the two groups were significantly different ($Mean_{con}$ = 38.32; $Mean_{exp}$ = 41.67). Once again the Pre/Post main effect is highly significant (F (1,90) = 33.97; p <.0001). Likewise, the Pre/Post by Experimental/Control interaction is also significant (F (1,90) = 5.96; p<.02). Thus, the significant interaction resulted from a lack of difference in imagery scores at the outset in contrast to higher imagery scores for experimental group subjects following their theatre attendance.

Conclusions

Results of both the total sample analysis and the more refined smaller stratified random sample analysis reveal the same pattern: students who attend theatre performances, in contrast to their counterparts who don't have this experience, show increases in imaginative activity as revealed by the Cognitive Visual Mental Imagery Test coded analysis of their stories. Presumably, this increase in imaginative activity is due to the intense imaginative and novel experience provided by this theatrical experience.

Table 2. Mean Imagery Scores: Small Sample

	Story Pre	Story Post
Experimental	36.15	41.67
Control	36.07	38.33

THE QUALITATIVE INVESTIGATION

The results of the quantitative study investigating the effects of theatre attendance on the visual mental imagery ability of children participating in the Massachusetts Arts Lottery Council Performing Arts Student Series, discussed above, provided the encouragement for a further investigation on the nature of the theatrical imagination of young people. That investigation suggested that as few as one theatre experience could positively increase the mental imagery skills of young people, particularly if those young people had limited prior theatre attendance and if that experience were a large-scale production, staged in a regular theatre during school time. The authors believe that the "as if" nature of the experience, particularly the "suspension of disbelief" aspect, was a major contributing factor in the positive contribution theatre made on the imagery abilities of these children. They wished to explore this premise further.
The following study is an attempt to describe the nature of the theatre-related imagery abilities of a small segment of the larger population. The focus is on general recall of theatrical moments, with attention to clarity, vividness and degree of detail. Also reported is the delineation of the theatrical aspects which are of particular importance to the development of the theatrical imagination, including production space, technical/artistic aspects of production (such as costumes and masks, for example), the "as if" nature of character, and pivotal moments in plot and/or action.

The Method

About the Sample. For this study, we targeted a very specific child, one that we felt would provide us with the broadest base of information. We wanted to talk to children who already said they liked attending theatre--in fact, it was their preferred leisure time activity selected from the following five activities: reading a book, attending a rock concert, viewing a movie, going to theatre, or attending an athletic event. Of the entire sample of 990 (discussed in the previous article), 66 children selected theatre as their favorite leisure time activity in November 1986 and 147 selected theatre as their favorite leisure time activity in June 1987. In November 1988, we were able to contact 94 of these theatre supporters, 23 boys and 71 girls. During the early part of 1989, we visited these children and administered the y test and asked them again to select their favorite leisure time activity. Of the 94 children, 82 again selected theatre.
The children we decided to talk with selected theatre all three times. What is interesting about their selection is that many of these children selected theatre as their favorite leisure-time activity before they had ever seen a professional performance. Not so surprising is the increased number of children who selected theatre immediately after they had seen a performance. On the other hand, what is surprising is the number of children who continued to select theatre even though they may not have seen any other performance for over a year. We believed that these children had a particularly vivid and powerful recall of the theatre experience and would provide some rich information. What ultimately characterized this sample, besides their limited or nonexistent prior theatre exposure, was their ease at discussing what they remembered about the experience and their enthusiasm at playing with these theatrical images.
During our 1989 return visit, twenty-six of these children, 18 girls and 8 boys, seemed to be eager and interested in talking to us about their experiences. These 26 children were invited to attend a shared theatrical experience. On May 7, 1989, thirteen children and their chaperons, together with the two interviewers (Dr. Rosenberg and Dr. Charles Combs) attended a production of *Androcles and the Lion* at Wheelock Family Theatre in Boston. Two weeks later, the interviewers returned to the children's schools and talked with each child for approximately forty-five minutes to an hour. All interviews were taped.
The Interview. Interviews were conducted face to face in a private room with either one or both of the interviewers present. The interview began with a general overview of why we were asking these questions. Following this general introduction, children were shown their drawings of the production viewed in 1987 (available for four of the thirteen) or production photos of the 1989 production. After each of the children viewed the photos, we proceeded to discuss various aspects of the production including x, y, and z.
The Analysis . All the tapes of the children were transcribed. The transcripts were scanned by two judges for all important imagery-related statements. Only if both judges agreed that a statement was important was the statement included. Once the imagery-related statements were identified, the first judge classified these statements into the theatre-related categories. Then, the second judge also classified the statements. Inter-rater agreement was .94 on the identification of statements and .95 on the classification of these statements into theatrical categories. Thirty-eight

significant theatre-related topics emerged during our conversations with these children; nineteen were deemed to be directly related to mental imagery and are discussed below.

The Results

The topics fall into four general groupings:

1. General recall (6 topics).
2. Imagery related to theatrical conventions (7 topics).
3. Transformational imagery (4 topics).
4. reality/imagination continuum (2 topics).

General Recall. Two weeks after they had seen the production of *Androcles and the Lion,* every single child was able to recall all or most of the major characters, the major action of the story, much of the actual dialogue, much of the detail of the technical aspects of the production, including costumes, lights, sets, and music. The major portion of the imagery described was either visual or aural, although two of the children did recall and describe their visceral response associated with a moment in the play. We classified responses like these as kinesthetic images:

EM: I remember when I went that my insides felt all excited and moving around.
DL: I had to lean forward and squinch up my ears to hear.
CP: They moved so close to me that I could touch them.

Within this grouping, the two most revealing topics have to do with children's responses to photographs of moments in the play and in their own drawing of favorite moments in the play. The photos helped spark the imagery recall. When we asked the children to name and describe the characters, only a few could do so. When we showed them the photographs, they were able to recall the character's personality, then his or her name, and finally to describe the action pictured in great detail. It seems, at least in terms of these thirteen children, that photographs of the actual production were very helpful in priming the pump, so to speak, of imagery recall.

Asking the children to draw their favorite moment (one that was not pictured in the photos) gave us much information about two aspects of the production: the recalled detail of the technical aspects of the production and the most important stage action of the play. Almost every one of the children was able to draw the patches on Androcles' costume (the Androcles character and his costume are drawn from the Commedia dell'arte character of Harlequin) in almost photographic detail. Likewise, the children were able to draw the symmetrical stage setting; their drawings accurately depicted the stage space, the detail of the rocks, and the colors of the curtains! Interestingly, most of the children drew actual moments of the play--they drew from memory images, not imagination ones.

While they were drawing, we complimented each child and asked him or her to describe their internal process. A typical imagery response described what was happening while drawing:

BK: I usually have a picture in my head and I try to draw from the picture.

Even when the children asked to see a photo before drawing and were refused, they still were able to draw with accuracy and enthusiasm.

Imagery Related to Theatrical Conventions. It is in this grouping that some interesting issues emerge, all of which are related to simultaneous modification of the experience, based on instinctual response to various aspect of the play. Research on the theatre experience (as well as our own first-hand experience) suggests that theatrical conventions are readily accepted by even the youngest theatre-goer. Members of the audience accept the premises, for example, that we can hear Viola's aside but Olivia can't, that the cherry tree about which the drama unfolds is really held up by a stand, that Peter Pan flies by the aid of wires, the actors really don't fly. In the theatre literature, this phenomenon is called suspension of disbelief; we actively involve ourselves in *not* allowing the illogic of the present situation to get in the way of our here-and-now experience.

Using an imagery framework to understand suspension of disbelief, however, helps to make more specific what these particular audience members experienced in terms of the various theatrical conventions in the production: sets, masks, costumes, scripts, lights, and music. In terms of experiencing conventions, it seems the children experienced three primary imagery strategies: overlay, blurring, and magnification. Many children merely overlayed one image on the reality of the experience, as these two children did:

HSR: How did you play that trick on yourself?
JR: Tell myself he's a person and then a lion and all that.
HSR: Did you believe it was a lion?
BK: I knew it wasn't a lion, but when I got into the play, I believed it was a lion talking.

Other children blurred the reality to allow themselves to go with the experience:

HSR: So was it a cave or not?
SK: I think it's a cave because you can see the opening and they had this cloth, but it's nothing like a cave, but I knew it was a cave. But it isn't clear. But I knew because the lion ran out.
HSR: Was that a real cave?
SM: I knew it was fake. It's hard. I don't know. . . But I decided to pretend.

Finally, children used the imagery strategy of magnification of images to make the experience *more* than the actual convention. In particular, children dealt with the conventions of masks in this very expansive manner; almost all of them thought the effect was to make the character "more so" and recalled the masks as uglier or more extensive than they were:

HSR: Do you know why they have on masks in the play?
TV: To show up meaner.

Transformational Imagery. The four groupings reflect specific "what if" or "as if" abilities as described in Rosenberg (1987). Children revealed that they were able to entertain dramatic possibilities. They were able to describe what happened before and what happened after the action of the play portrayed on the stage. All of these descriptions of course involve imagination images and are filled with the same detail as those images that provided the children with their recall ability.

When asked if they could change anything that took place onstage, the children were also able to use the here and now reality as a starting point and imagine from that point. Again detail is present in almost all the descriptions of how the play could be changed. Interestingly, the kinds of scenes or additions described seem to have their source in the related art form of the movies. Of the six children who wanted to add to the play, all six wished for aerial views, inside the houses which could only be pictured from the outside in the theatre, or cross-fades from one scene to another: all imagination images that have their source in the cinema. Clearly, the more common experience of attending the movies helped shape what the children hoped to see in the theatrical production.

Finally, when asked who they would like to be in the play, all five children who responded to the question described themselves dressed as the main character--Androcles. Whether watching television, movies, or theatre, these children all seemed to identify themselves in their minds' eyes with the main character.

Reality/Imagination Continuum. In this final grouping, the critical issue here is whether the children were able to discern that the theatrical reality is just that--an imaginative world different from the real world, but one that must be accepted for the purpose of having a total experience. Twelve of the thirteen children were open to talking about the degree to which this experience was like or different from reality, as well as how they could suspend disbelief, or at least allow themselves to go with the experience. Unlike the previous category of theatrical conventions, which deals primarily with the discussion of the convention itself, this category focuses on the discussion of the greater issue--the creation of an imaginative reality.

Interestingly, for these children at least, the most provocative questions concerned the real-life versus character life of the actors in the production of *Androcles and the Lion.* The autograph session after the production helped the children put this reality/imagination notion into perspective. Seeing the actors and comparing their personalities to their characters was of great interest. JR liked comparing both vocal and personality characteristics:

HSR: Was it different when you saw the person afterwards for autographs as opposed to when you saw them pretending to be someone else? Did it mess up your pretend?
JR: It was neat. . . He speaks different and all that.

HSR: Do you have an opinion about Pantilone, whether he was nice or bad, compared to the actor?
JR: He was a bad man. In the play, not for real. I met him for real afterwards. He seemed okay. It's neat.

EM remained fascinated by the vocal differences:

HSR: So they were different, in what ways?
EM: He didn't speak in a deep voice. . . He wasn't like aarrgh or anything.

Throughout the entire interview, she compared her aural images of the actors' voices with her images of the characters' voices. A related issue focused on casting--whether actors should or did play characters like themselves. JB seems to see an overlap of reality and illusion:

HSR: Do you think people should play characters that are like themselves or different from themselves?
JB: Probably somewhere in between.

SK thought that "good" people play characters like themselves, but bad characters are not played by mean people:

HSR: Were the personalities of those characters very much like the personalities of the characters they played?
SK: A little. Because she asked my name, and said that's a pretty little name and that makes people nice and she was nice in the play. So I guess she's a real nice person. But the person playing the Captain wouldn't be mean like that, he'd be very different.

All in all, these children explored the differences between reality and illusion and drew very personal conclusions about the created imaginative world of the theatre.

CONCLUSIONS

These two investigations represent some early attempts at describing and delineating the theatrical imagination. These studies suggest that the world of the theatre is a rich resource for the understanding of the artistic experience; those who watch provide us with as rich a body of material as those who create. Children, more than adults, seem eager to talk about their experiences. Our conversations with these children suggest that their collective theatre experience helped them learn about recalling, creating, exploring, and comparing a vast and interesting storehouse of mental images. It seems that Aristotle was correct; theatre both entertains and instructs.

BEFERENCES

Goldberg, P. (1983). Development of a Category System for the Analysis of the Responses of the Young Theatre Audience. *Children's Theatre Review, 32,* (2), 27-32.
Klein, J. (1987). Third Grade Children's Comprehension of *Monkey, Monkey* as a Function of Verbal and Visual Recall. *Youth Theatre Journal, 2,* (1), 9-13.
Klein, J., & Fitch, M. (1989). Third Grade Children's Verbal and Visual Recall of *Monkey, Monkey. Youth Theatre Journal, 4,* (2), 9-15.
Rosenberg, H. S. *Creative Drama and Imagination: Transforming Ideas into Action.* (1987). New York: Holt, Rinehart, and Winston.
Rosenberg, H. S. (1989). Transformations Described: How Twenty-Three Young People Think About and Experience Creative Drama. *Youth Theatre Journal, 4,* (1), 21-27.
Rosenberg, H. S., & Prendergast, C. (1983). *Theatre for Young People: A Sense of Occasion.* New York: Holt, Rinehart, and Winston.
Rosenberg, H. S., & Smith, J. K. (1981). The Effects of Advanced Organizers on Children's Responses to Theatre Viewing. *Children's Theatre Review Research Issue, 30,* (2), 17-24.
Saldana, J. (1989). A Quantitative Analysis of Children's Responses to Theatre from Probing Questions: A Pilot Study. *Youth Theatre Journal, 3,* (4), 7-17.

CHILDREN'S REACTIONS TO IMAGERY EXPERIENCES

Mary Elizabeth D'Zamko, Ed.D., and Lynne Schwab, Ph.D.

College of Education and Human Services
University of North Florida
Jacksonville, FL 32216

INTRODUCTION

Mental imagery and relaxation have been used in academic settings. One use of mental imagery has been to help students learn a concept like "circulatory system" by using an imaginary trip through the system. Mental imagery has been used as a readiness activity to prepare students for the academic day. Two ways this can be done are to have the student imagining himself or herself as a competent student, and practicing the ability to concentrate using an imagery activity. Stimulating creativity has been another use of mental imagery. For instance, mental imagery exercises have been used to precede brainstorming sessions. Another example of mental imagery in the classroom has been using transpersonal experiences to provide opportunities for students to improve communication skills.

Relaxation also has been used in academic settings to facilitate student learning. Relaxation prior to test taking has been a common practice. Teaching self control has been aided by the use of relaxation techniques. This, in turn, when practiced by the whole class has increased the ability of the teacher to maintain an ordered classroom.

While mental imagery and relaxation have been used in the classroom there appears to be a paucity of information about children's reactions to imagery and relaxation activities. Therefore, there was a need to do a preliminary field study to augment data collection in this area. The purposes of this study were (1) to collect data about the students' perceptions of the effects of imagery and relaxation activities in schools, and (2) to identify additional categories of information about their reactions that could guide further studies.

PROCEDURES

Data were collected from four public schools in Northeast Florida. Students in all school groupings experienced imagery and relaxation activities during the semester and, in half, preceding the administration of the survey. The topics and frequency of the activities varied from group to group. A description of the four groups follows.

Group 1. A second grade regular education classroom in a middle socio-economic neighborhood served as the setting for Group 1. The teacher was an innovative and energetic teacher who was a risk taker.

Group 2. A pull out gifted enrichment program for second graders from an upper middle socio-economic neighborhood was Group 2. The teacher gave the appearance of being a traditional teacher, but was very innovative and has been the Florida Special Education Teacher of the Year.

Mental Imagery, Edited by R.G. Kunzendorf
Plenum Press, New York, 1990

Group 3. A recently assembled group of fourth and fifth graders from a lower socio-economic neighborhood, with one of the investigators, as teacher, constituted Group 3.

Group 4. A sixth grade homeroom from a lower socio-economic neighborhood, with an innovative male teacher who has a casual teaching style, formed Group 4.

The survey instrument, see Table 1, was developed to provide opportunities for students to express their perceptions both in structured and in unstructured formats. The unstructured format allowed students to express thoughts and feelings in an unrestricted fashion.

The survey contained 25 items. The first sixteen were open-ended. The remaining items required the student to indicate which of three rankings represented their reactions to the items.

Table 1. Relaxation and Imagination Reaction Survey

Name:	School:

Directions. You have been doing some relaxation and imagination activities. Please think about these activities when you answer the questions below. Tell how you really feel about these activities. We are trying to find out how helpful using relaxation and imagination is to students.

1. The things I saw in my imagination were:
2. The things I heard in my imagination were:
3. The things I smelled in my imagination were:
4. The things I liked least about relaxation and imagination activities were:
5. When we did those activities I felt:
6. When we did those activities I thought:
7. After we started doing these activities, I felt:
8. After we started doing these activities, I thought:
9. After we started doing these activities, I could:
10. Before we started doing these activities, I felt:
11. Before we started doing these activities, I thought:
12. Before we started doing these activities, I could:
13. I'd like my friends to do these activities because:
14. When we do these activities my classmates:
15. The subject this helped me learn best is:
16. I think/feel doing this helped me learn: because:

For each of the following, circle the phrase that you would use to answer the question (the phrase that you like best).
For example: I like chocolate 1. a lot 2. some 3. not much.

17. When we do these activities my friends understand me
    1. better   2. about the same   3. worse
18. When we do these activities my mind works
    1. better   2. about the same   3. worse
19. When we do these activities I can learn
    1. better   2. about the same   3. worse
20. When we do these activities schoolwork is
    1. better   2. about the same   3. worse
21. When we do these activities it is
    1. more fun   2. fun   3. no fun
22. When we do these activities school is
    1. better   2. about the same   3. worse
23. When we do these activities I can work
    1. better   2. about the same   3. worse
24. I would like to do these relaxation and imagination activities
    1. more   2. don't care   3. less
25. When we do these activities my brain/mind works
    1. better   2. about the same   3. not as good

RESULTS

All responses were interpreted by the investigators as being "positive, neutral or negative" in nature. Responses where students did not express that they liked, disliked or perceived a change were considered neutral responses. See Table 2.

To simplify the data analysis, items five through sixteen clustered into five sets of scores. Items were based on similarity of content. For example, responses to items five and six indicated the students' feelings and thoughts when the activity occurred. Responses within clusters had internal consistency in all cases.

There were several major trends as perceived by the students. The students validated by providing information about their experiences that they, in fact, did have imagery experiences, and that for most students these experiences were very positive. During and after the imagery and relaxation experiences 70% - 95% of the students expressed positive responses about their feelings, thoughts and what they could do.

The majority of responses were positive regarding wanting friends to share these experiences; this was true even in the group that gave the most negative responses. This trend was also noted in the students' perceptions of how imagery and relaxation affect their school work. Regarding perceptions about whether their "minds worked better", there was only one negative response. The majority of the responses were positive and the remaining responses were neutral.

When asked to select a ranking of "more fun," "fun" or "no fun," with regard to doing these activities, two groups, the youngest, thought it was "more fun." Of the other two groups, the majority response was that it was "fun." Of the oldest group, one them considered it "no fun." Three of the four groups wanted to have more relaxation and imagination activities. In Group 4, the majority did not care whether or not they had more of these activities.

In addition to these structured rankings, students were asked to provide comments in an open ended and unstructured format. In response to the item where students were asked what they liked least about relaxation and imagery activities, the most frequent responses students gave were positive. "Nothing" or "I like everything" were common comments for this question. Younger children expressed difficulty with keeping their eyes closed for a period of time. There were 3 instances reported of being scared during the activity-- all within the sixth grade homeroom group. There were other comments that occurred only one time which were negative such as "it takes too much time," and "I might fall asleep." In two cases, the choice of background music did not facilitate the imagery.

DISCUSSION

These preliminary data support using imagery activities in schools since students perceive these activities in a positive way. The activities were perceived as fun, students want their friends to experience the activities and overall the students felt the activities helped their school performance.

Despite the positive results of this pilot study, there remain potential cautions to be explored. The choice of topic for the imagery experience should be carefully considered with regard to the characteristics of the students involved. For instance the socio-economic level, cultural background and emotional stability of the students might impact on the selection of the topic. The topic of the imagery experience may have the possibility of eliciting fear or some other negative response from certain students.

While the focus of this study was the perceptions of students about their imagery experiences, studies based on perceptions need to be substantiated by additional data. These data might include standardized test scores, observation scales and teacher and parent opinions.

There are additional areas that warrant further inquiry. What are the effects of the amount of imagery activities used in the classroom? What frequency of these activities is most effective? Which content is most suitable for which purposes? What are the most effective ways to integrate the mental imagery experiences with the content? What are the impacts of different socio-economic levels, cultural backgrounds and ages of students on the use of mental imagery in the classroom? What are the variables related to the teacher's characteristics that affect children's reaction to the experience?

In conclusion, research in the area of students' perceptions of imagery experiences should be expanded. The results of this type of research can lead to more positive and effective educational experiences for students.

Table 2. Summary of Reactions to Relaxation and Imagination Activities

	Positive Groups				Neutral Groups				Negative Groups			
	1	2	3	4	1	2	3	4	1	2	3	4
1. The things I saw in my imagination were ____.	96	100	91	96	---	---	---	---	4	0	9	4
2. The things I heard in my imagination were ____.	88	100	100	83	---	---	---	---	13	0	0	17
3. The things I smelled in my imagination were ____.	48	93	100	79	---	---	---	---	52	7	0	21
5-6. When we did those activities I felt; thought ____.	80	91	81	73	16	5	14	5	4	4	5	23
7-9. After we started doing these activities I felt; thought____.	95	92	85	70	7	6	15	18	2	2	0	14
10-12. Before we started doing these activities I felt, thought, could ____.	29	43	23	40	17	17	23	23	55	40	54	38
13-14. I'd like my friends to do these activities because____. When we do these activities my friends____.	76	91	71	52	14	9	23	41	10	0	6	7
15-16. The subject this helped me learn best is ____.	84	98	90	74	14	0	0	0	2	2	10	26
17. When we do these activities friends understand me____.	48	55	45	8	52	41	55	92	0	3	0	0
18. When we do these activities my mind works ____.	76	87	45	52	20	13	55	48	4	0	0	0
19. When we do these activities I can learn ____.	48	81	55	36	52	19	45	64	0	0	0	0
20. When we do these activities schoolwork is ____.	64	77	45	24	32	16	55	72	4	6	0	4
21. When we do these activities it is ____.	60	68	36	12	32	32	55	54	8	0	9	35
22. When we do these activities school is ____.	40	77	36	12	52	23	64	88	8	0	0	0
23. When we do these activities I can work ____.	60	23	45	36	40	16	45	64	0	3	9	0
24. I would like to do these relaxation and imagination activities ____.	64	90	82	21	28	3	9	50	8	6	9	29
25. When we do these activities my brain/mind works ____.	56	100	36	36	36	0	64	64	8	0	0	0

THE ROLE OF GUIDED IMAGERY IN EDUCATIONAL REFORM:

THE INTEGRATIVE LEARNING SYSTEM

Laurence D. Martel, Ph.D.

105 Reid Hall   and   The National Academy of Integrative Learning
Syracuse University   2550 M Street NW, Suite 500
Syracuse, NY 13244   Washington, DC 20037

This article reviews the Role of Guided Imagery as a part of the innovative Integrative Learning System which is based on a revolutionary Philosophy of Education and is causing outstanding success in learning results in schools, corporations and government agencies. It unveils several major paradigm shifts, including the shift from "manpower" to "mindpower".

INTRODUCTION

Since 1983 the United States has been defined, talked about, and read about as a "nation at-risk". We have been given approximately 30 National and State reports that define the problem and restate the problem of the failure of our children to perform at levels needed to live and work in our society. What seems to be happening is that both uncertain policy-makers with illiterate workforces and confused parents with fourth graders are questioning the value of education and schools. In a world in which what you know today can be outmoded in a year, new questions and alarms are being raised but not resolved. In the entire sphere of flux, people are wondering, "Do we know enough to get ourselves into a new direction? Is there a new vision, purpose, and direction toward which we can go as a people?"

When we speak about vision, purpose, and direction, how do we establish imagery in education in a way in which we can enhance people's performance? Perhaps one can begin with a view from Alvin Toffler, "*All education springs from some image of the future. If the image of the future held by a society is grossly inaccurate, its education system will betray its youth.*" How then can we be accurate about our "image" and what mechanism do we have to assure the appropriate application of that image for the future of society?

FIVE APPLICATIONS OF THE ROLE OF IMAGERY

We happen to live in a society in which not too long ago you used to go to school in order to go to work. Now we live in a society in which the activity of work is an activity of continuous learning. How we look anew at different concepts of education and learning can bring us into a new vision, purpose and direction with regard to learning and our view of the future. What I would like to suggest to you is that imagery is going to play a key role in the accuracy of our vision of the future. And in playing that key role it might be useful to explore at least five applications or variations of imagery, all related to each other, with which we must deal, if we are to be as successful as Toffler and other forecasters suggest we must be.

Mental Imagery, Edited by R.G. Kunzendorf
Plenum Press, New York, 1990

The Social Suggestive Norm

The first application expressed by Max Weber is that of the social suggestive norm that people attempt to do things or not as a result of the suggestive norms that are within their groups and their culture. There is a reason why every seventh grader in the United States for example, can hold up a diploma. It's an imaginary diploma and it's a diploma in "I-can't-ology". Why is it that seventh and eighth graders can tell you not what they can do but all the things they can't do? Why is it that they say, I *can't* do math, I *can't* get up and give a speech? Why is it that there is such negativity within the framework of social suggestion within their school that only a few succeed? Is it not true that only a few do succeed relative to the standard deviations which we impose in our "bell curve" mindset? As water rises to its own level within the physical world, research on expectancies indicates that performance is influenced by our suggested expectancy. The key point is that the dynamic of culture is influenced by "what we think about it".

The Paradigm

The second application deals with preconscious archetypes which order reality and give coherence to the way we organize information and perception. At the paradigm level, we deal in discrete boundaries of meaning which determine the categories of truth, reality, behavior, and lifestyle. For example, the industrial paradigm is in juxtaposition to the agrarian paradigm. Likewise, the paradigm of the "bell curve" is in juxtaposition to a new, paradigmatic image in which there are no acceptable levels of educational failure.

The Directional Level

The third application in which imagery plays a fundamental role in educational reform and learning is the level of being *able* to articulate vision, purpose and direction. It is the capacity to imagine, as Toffler is talking about, a future which can be otherwise. It is, for example, to speak not about a nation at-risk but to speak about a nation of promise with very clear goals, interests and direction that can deal with the other two categories: the paradigms and the social suggestive norms under which we operate. This level chooses to use imagery as a vehicle to get direction and to focus social suggestive norms and paradigms.

The Personal Level

Fourthly, we have found in our work throughout the world in both schools and in the workplace that imagery is a personal and professional working tool for learning, for working, for healthiness, and hardiness. We have found people to exponentially increase their ability to learn all kinds of things, such as, calculus, genetics in medical school, immunology, electronics and cognitive rehabilitation of the head injured. We have, for example, in Chicago's south side an all Black school which is in the poverty area of Morgan Street and 71st Street. Last year in 7 months of instruction, the first grade received an average 16 month gain in reading and 11 months gain in Math as measured by standardized tests. The first grade teachers are now saying publicly that they will never have a child leave them that is not on or above grade level. In an entry level program at Bell Atlantic for telephone operators using imagery techniques and other learning technologies, Bell Atlantic was within a very brief period of six months able to cut their entry level training programs in half. They are now publishing that they are saving a million dollars a year in just reduced training costs that have nothing to do, for example, with calculating the hourly wages of the people who are now back into the workforce. A very vivid example of what this means is that when I spoke with the supervisor a month ago, a supervisor who manages 90 people, she said that she used to certify people as being independent after about 30 days of observation. Now she is signing off on people within a week and often in two to three days. This is a powerful revolution in being able to do two things: to look at the personal and professional development of people in giving them new tools. Abraham Maslow once said, "if the only tool you had was a hammer, you tend to go around treating everything as if it is a nail." What we see here and what the great promise of the work that you are doing and that many of our other colleagues around the world are doing with regard to guided imagery is that it offers to us an expanded harvest of tools available for the practitioner.

64

The fifth application of imagery can help us move away from the single mindedness of dogmas such as "no pain, no gain" or "if it ain't broke, don't fix it." Integrative learning establishes that "if it's not joyful, it isn't learning" and "If it's not perfect, make it better." Also, there are other dogmas like the "uniformist" theory of efficiency in which there is "one best way" of doing things. Usually, that one best way of doing things is "my way". Imagery helps us establish the connections and the connectedness of diverse linkages and collaborations. And finally, I want to suggest that guided imagery has a tremendous role to play in helping us deal with diversity and pluralism, which is basically what democracies do. It is how they handle diversity of opinion, of ages, of political views and that is ultimately one of the issues that we are dealing with. How do we deal with diversity and pluralism? We must revisit "E pluribus unum". In this century we have created the industrial image of "one out of many;" whereas the agrarian image was "out of many: one." We have an imagery distinction between uniformity versus diversity. The twentieth century view that we have held is to take different people and reinvent them into a unified structure of doing business. (Example: This is the way you read. This is the way you do algebra. This is the way you count.) These uniformed methodologies in teaching and in training will ultimately get us a bell curve. Indeed, it is this disregard for individuality, culture and character which creates stupidity as a "learned behavior". Yet, because of Integrative Learning and Guided Imagery, we can look at diversity in a very different way, a way that allows us not to reinvent people, but to respect diversity, and to respect multiculturalism. We have a unique opportunity, I think, for the first time in this country to move from a nation of standardization to a nation that truly regards diversity, multilinguilism, and multiculturalism in a truly multinational way. And that, I think, is a great promise for us all.

Those are the five applications in which we are looking at imagery in terms of advanced learning technologies. Perhaps now more than at any other time in looking at the paradigm shifts that we are undergoing, we can be less victims of the shifts and more leaders and provocatures in helping to move those shifts into some sort of rational and moral structure as we move forward.

PRIMARY SHIFTS WHICH INCLUDE THESE APPLICATIONS

Taking the above applications into consideration, there are at least three primary shifts which have influenced our work. One very clearly is a major paradigm shift in western medicine: from the notion that disease is mechanistic and is located only in the machine, to a view that there is a symbiotic synchronization relationship between "mind and body" and that "disease" is a new process we call being a "human being". This is a shift from Newton's World of Physics to Einstein's World of Physics. One separates the mind from the body and the other integrates mental and bodily functions.

The second shift is in economic theory. We have had a substantial paradigm shift in what it is to capitalize western economies. In the 19 industrialized nations, as well as in the developing nations, we are having severe questions about how we move forward from a manufacturing society, a smokestack society, to not only an information society but a post-business society. This is a transition which is very important because in producing wealth in the 19th and 20th century, how many of you think that people were held in very high regard? We operated an economy that was based on a principle of a punchpress operator: you just hammered out your time; you just got in and did your work. In Frederick Winslow Taylor's view, who was the guru of management theory from the 20th century, workers didn't have minds. It fit very classically into logical positivism--the western tradition of Wittgenstein, Russell, Pavlov, Watson, and Skinner--that mental performance has no bearing on what people do. Before us today we have a shift from "manpower" to "mindpower". Corporations, such as Eastman Kodak, Xerox and Alcan, are looking anew at the only asset they have that grows in value over time: namely, the mental performance of employees.

The third area is in education where we have a major shift from the structure and curriculum of teaching to the process of learning. We are slowly moving from the belief that "teaching causes learning" to the notion that teaching "can allow learning to occur". The Integrative Learning System developed by Peter Kline and me, in combination with the exceptional work of many scholars, researchers, and practitioners, has opened the way for a new view that moves beyond the "bell curve" and has no acceptable level of failure in learning. By eliminating the "no pain, no gain" dogma, a revitalization of learning is occurring at all levels through the use of imagery which restores the joy of learning.

We are moving towards and have really shifted to a *mind-power* society. The idea that mental performance has no role in most medical results or in most work products has been totally castigated. We are moving from, and have shifted from, a narrow view of intelligence which is defined largely in terms of IQ testing (Alfred Benet's view of intelligence) to an expansive theory of multiple intelligences as expressed by the works of Howard Gardner (Harvard) and Robert Sternberg (Yale). "The Theory of Multiple Intelligence" is allowing us to think, at least, metaphorically, about how diversity can be incorporated into the learning place. Indeed, what we know about differences in students can be accommodated to get significant gains in learning and retention over time. May I refer you to Drs. Kenneth and Rita Dunn whose profound work is gaining worldwide acceptance and adoption.

There are several other shifts that we are clarifying to help lead in those new challenges. The industrial age was a teacher centered, authoritarian hierarchy - "I know all the information, and now I am going to give it to you." That is the mind set. It is competitive. We have a Nobel Prize mentality in the West in terms of anything that happens must be done by individuals. Anything else is cheating. For example: *Don't cheat. Are you paying attention? What do I have to do, draw you a picture?* In all of the research that we have, it shows that a large percent of the people get it *first* by getting a picture--a concrete image of a graphic design or a visual image that allows them to translate it into linguistics and then to perhaps abstraction in problem solving. Rather than a hierarchal system that pushes everything concrete to the bottom, we are moving toward a geodesic structure. Imagine a geodesic dome. A geodesic dome looks like the round disc structure we see on school playgrounds that is put together with linkages. Imagine that kind of structure for organizations as "Learner" centered. Every "learner" becomes a teacher and every teacher *assumes* and *accepts* the role of being a continuous lifelong learner.

Another thing that I think is very important is that the Greek word for education is "paideia". This can mean "play". I used to think it meant "to play". As a serious scholar I thought we could not "play" if it were "learning". (Remember, "no pain, no gain".) I have reconsidered what was meant in the sense of "the play". In Integrative Learning, the teacher is someone who stages the environment to allow all of the players to learn. For example, Nancy Ellis is an eighth grade teacher at the Guggenheim Elementary School in Chicago administered by Michael Alexander, Principal. The Board of Education in Chicago requires that all eighth graders take an outlining course. When Nancy Ellis first went through training in Integrative Learning four years ago, she decided that she would try using imagery and using a variety of other techniques that tied into the multiple intelligences. That is, she tied into references to interpersonal intelligence, intrapersonal intelligence, musical intelligence, the rhythms of learning, spacial intelligence and the traditional logical and linear intelligences upon which many of us rose or fell on the GRE's and the rest of our exams. In any event, the keypoint is that Nancy went back and rewrote the four-week course in which, previously, 80% of the class failed. In that four-week course, Nancy observed the students did not smile throughout the time in which they were taught. She changed the structure of the course to be taught in one week and restored the joy in the learning process. After one week, the students took the same exam that was given after four weeks. All of the students passed the course at an 80% proficiency. Nancy staged the environment in such a way as to enable things to create the play of learning to occur, and secondly, it was fun. Students enjoyed it. They began to communicate collaboratively with one another and it was exciting. Nancy realized that "teaching does not cause learning"; rather, "learning is allowed to occur" through wonder, amazement, and joy as well as through the social context of bonding and connectedness. I think most everyone can accept and hold on to certain kinds of notions, like affection, caring, trust, pride, and high regard and respect for the intelligence of each individual. And when this gets introduced in terms of multiple intelligences, people seek each other out. They begin to work toward collaboration as opposed to isolated learning and thinking.

THE INTEGRATIVE LEARNING SYSTEM

Based on the principles embodied in these changing images of education, the Integrative Learning System employs innovative, tested, teaching strategies that dramatically increase the rate of learning and retention for any age learner in any learning community. Focusing on the way information is presented in the classroom, it tailors learning to the individual, rather than forcing an individual to adapt to a single learning method. As a model of training and staff development, it disseminates innovative learning and teaching techniques that empower teachers and trainers to achieve far more from their students, in less time, and with greater results.

Integrative Learning Principles:

1. Respect for individuality
2. Strategic opportunities for learning
3. High regard for diversity as a resource capacity
4. The pursuit of excellence
5. Total quality leadership

The benefits of Integrative Learning:

1. Substantially reduces training costs
2. Teaches more material in less time
3. Creates a joyful, learner-centered environment
4. Increases creativity and inventiveness
5. Increases collaboration and corporate productivity
6. Reduces drop-out rates and teacher burn-out
7. Significantly increases student achievement and teacher motivation
8. Increases employability
9. Accelerates learning in education and business

The Integrative Learning System is based on the theoretical work of Dr. Laurence Martel and Peter Kline of the National Academy of Integrative Learning. It has an impressive rate of success in schools, corporations, and public and private agencies across the country and around the world. For more information contact, Dr. Laurence D. Martel or Mr. Morgan Doughton, The National Academy of Integrative Learning, 2550 M Street NW, Suite 500, Washington, DC 20037 (202/862-0124).

PRIVATE IMAGES BEHIND PERSONALITY TRAITS AND INTERPERSONAL DYNAMICS

THIN AND THICK BOUNDARIES: PERSONALITY, DREAMS, AND IMAGINATION

Ernest Hartmann, M.D.

Department of Psychiatry   and   Sleep Disorders Center
Tufts University School of Medicine   Newton-Wellesley Hospital
Boston, MA 02111   Newton, MA 02162

In this paper I will introduce a broad new personality dimension: Thin and Thick Boundaries in the Mind, and discuss its relationship with dreaming, with hypnotizability, and with imagery and imagination.

I will first define what I mean by thin and thick boundaries in its broadest sense; however, the concept is unlikely to become meaningful until we discuss clinical research and clinical cases that led to it, in the following pages.

Our minds are obviously complex entities. We may think of our minds as consisting of thoughts, feelings, moods, memories; of ego, id, superego, or conscious, preconscious, unconscious; or of distributed processing modules dealing with linguistics, semantics, memory storage, etc. No matter which of these views we adopt, our minds appear to be made up of parts, functions or processes which are in a sense separate from one another, and yet in communication with one another. We can consider them separated by a "boundary"; the degree of separateness is considered boundary thickness, the degree of communication boundary thinness. We also think of some kind of boundary around our whole selves, separating us from others and from the world; again this boundary may be relatively thick or thin.

As a first "clinical" approximation, we think of some individuals for whom everything is kept separate and in its place: order, organization; thoughts are one thing, feelings another; such a person may be seen as solid, perhaps somewhat rigid, well-defended or even "armored"; "thick-skinned". This is a person with thick boundaries in many senses. At the other extreme are people in whose minds things are fluid; thoughts, images, feelings merge readily; they are unusually sensitive, open, vulnerable. These people can be thought of as having thin boundaries.

To make this concept more understandable, to put some flesh on its bones, let me discuss how my collaborators and I derived it from our studies of people with frequent nightmares (Hartmann et al 1981; Hartmann 1984; Hartmann et al 1987).

Nightmares are among the most vivid and intense dreams experienced by most people. We were interested for many reasons in what might produce or affect nightmares. Among other things we examined the chemistry of the nightmare; many pharmacological agents increase or decrease the incidence of nightmares (Hartmann 1984), and we were able to show experimentally that a small dose of l-DOPA could increase the incidence of nightmares, as well as making dreams more vivid and detailed (Hartmann et al 1978). During these studies we also became interested in the question of "who has nightmares"-- the personality of the nightmare sufferer.

In order to study their personality systematically, we chose not to examine our patients coming for help with nightmares, since there were always complicating factors involved in the specific pathology (usually *not* nightmares) for which the patient sought help. We chose instead to study subjects with nightmares obtained through newspaper advertisements. (Which is also not perfect, since obviously we can study only those who have nightmares, see the ads, and decide to come in and talk about their nightmares.)

Summarizing two separate investigations, a total of 50 subjects with nightmares were studied. In one of the studies twelve subjects with frequent nightmares were compared to twelve

Mental Imagery, Edited by R.G. Kunzendorf
Plenum Press, New York, 1990

vivid dreamers with no nightmares and twelve non-vivid dreamers without nightmares. (Six males and six females in each group). In both studies "frequent nightmare" subjects were chosen on the basis that they reported at least one nightmare per week at home (the mean was actually over three per week) for over one year, and reported a history of lifelong nightmares, or at least "off and on since childhood". We wanted to study nightmares in "pure culture", and thus took only subjects who described their nightmares as long, frightening dreams which woke them usually during the second half of the night. This was to obtain a group with definite nightmares (REM-nightmares) as opposed to night terrors or mixed pictures. Some, but not all these subjects also took part in laboratory studies enabling us to confirm that they had REM-nightmares. (See Hartmann 1984 for details.)

Every subject had at least two detailed psychiatric interviews and took the MMPI and other psychological tests. In the three-group controlled study all were given a Rorschach test and five cards of the TAT, all scored on a blind basis.

Our findings, comparing the nightmares subjects with the controls, and also with population norms on various tests can be summarized as follows.(Only the points that clearly differentiated the nightmare subjects from other groups will be mentioned). On interview the nightmare subjects described not only nightmares but frequent dreams, and very long, detailed dreams in general. They woke from one dream into another; they described figures in their dreams changing and merging; and they themselves could be another person, someone of the opposite sex, or an animal in their dreams. Often they described not knowing they were really awake for a long time after waking, especially if they had had an intense dream. They described spending a great deal of time in drowsiness, or reverie, or day-dreaming; some described "daymares"-- daydreams that seemed to get out of control and become frightening. They described vivid imagery in general, often so vivid that they had some trouble differentiating it from reality.

Their thoughts flowed readily from one thing to another-- they seemed to free associate without being asked to, so that it sometimes took them five or ten minutes to answer a simple question. Along with this they were immensely trusting and open, much more so than the control groups. The nightmare sufferers would share all kinds of intimate details of their lives with me or other interviewers within a few minutes. They also appeared to be open and trusting in their other relationships, sometimes too much so, becoming involved with difficult and inappropriate partners; and several had actually been attacked when they trustingly walked alone in parts of town that others usually shunned.

They all described their childhoods, and their adolescences, as difficult or complicated. However, they were very seldom referring to gross trauma or abuse. (It is difficult to be certain about such childhood trauma, but even on detailed questioning, they did not report more trauma than the other groups.) In desciding their difficult childhoods they would discuss problems such as the birth of a younger sibling which disturbed them greatly, or interpersonal problems among the family members, which they reported feeling more, or being disturbed by more, than the others. It appeared that they felt unusually sensitive or vulnerable, and in fact they would often use the word "sensitive" in a number of different senses to describe themselves. The common descriptions were: "I was easily hurt" and "Everything got to me." This continued through their lives, and in adolescence they usually described painful relationships and breakups, sometimes with suicide attempts.

Also they described themselves as artistic or creative in some way. As adults (they were 20 to 40 at the time of the study) most were working or studying in fields that included the arts, teaching, and therapy of various kinds. It was striking that none of the nigtmare group had ordinary blue-collar or white-collar eight-hour-a-day jobs.

Some of these characteristics seem to suggest psychopathology. However, trying to assign formal DSM III diagnoses to the 50 nightmare subjects, we found that less than one third could be given a diagnosis. (No one among the 24 vivid or non-vivid dream control groups qualified for a DSM III diagnosis.) When a diagnosis was applicable it was usually a personality disorder: most commonly schizotypal personality disorder, next borderline personality disorder; two could be diagnosed as probably schizophrenic. Interestingly no one qualified clearly for a diagnosis of the anxiety disorders. Overall, considering that these people had very frequent nightmares for many years, I was struck by the absence of pathology compared to what one might have expected; over two thirds could be given no psychiatric diagnosis.

The MMPIs showed significant elevations, compared to the control groups, on the "psychotic" side of the profile (Pa,Pt,Sc,Ma) but no elevations on the "neurotic" side, usually associated with various forms of anxiety and depression. This again suggests that the nightmare sufferers were not a "sick" group in an overall sense. Elevations on the psychotic side of the

72

profile are found to characerize people with borderline personality, and groups of art students, as much as actual psychotic patients.

The Rorschachs showed a great deal of interesting vivid, emotional, and "primary process" material in the protocols of the nightmare subjects. However they did not differ from the other groups on any of the standard Exner measures. Only one quantitative measure showed a difference: this was a detailed scoring of "permeable boundaries" (Sivan 1983), based on the work of Blatt and Ritzler (1974) and the work of Fisher and Cleveland (1958). The nightmare group scored significantly higher (p<.01) than the two control groups on this measure.

The TAT cards were used to look for interpersonal aggression or hostility (Cooper et al 1986). The nightmare groups did not show any more hostility than the control groups. In fact (and of interest in itself) the highest hostility ratings were found in male non-vivid dreamers.

Overall, in summarizing the findings on frequent nightmare subjects, we concluded that they could not be described globally as a group of anxious people, nor of hostile people; nor was there much overall pathology, though there was some, along the lines we have discussed. The words that kept recurring in our desriptions were "open", "vulnerable","vivid" (in terms of their imagery and also their behavior in the interview), "tendency to merge", "undefended". It seemed to me that the best way to describe them overall was to say that they had "thin boundaries" in many senses, possibly in all senses in which the term boundaries has been used.

Table 1 represents my best current effort to summarize the different types of boundaries in the mind, which I am discussing. I hope the terms are relatively clear, since space does not

Table 1: Types of Boundaries

Perceptual Boundaries
        Sensation; sensory input
        Sensory focus or bandwidth
        Contents of perception (percepts)
Boundaries between two thoughts, or between two feelings
Boundaries between thought and feeling
Associative Process: free association
Boundaries between states of awareness or states of consciousness
Sleep-Dream-Wake Boundaries
        Between sleep and waking
        Between dreaming and waking
        Boundaries around the dream
        Daydreaming
Play
Boundaries related to memory:
        Early memories
        Recent memories, and memory organization
        The personal past
        Future plans
Boundaries around oneself: body boundaries
        Barrier against stimuli
        Body boundary; skin
        Body boundary in posture or musculature
        Space around oneself; body space
Interpersonal boundaries
Boundaries between conscious and unconscious, or between id, ego, and superego
Defense mechanisms as boundaries
The boundaries of Identity
        Sexual identity
        Age identity. Adult vs child
        Constancy of identity
Group boundaries
Organization of one's life
Opinions, judgements about the world and the nature of the true, the beautiful, the good
Preferences
Decision-making; action

permit a discussion of each type (see Hartmann 1991). (The questions listed later may also foster understanding of types of boundaries.) In any case it appeared to us that our groups of subjects with lifelong frequent nightmares were on the "thin" side of the continuum in all these senses. Clinical cases I have seen-- patients suffering from frequent niightmares-- also appear to fit this pattern. However, patients or research subjects who have pure night terrors rather than nightmares are quite different (Hartmann et al. 1982), as are patients who do not report nightmares in childhood or adolescence, but develop post-traumatic nightmares after a wartime experience (Van der Kolk et al. 1984).

I became very interested in the concept of boundaries in the mind as a general description or dimension of personality. It was easy to find cases that appeared to have the opposite characteristics -- thick boundaries. These were people who kept things very separate: thoughts are one thing, feelings another; men are men, women are women, vive la difference; they were asleep or awake,period (no half-asleep states, no uncertain states, little daydreaming); they did not become overinvolved in relationships; they had strong defenses and a strong sense of self; they were dependable, organized, perhaps rigid, unbending. Mostly they could not be given a diagnosis, but if any diagnosis fit them it was obsessive-compulsive personality disorder.

In an attempt to study the concept of boundaries further, we developed a 145-item pencil-and-paper test, the Boundary Questionnaire, which included questions on all the aspects of boundaries we could think of. The questions fall into twelve general content categories:

1. Sleep/Wake/Dream (14 items)
   Example: "When I wake in the morning I am not sure whether I am awake for a few minutes."
2. Unusual Experiences (19 items)
   Example: "I have had deja vu experiences."
3. Thoughts, Feeling, Moods (16 items)
   Example: "Sometimes I don't know whether I am thinking or feeling."
4. Childhood, Adolescence, Adulthood (6 items)
   Example: "I am very close to my childhood feelings."
5. Interpersonal (15 items)
   Example: "When I get involved with someone, we sometimes get too close."
6. Sensitivity (5 items)
   Example: "I am very sensitive to other people's feelings."
7. Neat, Exact, Precise (11 items)
   Example: "I keep my desk and worktable neat and well organized."
8. Edges, Lines, Clothing (20 items)
   Example: "I like houses with flexible spaces, where you can shift things around and make different uses of the same rooms."
9. Opinions about Children (8 items)
   Example: "I think a good teacher must remain in part a child."
10. Opinions about Organizations (10 items)
    Example: "In an organization, everyone should have a definite place and a specific role."
11. Opinions about People, Nations, Groups (14 items)
    Example: "There are no sharp dividing lines between normal people, people with problems, and people who are considered psychotic or crazy."
12. Opinions about Beauty, Truth (7 items)
    Example: "Either you are telling the truth or you are lying; that's all there is to it."

Within each category, questions cover as wide a range as possible. For instance, in the first category Sleep/Wake/Dream, there are questions about sleep-wake boundaries: "When I awake in the morning, I am not sure whether I am really awake"; questions about dreams: "In my dreams, people sometimes merge into each other or become other people"; questions about dreams and waking: "My dreams are so vivid that even later I can't tell them from waking reality"; questions about daydreams: "My daydreams don't always stay in control"; and questions about a number of in-between experiences: "I spend a lot of time daydreaming, fantasizing, or in reverie."

Respondents taking the questionnaire are instructed to respond to each item on a 5 point scale from 0 (Not at all true of me) to 4 (Definitely true of me). About two-thirds of the items are worded so that 4 is "thinnest" (for instance, "When I get involved with someone we sometimes get too close."); one-third are worded in the opposite direction, where 4 is "thickest" and "0" is "thinnest" (for instance, "In an organization, everyone should have a definite place and a specific role".) In scoring the questionnaire, the score on the "thin" items is added directly, while the score on the "thick" items is inverted (0=4, 1=3, etc.) and then added.

Each person receives a subscore on each of the 12 categories, a total score for the first 8 categories (called "Personal Total"), a total for the last four categories (called "World Total"), and an overall total boundary score ("Sum Bound").

The boundary questionnaire has been refined and tested for reliability and validity in several ways. It has good split-half reliability: coefficient alpha = .925. It has face validity, in that five groups we chose on the basis of an a priori prediction that they would score thick or thin did score in this way: two new groups of nightmare sufferers, a group of museum school art students and a group of university music students all scored much thinner than the overall mean; a group of naval officers scored much thicker than the mean.

Three hundred people--patients , students and research subjects--have taken the MMPI as well as the Boundary Questionnaire. The relationships between SumBound, the overall measure of thinness, and the MMPI scales was almost exactly as I had predicted: There was a strong positive correlation between Sumbound and the "psychotic scales: (.41 with Pa; .21 with Pt; .25 with Sc; .31 with Ma. All significant at $p<.001$). There was basically no correlation, with Hs(-.08), D(.02), Hy(.02), and Si(.07). SumBound correlated .32 with the F-scale -- almost certainly a valid F-measure suggesting unusual experiences and reports. SumBound correlated negatively with the L-scale (-.31) and with the K-scale (-.37). All these correlations were significant at $p<.001$. The correlation with K makes perfect sense since K measures "defensiveness"; and the relatively high F/low K pattern (correlating with thin boundaries) is usually read to mean openness and lack of defensiveness. The correlation with L (lying or wanting to appear too good) is consistent with the correlation with K, but I had not predicted such a strong correlation.

An exploratory factor analysis of the Boundary Questionnaire resulted in a best solution of 13 orthogonal factors, the first 12 of which were easily interpretable in common-sense or clinical terms. The first four most reliable factors accounting for most variance were: Factor I (by far the strongest and most reliable), which was called Primary Process. It describes a person with experiences of merging, of fluctuating identity, vivid imagery difficult to distinguish from reality, and synesthesia.

Factor II described a preference for clear borders and demarcations in nations, houses, pictures, stories, and relationships. Factor III describes identification, especially with children. Factor IV refers to fragility or vulnerability. See Harrison et al (1990) for further detail and discussion.

In any case we were satisfied that the Boundary Questionnaire was measuring thin and thick boundaries more or less as we had expected it to do. I will mention a few general results we have obtained with the Boundary Questionnaire, before discussing its relationship to imagery.

Overall women tended to score "thinner" on the questionnaire than men, despite the absence of any questions that would call for obviously different answers from the two sexes. In our total sample of over 980 subjects, the overall mean for SumBound (thinness) was 273;the mean for women's scores was 285, for men 261 (p<.001). Women also scored significantly thinner on most of the factors, with a single exception: women scored significantly thicker than men on factor VIII, called "Belief in impenetrable intergroup boundaries."

One study (Bevis 1987) demonstrated in a subgroup of 38 students taking the Boundary Questionnaire and a number of other measures, that women scored thinner than men, and also that women valued "thinness" in terms of closeness, interdependence etc. more than men, whereas men scored thicker and valued "thickness" in terms of independence, solid sense of self, etc. more than women.

We also found that in our total sample, which included people aged 18 to 65, there was a significant negative correlation between SumBound and age; older people scored slightly thicker. This is an intereesting finding but its interpretation is not certain. It is possible that we all tend to "thicken" with age; but it is also possible that the younger subjects -- predominantly students born in the late 1960s-- scored thinner than people born in the fifties or earlier because of cultural factors relating to that period, when "thinness" seemed to be valued more by society than in earlier decades; in that case these students may well remain relatively "thin" and the older subjects may have been relatively "thick" all along.

Another finding was that although art students scored very thin on the Boundary Questionnaire, established artists of several kinds scored very much in the average range. However, there were interesting differences between artists: thinner scores were found in "pure creative" artists -- sculptors and composers-- than in "interpretive artists"--instrumentalists, and instrument makers (S. Beal, 1988).

I hope the reader now has some sense of the concept of thin and thick boundaries in the mind, and the Boundary Questionnaire as an attempt to quantify the concept. Let me end by addressing the question of the relationship of boundaries to imagery.

Clearly I believe there is a relationship; one of the early findings in the nightmare studies was that the subjects with lifelong frequent nightmares reported vivid imagery, sometimes difficult to distinguish from reality, and also reported merging of thought, feeling and imagery. Thus right from the beginning vivid or pervasive imagery appeared to form part of the concept of thin boundaries, and accordingly the Boundary Questionnaire contains several questions dealing with imagery.

Data from an internal analysis of the Boundary Questionnaire clarifies the strength of this relationship. The first and strongest orthogonal factor, on which over one third of the questions have a loading of .25 or more, represents " merging or fluctuating identity, imagery so vivid it is hard to distinguish from reality, and synesthesia...". Also, an examination of the item-total correlations (how well does each of the individual questions relate to overall "thinness" on the questionnaire) reveals that out of the 145 questions the single question with the highest correlations with overall thinness (+.49) deals with imagery and the difficulty of telling it from reality: "I have had the experience of someone calling me or speaking my name and not being sure whether it was really happening or whether I was imagining it."

Dreams are of course a form of mental imagery, and there is a strong relationship between thin boundaries and dream recall. Six hundred of the subjects who took the Boundary Questionnaire also filled out a brief data sheet containing twelve questions about occupation, education, usual amount of sleep, etc. and including the question" "Frequency of remembered dreaming (per week) ", as well as questions about nightmares and other sleep-related events. Only one of these questions showed a strong relationship with thinness (SumBound); this was not the frequency of nightmares (which showed only a weak positive correlation) but the question on frequency of dreaming, which correlated +.40 (p<.001) with SumBound. This relationship could have been in part tautological, since the questionnaire includes several questions about dreams; therefore the correlation was recalculated after removing all questions dealing with dreams, daydreams, nightmares, sleep or waking; it remained almost as high: r = +.36 (p<.001).

The relationship between boundary structure and frequency of dream recall was also examined by pulling out of the total sample the extreme groups in terms of dream recall. We found about sixty subjects who could be called "high frequency dreamers", reporting seven or more dreams per week, and about the same number of subjects who could be called non-dreamers, reporting either no dreams at all, or less than one per year. The frequent dreamers scored significantly thinner on SumBound and on all twelve content categories of the Boundary Questionnaire.

We were also interested in the relationship of boundary structure to the kinds of dreams experienced. This sort of data was not available for the overall sample. However, we obtained a written report of a recent dream in a standard format from ten subjects who scored very thin and ten who scored very thick on the Boundary Questionnaire (each group was half male and half female). Ratings by two blind judges on a number of established dream rating scales revealed that the "thin" scorers had significantly longer dreams, more vivid dreams, more "dreamlike" dreams, more emotional dreams, more nightmare-like dreams, and more bizarre dreams.

We also found that thinness on the Boundary Questionnaire was related to hypnotizability and absorbtion. Among a group of 200 college students (Barrett 1989), there was a correlation of r=+.19 (p<.01) between SumBound and the Harvard Group Scale of Hypnotic Susceptibility Scale, and a correlation of +.29 (p<.01) between SumBound and the Field Inventory. The first measures overt responses to hypnotic suggestion--arm raising and so on--while the latter measures the associated subjective experience, and thus is more related to imagerry. Sumbound showed an even higher correlation (+.54 , p<.001) with absorbtion, using Tellegen's absorbtion scale.

In another approach to imagery and boundaries, Kunzendorf and Mauer (1988-1989) demonstrated that in subjects who scored "thin" on the Boundary Questionnaire imaged emotion had a greater effect on perception (of pictures of faces) than in "thick" subjects. In addition, thin-scoring subjects, especially those who were highly hypnotizable, had greater difficulty determining whether they had experienced something in the auditory or the visual modality.

In another recent study we demonstrated that imagery altered skin temperature more in subjects with thin boundaries. A small group who scored either very thick or very thin took part in a study in which the subject imagined sitting by a fire, or imagined holding an ice cube, while a sensitive electronic skin thermometer measured temperature of the back of the subject's hand. There was considerable variability, and in fact some subjects had a temperature change in the reverse direction to what wqs expected; however the "thin" subjects showed a significantly greater absolute change in skin temperature.

Thus on many different measures thinness on the boundary questionnaire is related to hypnotizability, to dream-ability, and to image-ability. I feel certain that a relationship exists with other imagery-based measures. For instance it is likely that highly fantasy-prone persons, as described first by Wilson and Barber (1983) and studied in detail by Lynn and Rhue (1988) would score very thin on the Boundary Questionnaire.

I suggest that thin and thick boundaries may be a trait or a broad personality dimension underlying all these more specific "abilities" and "pronenesses". Of course the concept of thin and thick boundaries does not totally encompass each of them. Each is probably multifactorial; for instance dream recall involves not only thin boundaries but also some physiological factors such as soundness of sleep and amount of REM-sleep time. Hypnotizability probably involves several different factors as well.

However thin and thick boundaries can be considered at least an aspect of each of these abilities. And if thin and thick boundaries in the mind is a viable construct referring, as suggested earlier, to divisions or boundaries between any two mental processes or functions, then its relationshbip to these imagery abilities is understandable. In fact all of them involve "boundaries" of one sort or another: vivid imagery difficult to distinguish from reality is clearly a thin or indefinite boundary; ability of imagery to affect body temperature, or perception, involves crossing a boundary to the regions or processes controlling the autonomic nervous system; hypnotizability involves "letting in" the hypnotist or the hypnotic suggestion across a boundary; and dream recall is the ability to pull material experienced in one state (dreaming, usually in REM sleep) across a boundary, to be remembered in a different state (waking).

These issues, as well as a possible underlying biology of thin and thick boundaries, are discussed in detail elsewhere (Hartmann 1991).

REFERENCES

Barrett, D. (1989). *The relationship of thin vs. thick boundaries to hypnotic susceptibility.* Paper presented to the Eastern Psychological Association, Boston.
Beal, S. (1988). *The boundary characteristics of artists.* Doctoral dissertation, Department of Psychology, Boston University, Boston, MA.
Bevis, J. (1986). *Connectedness versus separateness: Understanding male/female differences in self and relationship.* Doctoral dissertation, Department of Psychology, Boston University, Boston, MA.
Blatt,S. and Ritzler, B. (1974). Thought disorder and boundary disturbance in psychosis. *Journal of Consulting and CLinical Psychology*, 42, 370-381.
Cooper, S.H., and Hartmann, E. (1986). Hostility levels of lifetime nightmare sufferers: a test of a clinical hypothesis. *Psychoanalytic Psychology*, 3, 373-377.
Fisher, S., and Cleveland, S. (1958). *Body image and personality.* Princeton, NJ: Van Nostrand.
Harrison, R., Hartmann, E., and Bevis, J. (1990). *The Hartmann Boundary Questionnaire: a measure of thin and thick boundaries.* Under editorial review.
Hartmann, E. (1984). *The nightmare: the psychology and biology of terrifying dreams.* New York: Basic Books.
Hartmann, E. (1991). *Boundaries in the mind.* New York: Basic Books.
Hartmann, E., Russ, D., Oldfield, M., Sivan, I., and Cooper, S. (1987). Who has nightmares? The personality of the lifelong nightmare sufferer. *Archives of General Psychiatry*, 44, 49-56.
Hartmann, E., Russ, D., van der Kold, B., Falke, R., and Oldfield, M. (1981). A preliminary study of the personality of the nightmare sufferer: relationship to schizophrenia and creativity? *American Journal of Psychiatry*, 138, 794-797.
Hartmann, E., Skoff, B., Russ, D., and Oldfield, M. (1978). The biochemistry of the nightmare: possible involvement of dopamine. *Sleep Research*, 7, 89.
Hartmann, E., Greenwald, D., and Brune, P. (1982). Night-terrors-sleep walking: personality characteristics. *Sleep Research*, 11, 121.

Kunzendorf, R., and Maurer, J. (1988-1989). Hyypnotic attenuation of the "boundaries" between emotional, visual, and auditory sensations. *Imagination, Cognition, and Personality*, 8, 225-234.

Lynn, S., and Rhue, J. (1988). Fantasy Proneness: Hypnosis, developmental antecedents, and psychopathology. *American Psychologist*, 43, 35-44.

Sivan, I., (1987). *Anxiety and ego function of nightmare dreamers*. Masters dissertation, Department of Psychology, University of Haifa, Haifa, Israel.

Van der Kolk, B., Blitz, R., Burr, W., Sherry, S., and Hartmann, E. (1984). Nightmares and trauma: a comparison of nightmares after combat with lifelong nightmares in veterans. *American Journal of Psychiatry*, 141, 187-190.

Wilson, S., and Barber, T. (1983). The fantasy-prone personality: indications for understanding imagery, hypnosis, and parapsychological phenomena. In A.A. Sheikh (Ed), *Imagery: Current theory, research, and application* (pp. 340-390). New York: Wiley.

IMAGERY, HYPNOSIS AND HYPNOTIZABILITY

Nicholas P. Spanos, Ph.D.

Department of Psychology
Carleton University
Ottawa, Ontario, Canada K1S 5B6

Imaginal processes have been associated with the topic of hypnosis since the report of the French Royal Commission on animal magnetism in the late eighteenth century (Franklin et al., 1784/1970). Much contemporary research on imagery and hypnosis has revolved around two empirical issues. One issue deals with the hypothesis that hypnotic procedures facilitate the vividness of imagery to a greater extent than do nonhypnotic procedures, and the second deals with the relationships between imaginal propensities and hypnotizability. This paper will review empirical evidence relating to these two issues.

HYPNOTIC ENHANCEMENT OF IMAGERY

Numerous investigators (see Holroyd, 1986 for a review) have suggested that hypnotic procedures facilitate the vividness and life-like quality of mental imagery to a greater extent than do nonhypnotic procedures. For instance, a number of clinical investigators (Astor, 1973; Dengrove, 1973; Fuchs, Hoch, Paldi, Abramovici, Brandes, Timor-Tritsch and Kleinhaus, 1973; Kroger and Fezler, 1976) employ hypnotic procedures in conjunction with other therapeutic interventions because they believe that hypnotic procedures heighten the vividness of therapeutic imagery. Despite such clinical claims, however, the available empirical evidence runs counter to this hypothesis.

A large number of studies conducted on nonclinical samples in experimental contexts (Barber and Wilson, 1977; Coe, St. Jean and Burger, 1980, Experiment 2; Ham and Spanos, 1974; Nilsson, 1990; Spanos, Bridgeman, Gwynn and Stam, 1983; Spanos, Ham and Barber, 1973; Spanos, Mullens and Rivers, 1979; Starker, 1974) found that ratings of imagery vividness following hypnotic procedures were not significantly higher (but were sometimes significantly lower) than ratings made under imagination control, task-motivation, relaxation or other control procedures.

In all of the above studies imagery and its effects were assessed in terms of verbal report. Bowers (1967) hypothesized that hypnotic subjects report their imaginal experiences accurately, while motivated control subjects tend to exaggerate the vividness of their imaginal experiences. This hypothesis implies that imagery suggestions will produce greater effects in hypnotic than in nonhypnotic subjects when the dependent variable is not under direct voluntary control. Two recent studies (Spanos and Brice, 1990; Spanos, Stenstrom and Johnston, 1988) provided data relevant to this issue. Spanos and Brice (1990) found that hypnotic and nonhypnotic subjects given suggestions to imagine sucking on a lemon reported equivalent levels of imagery vividness. However, nonhypnotic subjects exhibited significantly higher levels of salivation than hypnotic subjects. Spanos et al. (1988, Experiment 2) administered suggestions for wart regression to hypnotic and nonhypotic subjects. Subjects in these groups failed to differ in the vividness ratings assigned to their suggested imagery or in the degree of their wart regression. On the other hand, vividness of suggested imagery ratings in hypnotic and nonhypnotic subjects was significantly correlated with wart regression. In short, the data from these two studies fail to support the hypothesis that hypnotic imagery is more vivid than the nonhypnotic imagery generated by motivated control subjects.

Clinical investigators (e.g., Graham, 1986) sometimes suggest that laboratory findings should not be generalized to clinical settings. With respect to hypnosis and imagery, the implication of this caution is that regardless of the finding obtained in laboratory settings, hypnotic procedures may be more effective than nonhypnotic ones at generating imagery in clinical settings. The findings of Spanos et al. (1988, Experiment 2) concerning the equivalence of hypnotic and nonhypnotic imagery during wart regression suggestions fail to support this hypothesis. Recently, Nolan, Spanos, Haward and Scott (1989) examined this issue in the context of the cognitive-behavioral treatment of chronic headache. Hypnotic and non-hypnotic subjects administered an imagery-based cognitive-behavioral treatment reported equivalent levels of suggested imagery vividness during the treatment and equivalent levels of headache reduction following treatment. Thus, the available evidence from both laboratory and clinical settings indicates that hypnotic procedures are no more effective than nonhypnotic motivational procedures at enhancing the vividness of imagery. These findings are consistent with a large body of evidence which indicates that hypnotic subjects and motivated control subjects exhibit equivalent response to a wide range of suggestions in both laboratory settings (Barber, 1969; Barber, Spanos and Chaves, 1974) and clinical settings (Spanos, in press, b).

Despite the consistency of the above findings, the relationship between imagery enhancements and hypnotic procedures is more complex than it first appears. For example, experiments that use subjects as their own control sometimes obtain greater levels of reported imagery enhancement in hypnotic than in nonhypnotic subjects (e.g., Crawford and Allan, 1983). An interesting study by Coe, St. Jean and Burger (1980) examined the role of subtle social demands in producing this effect. In this study subjects rated the vividness of their imagery under both imagination control and hypnotic conditions. Half of the subjects were tested in the imagination condition first and the hypnotic condition second, and the remaining half were tested in the reverse order. Subjects tested under the imagination first hypnosis second order rated their imagery as more vivid following hypnosis. Those tested in the reverse order reported no differences in imagery vividness between conditions. Spanos, McPeake and Carter (1973) conducted a related study on suggested visual hallucinations. Subjects in one condition were administered a hallucination suggestion on pretest and then an equivalent suggestion following an hypnotic induction procedure (posttest). Those in a second condtion were never pretested, but were administered the posttest hallucination suggestion following an hypnotic induction procedure. Pretested subjects reported more intense hallucinations following the hypnotic procedure, than on pretest. However, non pretested subjects rated their hypnotic hallucinations as less intense than did pretested subjects. In fact, the hypnotic hallucinations of the nonpretested subjects did not differ in rated intensity from the pretest hallucinations of the pretested subjects. Subjects in a third condition were administered the pretest and posttest hallucination suggestions without an intervening hypnotic induction procedure, and reported no pretest to posttest increments in hallucination intensity.

The findings of the Coe et al. (1980) and Spanoes et al. (1973) studies indicate that assessing imagery vividness both before and after the administration of hypnotic procedures provides subjects with expectations for posttest improvement and also, with an objective baseline (i.e., subjects' own nonhypnotic rating of vividness) against which to define improvement. Subjects who are administered hypnotic procedures without baseline testing are provided with expectations for high levels of performance, but no objective standard against which to anchor their level of performance. Without a standard subjects are unable to convert expectations for high levels of performance into a rating that will reflect improvement. Consequently, these subjects perform no better following hypnosis than pretested subjects do before hypnosis.

In summary, the available evidence indicates that hypnotic procedures can sometimes bias subjects' estimation of imagery vividness. However, this evidence provides no support for the hypothesis that hypnotic procedures actually enhance imagery vividness to a greater extent than nonhypnotic motivational procedures. The findings in this area also underscore the important role played by contextual variables in influencing the expectations and interpretations that subjects develop, and the manner in which such expectations are translated into performance increments.

IMAGERY AND HYPNOTIZABILITY

The test suggestions used on standardized scales of hypnotizability usually invite subjects to imagine situations that are congruent with the overt response called for by the suggestions. For example, the "moving hands" suggestion on the Stanford Hypnotic Susceptibility Scale, Form C (SHSS:C: Weitzenhoffer and Hilgard, 1962) asks subjects to imagine that their hands are attracted like magnets, and the arm rising suggestion on the Carleton University Responsiveness to Suggestion Scale (CURSS: Spanos, Radtke, Hodgins, Stam and Bertrand, 1983) invites them to imagine a helium filled balloon tied to the wrist and lifting it into the air.

Performance on hypnotizability tests tends to be relatively stable even after long temporal intervals (Hilgard, 1987). Moreover, the various hypnotizability scales in common use correlate with one another to a substantial degree (e.g., Spanos, Radtke, Hodgins, Bertrand, Stam and Moretti, 1983). The cross-test and cross-time consistency associated with hypnotizability scores is interpreted by some investigators as reflecting a stable trait or capacity (Hilgard, 1987; Peryr, 1977). Relatedly, the prominence of the requests to imagine contained in hypnotizability test suggestions has led numerous investigators to hypothesize that hypnotizability is a trait closely related to subjects' propensities for engaging in imaginal activities (J. Hilgard, 1970; Sheehan, 1979; Tellegen and Atkinson, 1974).

Most of the empirical research attempting to relate hypnotizability to imaginal propensities has focused on imagery vividness as measured by some variation of the Betts questionnaire. The many studies which have assessed the relationship between imagery vividness and hypnotizability have yielded contradictory results (for reviews, see de Groh, 1989; Sheehan, 1979). A number of studies reported significant linear correlations of low to moderate magnitude between imagery vividness and hypnotizability (Farthing, Venturino and Brown, 1983; Hilgard, Sheehan, Monteiro and MacDonald, 1981; Shor, Orne and O'Connell, 1966; Spanos, Stam, Rivers and Radtke, 1980; Wagman and Steward, 1974). However, numerous other studies failed to find significant linear correlations between these variables (Katsanis, Bardnard and Spanos, 1988; Perry, 1973; Spanos, McPeake and Churchill, 1976; Van Dyne and Stava, 1981). Contradictory findings were obtained even between studies that used the same tests to assess hypnotizability and imagery, and between studies that assessed the relationships between these variables for the two sexes separately (Diamond and Taft, 1975; Hilgard, 1970; Sutcliffe, Perry and Sheehan, 1970).

Studies that assessed linear correlations between absorption and hypnotizability yielded positive findings more consistently than those that assessed imagery vividness and hypnotizability (de Groh,1989). Even here, however, several studies have failed to obtain significant correlations between absorption and hypnotizability (e.g., Perlini, Lee and Spanos, 1990), and in most studies the linear correlations between these variables, although significant, have been of low magnitude (e.g., Hoyt et al., 1989).

The studies described above assessed *linear* relationships between imagery vividness or absorption and hypnotizability. However, several investigators (de Groh, 1989; Hilgard, 1970; Sutcliffe et al., 1970; Spanos, Brett, Menary and Cross, 1987) have suggested that propensities for imaginal activities and hypnotizability may be nonlinearly related. For instance, Spanos, Brett et al. (1987) found that the relationship between absorption and hypnotizability was fan-shaped rather than linear. Subjects with very low absorption scores never attained high hypnotizability. As absorption scores increased, so did the proportion of subjects who scored high in hypnotizability. Nevertheless, substantial numbers of subjects with moderate and high scores on absorption scored low in hypnotizability. Relationships between imagery vividness and hypnotizability were also found to be fan-shaped rather than linear (de Groh, 1989; Katsanis et al., 1988).

The fan-shaped relationship between imaginal activity measures and hypnotizability obtained in these studies (de Groh, 1989; Spanos, Brett et al., 1987) may help to explain the low and sometimes nonsignificant *linear* correlations obtained between these variables in earlier studies. Many of these studies employed small sample sizes, and when samples are small even a relatively few subjects with high vividness but low hypnotizability scores can substantially lower the magnitude of a linear correlation. In fact, small variations in the proportion of such subjects due to chance or to minor variations in sampling procedures between studies can easily determine whether or not a linear correlation between, say imagery vividness, and hypnotizability attains statistical significance.

Interestingly, imaginal propensities are not the only variables that share a fan-shaped relationship with hypnotizability. Several studies (Katsansis et al., 1988; Spanos, Brett et al., 1987) indicate that attitudes toward hypnosis and expectations concerning hypnotic responding are also related to hypnotizability in a fan-shaped pattern. More specifically, subjects with negative attitudes and expectations concerning hypnosis usually score low in hypnotizability whereas subjects with moderate and high scores on these variables score at all levels of hypnotizability.

Taken together, these findings indicate that negative attitudes, negative expectations or the absence of imaginal propensities suppress hypnotic responding. However, positive attitudes, positive expectations or high levels of imaginal ability are not, in and of themselves, sufficient to engender high levels of hypnotizability. Several studies (de Groh, 1989; Spanos and McPeake, 1975; Spanos, Radtke, Hodgins, Bertrand, Stam and Dubreuil, 1983; Yancer and Johnson, 1981) examined the combined abilities of attitude, expectancy and imaginal propensity to predict hypnotizability. Although various combinations of these variables improved prediction, most of the variance in hypnotizability scores still remained unaccounted for. What then does account for the wide variability in hypnotizability socres seen among cooperative, imaginative subjects who hold positive attitudes and expectations concerning hypnotic responding? In the remainder of this paper I will review evidence which suggests that much of this residual variability is related to the tacit interpretations that subjects develop about the test suggestions they are administered.

Interpretations of Test Suggestions

Hypnotic test suggestions are ambiguous communications. Instead of instructing subjects to carry out behavioral responses, suggestions are worded in the passive voice and inform subjects that a response is occurring or will occur automatically and without their active participation (e.g., your arm is rising, feeling lighter and rising in the air). Thus, despite explicit instructions to imagine events that are congruent with the requisite response (e.g., imagine a pully raising your arm), the response itself is defined by the suggestion as a "happening" rather than a goal-directed action (Spanos, 1971, 1986b; Spanos, Rivers and Ross, 1977).

In a number of earlier papers I suggested that, despite the passive wording of suggestions, the behavioral phenomena traditionally associated with hypnosis (e.g., amnesia, catalepsy) are, in fact, goal-directed actions rather than involuntary happenings (Spanos, 1986b; 1989). According to this formulation many cooperative and imaginative subjects are misled by the passive wording of suggestions into believing that they are to wait passively for suggested effects to "happen by themselves." However, because hypnotic responses do not occur automatically these subjects tend to fail suggestions.

Other cooperative and imaginative subjects develop the tacit understanding that suggestions are to be interpreted metaphorically rather than literally (Sarbin and Coe, 1972). These subjects tacitly understand that they are required to behave *as if* the events suggested are real (e.g., as if their arm is pulled upward by a balloon). Some of these subjects carry out the requisite behavioral responses and, simultaneously become absorbed in suggestion-related imaginings. Absorption in suggestion-related imaginings implies that subjects are attending to their imaginings and, thereby, limiting their simultaneous involvement in such metacognitive processes as reflecting upon the fact that they are generating their own responses, or reflecting on the broader meaning of what they are doing. Subjects who carry out the requisite responses while remaining absorbed in their suggestion-related imaginings tend to experience their goal-directed responses to suggestions as involuntary happenings (Spanos and McPeake, 1974).

Several recent studies (Gorassini, 1989; Katsanis et al., 1988; Spanos, Gwynn, Gabora and Jarrett, 1989; Spanos, Gabora and Hynford, 1990) have examined these ideas by assessing the interpretations that subjects held of test suggestions. In several studies (e.g., Gorassini, 1989; Spanos, Gwynn et al., 1989) subjects were administered a questionnaire assessing their interpretations *after* they had responded to the test suggestions. The questionnaire described several possible interpretations of suggestions; the two most important being (a) waiting passively for suggested effects to happen by themselves (i.e., passive interpretation), and (b) carrying out the requisite responses while engaging in suggestion-related imagery (i.e., active interpretation). In other studies (Katsanis et al., 1988; Spanos,Gabora et al., 1990) the interpretation questionnaire asked subjects about how they intended to respond, and was administered *before* they were given the test suggestions. Regardless of when the interpretation questionnaire was administered, subjects who adopted (or planned to adopt) active interpretations of suggested demands scored significantly higher on behavioral and subjective indexes of hypnotizability than those who adopted (or planned to adopt) passive interpretations. Furthermore, the findings of several studies (Katsanis et al., 1988; Spanos, Gwynn et al., 1989) indicated that the degree to which subjects adopted an active interpretation predicted their hypnotizability even when attitudes toward hypnosis and expectations of hypnotic responding were statistically controlled.

Katsanis et al. (Study 2, 1988) reasoned that an active interpretation of suggestions would be most useful for subjects who possessed the ability to generate the requisite imaginings with a high degree of vividness. In order to test this hypothesis Katsanis et al. (Study 2, 1988) assessed subjects' ability to generate vivid imagery with a modification of the Betts questionnaire, as well as assessing their interpretations of suggested demands. Among subjects who attained very low imagery scores there was no significant relationship between degree of adopting an active interpretation and hypnotizability socres. On the other hand, among subjects with high imagery vividness scores, the correlation between adoption of active interpretations and hypnotizability was substantial and highly significant.

In summary, a number of studies now indicate that hypnotic responsiveness is substantially influenced by the way in which subjects interpret suggestions. Subjects who adopt a passive interpretation of suggested demands tend to score lower in hypnotizability than those who adopt an active interpretation. Importantly, these findings hold even among subjects with positive attitudes and expectations concerning hypnosis, and with the ability to generate vivid imagery. One hypothesis implied by these findings suggests that it should be possible to produce substantial enhancements in hypnotic responsiveness by teaching low hypnotizables to adopt an active interpretation of suggested demands. However, the degree to which such teaching is effective is likely to be influenced by subjects' imaginal skills on the one hand, and by their attitudes toward hypnosis on the other.

Is Hypnotizability a Stable Trait?

As described earlier, hypnotizability is conceptualized by some investigators as a stable trait or disposition (Hilgard, 1987; Perry, 1977). To support the trait view investigators usually cite evidence for the cross-test and cross-time stability of hypnotizability and evidence that a wide variety of treatment interventions, which were designed to enhance hypnotizability (e.g., individualized induction procedures, meditation training, sensory restrictions, EEG biofeedback) failed to achieve large or consistent hypnotizability gains (Perry, 1977).

A sociocognitive alternative to the trait view suggests that hypnotizability involves modifiable sets of attitudes, interpretations and expectations as well as imaginal abilities. According to this view the high cross-test and cross-time correlations obtained with hypnotizability scales reflect stability in the attitudes, expectations, and interpretations which subjects bring to the hypnotic test situation. Relatedly, for a socio-cognitive view, the failure of interventions like meditation training or sensory restriction to produce stable enhancements in hypnotizability may simply indicate that such treatments fail to influence the most important contextual determinants of hypnotic responding--subjects' attitudes and expectations toward hypnosis, and their interpretation of suggested demands.

Recently, Spanos, Gabora, Jarrett and Gwynn (1989) illustrated the important role of context-specific variables in influencing the cross-test stability of hypnotizability. All subjects were tested on two different hypnotizability scales. For half the subjects both scales were defined as tests of hypnosis. For the remaining subjects only the first scale was defined as hypnotic. The second scale (ostensibly administered as part of a different study) was defined as an index of creative imagining, and the hypnotic induction on that scale was replaced by brief instructions encouraging imaginative responding.

A high correlation was obtained btween scores on the two scales when both were defined in terms of hypnosis. However, a significantly lower correlation was obtained between the two scales when one was defined in terms of hypnosis and the other in terms of imagination. These findings suggest that the cross-test stability in hypnotizability that is usually attributed to a trait (e.g., Hilgard, 1987) may, instead, reflect stability in the understandings and interpretations that subjects hold about hypnosis.

Skill Training and Hypnotizability

Contrary to trait conceptualizations, studies conducted in five independent laboratories now indicate that training procedures based on social learning principles can produce large gains in hypnotizability (Bertrand, Stam and Radtke, 1990; Diamond, 1972; Gfeller, Lynn and Pribble, 1987; Sachs, 1971; Spanos, 1986a). For example, Gorassini and Spanos (1986) employed a three-component skill training package aimed at teaching (a) positive attitudes toward hypnosis, (b) the use of imagery strategies for experiencing suggested effects, and (c) the adoption of an active interpretation toward suggested demands. A large number of experiments using this skills training package has now been completed, and these experiments clearly demonstrate that low hypnotizables who undergo skill training typically exhibit large increments on both behavioral and subjective indexes of hypnotizability (for reviews see Spanos, 1986a, in press). Furthermore, training induced gains generalized to novel suggestions that were not included as practice items during training, and to particularly difficult and unusual items such as those for selective amnesia, posthypnotic responding and "trance logic" (Gfeller et al., 1987; Spanos, Lush and Gwynn, 1989). Relatedly, Spanos, Cross, Menary and Smith (1988) found that skill training gains were maintained more than a year and a half following training.

Components in skill training. In a number of studies (Spanos, Flynn and Niles, in press; Spanos, Robertson, Menary and Brett, 1986) we have attempted to delineate the components of our skill training package that produce large hypnotizability gains. For example, Spanos, Robertson et al. (1986) gave one group of low hypnotizables our full three component skill training package while lows in a second group received information designed to enhance attitudes and teach imagery strategies, but no information about how to interpret suggestions. Subjects in the two groups showed equivalent increments in their attitudes toward hypnosis, but only those given the interpretation information exhibited large hypnotizability gains.

Bates, Miller, Cross and Brigham (1988) suggested that skill training induced gains in hypnotizability resulted from high rapport between trainer and subject which led subjects to comply with suggested demands in order to avoid disappointing the trainer. According to this hypothesis the specific information included in skill training is irrelevant to treatment gain. Supposedly, and treatment which builds subject/trainer rapport, and which contains explicit demands for enhanced performance, should lead to large hypnotizability increments in low hypnotizables. It is difficult to see how the Bates et al. (1988) hypothesis can account for the findings of the Spanos, Robertson et al. (1986) study. Both groups of lows in that study were taught by the same trainer and both were informed that their training would enhance hypnotizability. Nevertheless, only those given the interpretation information showed large hypnotizability gains. Recently, Spanos, Flynn et al. (in press, Experiment 1) tested the Bates et al. (1988) hypothesis by administering skill training to low hypnotizables in one condition, and a relaxation procedure designed to enhance rapport and create demands for enhanced responsiveness to lows in a second condition. Importantly, the relaxation training procedure did not teach subjects to develop an active interpretation of suggestions. Subjects in the two conditions reported equivalent levels of rapport with and liking for their trainer. Nevertheless, only those given skill training exhibited large hypnotizability gains.

The findings just reviewed do *not* indicate that attitudes toward hypnosis and trainer/subject rapport are irrelevant to skill-training induced gains in hypnotizability. Instead these findings, like those reviewed earlier in this paper, indicate that positive attitudes and rapport are not sufficient for producing large hypnotizability gains. In fact, several studies (Cross and Spanos, 1988; Gfeller et al., 1987; Spanos, Cross, Menary, Brett and de Groh, 1987; Spanos, Flynn et al. in press, Experiment 2) indicate that rapport, attitudes toward hypnosis, and imagery vividness are important moderators of the degree to which skill training enhances hypnotizability.

Moderators of skill training induced gain. Not all subjects who undergo skill training exhibit large gains in hypnotizability, and substantial variability remains in the posttraining hypnotizability scores of skill trained subjects (Spanos, 1986a). Spanos, Cross et al. (1987) found that the extent to which subjects benefited from skill training was correlated with the degree that their attitudes toward hypnosis became positive as a result of training, and Cross and Spanos (1988) and Gfeller et al. (1987) found that training induced gains were correlated with the degree to which subjects developed rapport with their trainer. In other words, subjects who do not like their trainer or who, despite skill training, retain negative attitudes toward hypnosis, benefit little from training information about how to interpret suggested demands.

Two studies (Cross and Spanos, 1988; Spanos, Cross et al., 1987) found that subjects' scores on the Betts imagery questionnaire correlated with the extent to which they benefited from skill training. Subjects with little ability to generate vivid imagery were relatively unsuccessful at enhancing their hypnotizability with skill training. On the other hand, subjects who possessed the ability to generate vivid imagery and who developed positive attitudes toward hypnosis, were particularly likely to exhibit large hypnotizability gains following skill training. These results are consistent with those of Katsanis et al. (1988) who found that [in untrained subjects] an active interpretation of suggested demands was associated with relatively high hypnotizability only among subjects with relatively high levels of imagery ability.

SUMMARY AND CONCLUSIONS

Taken together, the findings reviewed in this paper suggest that hypnotic procedures are no more effective at enhancing imaginal activities than are numerous nonhypnotic procedures that enhance subjects' motivations and expectations. However, these findings also indicate that imaginal abilities play an important albeit complex role in influencing the extent to which subjects respond to hypnotic suggestions.

Hypnotic test suggestions invite subjects to create imaginary scenes, and subjects with little ability to imagine are restricted in their ability to generate the subjective experiences called for by these suggestions. On the other hand, many subjects with the requisite imaginal abilities fail to respond to hypnotic suggestions either because they hold negative attitudes and expectations about hypnosis, or because they develop passive interpretations of suggested demands which are not conducive to high levels of hypnotic responding. When low hypnotizable subjects with the requisite imaginal skills learn positive attitudes toward hypnosis and active interpretations of suggested demands, they tend to exhibit large hypnotizability gains. On the other hand, subjects who have difficulty generating and becoming absorbed in imaginings also have difficulty responding to suggestions even after exposure to skill training.

REFERENCES

Astor, M. H. (1973). Hypnosis and behavior modification combined with psychoanalytic psychotherapy. *International Journal of Clinical and Experimental Hypnosis, 21,* 18-24.

Barber, T. X. (1969). *Hypnosis: A scientific approach.* NY: Van Nostrand Reinhold.

Barber, T. X., Spanos, N. P., & Chaves, J. F. (1974). *Hypnosis, imagination and human potentialities.* NY: Pergamon.

Barber, T. X., & Wilson, S. C. (1977). Hypnosis, suggestion and altered states of consciousness: Experimental evaluation of the new cognitive-behavioral theory and the traditional trance-state theory of "hypnosis." *Annals of the New York Academy of Sciences, 296,* 34-47.

Bates, D. L., Miller, R. J., Cross, J. J., & Brigham, T. A. (1988). Modifying hypnotic suggestibility with the Carleton Skills Training Program.*Journal of Personality and Social Psychology, 55,* 120-127.

Bertrand, L. D., Stam, J. J., & Radtke, H. L. (1990). *The Carleton Skill Training Package for modifying hypnotic susceptibility: A replication and extention.* Unpublished manuscript, University of Calgary.

Bowers, K. S. (1967). The effects of demands for honesty on resorts of visual and auditory hallucinations. *International Journal of Clinical and Experimental Hypnosis, 15,* 31-36.

Coe, W. C., St. Jean, R. L., & Burger, J. M. (1980). Hypnosis and the enhancement of visual imagery. *International Journal of Clinical and Experimental Hypnosis, 28,* 225-243.

Crawford, H. J., & Allan, S. N. (1983). Enhanced visual memory during hypnosis as mediated by hypnotic responsiveness and cognitive strategies. *Journal of Experimental Psychology: General, 112,* 657-680.

Cross, W., & Spanos, N. P. (1988). The effects of imagery vividness and receptivity on skill training induced enhancements in hypnotic susceptibility. *Imagination, Cognition and Personality, 8,* 89-103.

de Groph, M. (1989). Correlates of hypnotic susceptibility. In N. P. Spanos & J. F. Chaves (Eds.), *Hypnosis: The cognitive-behavioral perspective* (pp. 32-63). Buffalo, NY: Prometheus.

Dengrove, E. (1973). The uses of hypnosis in behavior therapy. *International Journal of Clinical and Experimental Hypnosis, 21,* 13-17.

Diamond, M. J. (1972). The use of observationally presented information to modify hypnotic susceptibility. *Journal of Abnormal Psychology, 79,* 174-180.

Diamond, M. J. (1977). Hypnotizability is modifiable: An alternative approach. *International Journal of Clinical and Experimental Hypnosis, 25,* 147-166.

Diamond, M. J., & Taft, R. (1975). The role played by ego permissiveness and imagery in hypnotic responsiveness. *International Journal of Clinical and Experimental Hypnosis, 23,* 130-138.

Farthing, G. W., Venturino, M., & Brown, S. W. (1983). Relationships between two different types of imagery vividness questionnaire items and three hypnotic susceptibility scale factors: A brief communication. *International Journal of Clinical and Experimental Hypnosis, 31,* 8-13.

Franklin, B. et al. (1984/1970). Report of Dr. Benjamin Franklin and the other commissioners, charged by the King of France with the examination of the animal magnetism as now practiced at Paris.
Reprinted in M. M. Tinterow (Ed.), *Foundations of hypnosis: from Mesmer to Freud* (pp. 82-128). Springfield, IL: C. C. Thomas.

Fuchs, K., Hoch, A., Palid, E., Abramovici, H., Brandes, J. M., Timor-Tritsch, I., & Kleinhaus, M. (1973). Hypno-desensitization therapy of vaginismus: Part I: "In vitro" method. *International Journal of Clinical and Experimental Hypnosis, 21,* 144-156.

Gfeller, J., Lynn, S. J., & Pribble, W. (1987). Enhancing hypnotic susceptibility: Interpersonal and rapport factors. *Journal of Personality and Social Psychology, 52,* 586-595.

Gorassini, D. R. (1989). The relationship between planned and actual responses to hypnotic suggestions. *Imagination, Cognition and Personality, 8,* 283-294.

Gorassini, D. R., & Spanos, N. P. (1986). A social-cognitive skills approach to the successful modification of hypnotic susceptibility. *Journal of Personality and Social Psychology, 50,* 1004-1021.

Graham, K. (1986). Explaining "virtuoso" hypnotic performance: Social psychology or experiential skill? *Behavioral and Brain Sciences, 9,* 473-474.

Ham, M. W., & Spanos, N. P. (1974). Suggested auditory and visual hallucinations in task-motivated and hypnotic subjects. *American Journal of Clinical Hypnosis, 17,* 94-101.

Hilgard, E. R. (1987). Research advances in hypnosis: Issues and methods. *International Journal of Clinical and Experimental Hypnosis, 35,* 248-264.

Hilgard, E. R., Sheehan, P. W., Monteiro, K. P., & MacDonald, H. (1981). Factorial structure of the Creative Imagination Scale as a measure of hypnotic responsiveness: An international comparative study. *International Journal of Clinical and Experimental Hypnosis, 29,* 66-76.

Hilgard, J. R. (1970). *Personality and hypnosis.* Chicago: University of Chicago Press.

Holroyd, J. (1985). Hypnosis applications in psychological research. *Imagination, Cognition and Personality, 5,* 103-116.

Hoyt, I. P., Nadon, R., Register, P. A., Chorny, J., Fleeson, W., Crigorian, E. M., Otto, L., & Kihlstrom, J. F. (1989). Daydreaming absorption and hypnotizability. *International Journal of Clinical and Experimental Hypnosis, 37,* 332-342.

Katsanis, J., Barnard, J., & Spanos, N. P. (1988). Self-predictions, interpretational set and imagery vividness as determinants of hypnotic responding. *Imagination, Cognition and Personality, 8,* 63-67.

Kroger, W. S., & Fezler, W. D. (1976). *Hypnosis and behavior therapy: Imagery conditioning.* Philadelphia: Lippincott.

Nilsson, K. M. (1990). The effect of subject expectations of "hypnosis" upon vividness of visual imagery. *International Journal of Clinical and Experimental Hypnosis, 38,* 17-23.

Nolan, R., Spanos, N. P., Hayward, A., & Scott, H. (1989). *Hypnotic and nonhypnotic imagery-based strategies in the treatment of tension and mixed tension/migraine headache.* Unpublished manuscript, Carleton University.

Perlini, A. H., Lee, A., & Spanos, N. P. *The relationship between imaginal and hypnotic susceptibility: Conceptual artifact or essence.* Unpublished manuscript, Carleton University.

Perry, C. W. (1973). Imagery, fantasy and hypnotic susceptibility: A multi-dimensional approach. *Journal of Personality and Social Psychology, 26,* 217-221.

Perry, C. W. (1977). Is hypnotizability modifiable? *International Journal of Clinical and Experimental Hypnosis, 25,* 125-146.

Sachs, L. B. Construing hypnosis as modifiable behavior. In A. Jacobs & L. B. Sachs (Eds.), *The psychology of private events* (pp. 65-71). NY: Academic Press.

Sarbin, T. R., & Coe, W. C. (1972). *Hypnotic behavior: The psychology of influence communication.* NY: Holt.

Sheehan, P. W. (1967). A shortened version of the Betts Questionnaire upon Mental Imagery. *Journal of Clinical Psychology, 23,* 386-389.

Sheehan, P. W. (1979). Hypnosis and the process of imagination. In E. Fromm & R. E. Shor (Eds.), *Hypnosis: Developments in research and new perspectives* (pp. 381-411). NY: Aldine.

Shor, R. E., Orne, M. T., J & O'Connell, D. N. (1966). Psychological correlates of plateau hypnotizability in a special volunteer sample.*Journal of Personality and Social Psychology, 3,* 80-95.

Spanos, N. P. (1971). Goal-directed fantasy and the performance of hypnotic test suggestions. *Psychiatry, 34,* 86-96.

Spanos, N. P. (1986a). Hypnosis and the modification of hypnotic susceptibility: A social psychological perspective. In P. L. N. Naish (Ed.), *What is hypnosis?* (pp. 85-120). Philadelphia, Open University Press.

Spanos, N. P. (1986a). Hypnosis, nonvolitional responding and multiple personality: A social psychological perspective. In B. Maher & W. Maher (Eds.), *Progress in experimental personality research,* (Vol. 14, pp. 1-62). NY: Academic Press.

Spanos, N. P. (in press, a). A sociocognitive approach to hypnosis. In S. J. Lynn (Ed.), *Theories of hypnosis.* NY: Pergamon.

Spanos, N. P. (in press, b). Hypnosis, hypnotizability and hypnotherapy: A socio-cognitive perspective. In C. R. Synder (Ed.), *Handbook of social and clinical psychology.* NY: Pergamon.

Spanos, N. P., & Brice, P. (1990). *Hypnotic and nonhypnotic suggested imagery and ethe elicitation of salivation.* Unpublished manuscript, Carleton University.

Spanos, N. P., Bridgeman, M., Stam, H. J., Gwynn, M. I., & Saad, C. (1983). When seeing is not believing: The effects of contextual variables on the reports of hypnotic hallucinators. *Imagination, Cognition and Personality, 2,* 195-209.

Spanos, N. P., Brett, P. J., Menary, E. P., & Cross, W. P. (1987). A measure of attitudes toward hypnosis: Relationships with absorption and hypnotic susceptibility. *American Journal of Clinical Hypnosis, 30,* 139-150.

Spanos, N. P., Cross, W. P., Menary, E. P., Brett, P. J., & de Groh, M. (1987). Attitudinal and imaginal ability predictors of social cognitive skill-training enhancements in hypnotic susceptibility. *Personality and Social Psychology Bulletin, 13,* 379-398.

Spanos, N. P., Cross, W. P., Menary, E. P., & Smith, J. (1988). Long term effects of cognitive skill training for the enhancement of hynotic susceptibility. *British Journal of Experimental and Clinical Hypnosis, 5,* 73-78.

Spanos, N. P., Flynn, D. M., & Niles, J. (in press). Rapport and cognitive skill training in the enhancement of hypnotizability. *Imagination,Cognition and Personality.*

Spanos, N. P., Gabora, N. J., & Hynford, C. (1990). *Self-predictions and interpretations of suggested demands as predictors of hypnotizability.* Unpublished manuscript, Carleton University.

Spanos, N. P., Gabora, N. J., Jarrett, L. E., & Gwynn, M. I. (1989). Contextual determinants of hypnotizability and of relationships between hypnotizability scales. *Journal of Personality and Social Psychology, 57,* 271-278.

Spanos, N. P., Gwynn, M. I., Gabora, N. J., & Jarrett, L. E. (1989). *Response expectancies and interpretational sets as determinants of hypnotic susceptibility.* Unpublished manuscript, Carleton University.

Spanos, N. P., Ham, M. W., & Barber, T. X. (1973). Suggested ("hypnotic") visual hallucinations: Experimental and Phenomenological data. *Journal of Abnormal Psychology, 81,* 96-106.

Spanos, N. P., Lush, N. I., & Gwynn, M. I. (1989). Cognitive skill training enhancement of hypnotizability: Generalization effects and trance logic responding. *Journal of Personality and Social Psychology, 56.* 795-804.

Spanos, N. P., & McPeake, J. D. (1974). Involvement in suggestion related imaginings, experienced involuntariness and credibility assigned to imaginings in hypnotic subjects. *Journal of Abnormal Psychology, 83,* 687-690.

Spanos, N. P., McPeake, J. D., & Carter, W. (1973). The effects of pretesting on response to a visual hallucination suggestion in hypnotic subjects.*Journal of Personality and Social Psychology, 28,* 293-297.

Spanos, N. P., McPeake, J. D., & Churchill, N. (1976). Relationships between imaginative ability variables and the Barber Suggestibility Scale. *American Journal of Clinical Hypnosis, 19,* 39-46.

Spanos, N. P., Mullens, D., & Rivers, S. M. (1979). The effects of suggestion structure and hypnotic vs. task-motivation instructions on response to hallucination suggestions. *Journal of Research in Personality, 13,* 59-70.

Spanos, N. P., Radtke, H. L., Hodgins, D. C., Bertrand, L. D., Stam, H. J. & Dubreuil, D. L. (1983). The Carleton University Responsiveness to Suggestion Scale: Stability, reliability and relationships with expectancies and hypnotic experiences. *Psychological Reports, 53*, 555-563.

Spanos, N. P., Radtke, H. L., Hodgins, D. C., Bertrand, L. D., Stam, H. J. & Dubreuil, D. L. (1983). The Carleton University Responsiveness to Suggestion Scale: Relationships with other measures of susceptibility, expectancies and absorption. *Psychological Reports, 53*, 523-535.

Spanos, N. P., Rivers, S. M., & Ross, S. (1977). Experienced involuntariness and response to hypnotic suggestions. *Annals of the New York Academy of Sciences, 296*, 208-221.

Spanos, N. P., Robertson, L. A., Menary, E. P., & Brett, P. J. (1986). A component analysis of cognitive skill training for the enhancement of hypnotic susceptibility. *Journal of Abnormal Psychology, 95*, 350-357.

Spanos, N. P., Stam, H. J., Rivers, S. M., & Radtke-Bodorik, H. L. (1980). Meditation, expectation and performance on indices of nonanalytic attending. *International Journal of Clinical and Experimental Hypnosis, 28*, 244-251.

Spanos, N. P., Stenstrom, R. J., & Johnston, J. C. (1988). Hypnosis, placebo and suggestion in the treatment of warts. *Psychosomatic Medicine, 50*, 245-260.

Starker, S. (1974). Effects of hypnotic induction upon visual imagery. *Journal of Nervous and Mental Disease, 159*, 433-437.

Sutcliffe, J. P., Perry, C. W., & Sheehan, P. W. (1970). The relation of some aspects of imagery and fantasy to hypnotizability. *Journal of Abnormal Psychology, 76*, 279-287.

Tellegen, A., & Atkinson, G. (1974). Openness to absorbing the self-altering experiences ("absorption"), a trait related to hypnotic susceptibility. *Journal of Abnormal Psychology, 83*, 268-277.

Van Dyne, W. T., & Stava, L. J. (1981). Analysis of relationships among hypnotic susceptibility, personality type and vividness of mental imagery. *Psychological Reports, 48*, 23-26.

Wagman, R., & Stewart, C. G. (1974). Visual imagery and hypnotic susceptibility. *Perceptual and Motor Skills, 38*, 815-822.

Weitzenhoffer, A. M., & Hilgard, E. R. (1962). *The Stanford Hypnotic Susceptibility Scale, Form C.* Palo Alto, CA: Consulting Psychologists Press.

Yanser, R. J., & Johnson, H. L. (1981). Absorption and attitude toward hypnosis: A moderator analysis. *International Journal of Clinical and Experimental Hypnosis, 29*, 375-382.

HYPNOTIC SUSCEPTIBILITY, IMAGING ABILITY, AND INFORMATION PROCESSING: AN INTEGRATIVE LOOK

Benjamin Wallace, Ph.D.

Department of Psychology
Cleveland State University
Cleveland, OH 44115

INTRODUCTION

At the beginning of the 19th century, Jose Custodi di Faria advocated a psychological explanation of what was then known as mesmerism. He stressed that so-called lucid sleep was taking place during this manipulation and that this was produced solely by the subject's heightened expectations and receptive attitudes. Since the subject wanted to be mesmerized and expected something to happen as a result, the expectations were in fact realized. With the emphasis on psychological factors during the mesmeric process, Faria developed what might be called a standard procedure for inducing lucid sleep. He used a series of soothing and commanding verbal suggestions while the subject was in the receptive mesmeric state. Faria then realized, as did others to follow such as Ambroise August Liebeault and Hippolyte Marie Bernheim, that verbal suggestion played a major role in mesmerism (Wallace and Fisher, 1987).

Since in those days, mesmerism was receiving an unfavorable reception from the medical community, a British physician, James Braid offered in 1826 a change in name from mesmerism to neurohypnotism (the prefix was later dropped). With this name change, Braid also offered an explanation as to what he believed was occurring during hypnosis. Specifically, he suggested that hypnosis involved a process that he called monoideism. Basically, this term referred to a process of focused attention or concentration on a single idea or image during a state of relaxation. During hypnosis, Braid believed, a subject's attention was focused only on a given thought while all other thoughts were being attenuated. This concept may be comparable to what is today referred to as selective attention (Haber and Hershenson, 1980; Treisman and Geffen, 1967). According to Braid, the ability to selectively attend to a single idea, thought, or image was limited to about 10 percent of his subjects.

As is evident from this brief historical introduction, hypnosis has traditionally been associated with different levels of subject susceptibility and the notions that imagery and attention play integral roles. The focus of this chapter will be to examine these possibilities and to present experimental evidence that hypnotic susceptibility, imaging ability, and attention are related phenomena.

HYPNOTIC SUSCEPTIBILITY

While Braid made the observation that approximately 10 percent of his subjects were susceptible to hypnotic suggestion, he did not have at his disposal the necessary tool to verify his belief. Fortunately, contemporary research in hypnosis does not need to rely on an estimate. There are a number of standardized, reliable, and valid tests to determine hypnotic susceptibility. The most commonly used tests include the Stanford Hypnotic Susceptibility Scale (Weitzenhoffer and Hilgard, 1959, 1962), the Barber Suggestibility Scale (Barber and Glass, 1962), and the Harvard Group Scale of Hypnotic Susceptibility (Shor and Orne, 1962). The first two are individually administered; the latter is typically administered in a group setting. Each hypnotic susceptibility test consists of a number of items or suggestions with which subjects are asked to comply. The more suggestions with which subjects comply, the greater is judged to be their level of hypnotic susceptibility. And while there are reports that the various susceptibility tests do not always correlate highly with each other (e.g., Register and Kihlstrom, 1986), there are also reports showing that the tests do highly correlate (e.g., Wallace, 1990a). Further, there have been many reports concerning various cognitive correlates of hypnotic susceptibility.

Mitchell (1970) reported that subjects classified as high in hypnotic susceptibility (highs) were better able than those classified as low in such susceptibility (lows) to resist distractions in a tracking task. Van Nuys (1973) found highs better able to concentrate and to attend to their own breathing or to concentrate on a candle flame. Additionally, a positive relationship was reported between hypnotic susceptibility level and performance in a selective listening task (Karlin, 1979), in the ability to call out or write random numbers (Graham and Evans, 1977), in reports of the perception of the Ponzo illusion (Miller, 1975), in perception of the autokinetic illusion (Wallace, Garrett, and Anstadt, 1974), and in reports of Necker cube and Schroeder staircase apparent reversals (Wallace, Knight, and Garrett, 1976). In general, these results have been discussed in terms of the ability of high hypnotics to be better able to concentrate or to fixate their attention during a task requiring such an ability. The better they are able to utilize their attentional processes, the better their performance.

There have also been a number of reports of hypnotic susceptibility level being related to performance in a number of visual search tasks. And in accordance with previous studies that have examined the relationship between hypnotic susceptibility and performance, if high hypnotics are better able to selectively attend in an environment of perceptual complexity, then their performance should exceed that of low hypnotics. Some studies that have examined the attentional processes of high and low hypnotics include those by Wallace and Patterson (1984), Priebe and Wallace (1986), Crawford (1981), and Crawford and Allen (1983).

Wallace and Patterson (1984) examined the ability of subjects to find an embedded letter within a 6 x 50-letter array. Subjects were requested to search for a specific letter, contained only once in the array, until it was located. When it was found, subjects were requested to so indicate by circling it with a pencil. Other than this simple instruction, the manner in which subjects went about performing their search was left to their discretion. Thus, during the search, the experimenter was not only concerned with whether the letter was found, but also with the processes involved in finding the letter. Since this task is not very difficult, all subjects eventually found the letter. However, those classified high in hypnotic susceptibility found the letter more quickly than those judged low in susceptibility. In addition, most highs searched for the letter in a manner that was distinguishable from the manner used by lows.

Highs performed the visual search for a letter by one of two methods. Either they used their pencil as a guide, placing it beneath each 6-letter string, and then searched for the embedded letter in what might be termed a row-by-row or parallel manner. Another method consisted of placing two fingers, one from each hand, at the left and right of each 6-letter string and then proceeding to search in the row-by-row manner. In any case, visual search for most highs consisted of examining rows in pursuit of the embedded letter.

Lows exhibited search behavior that differed from the highs. While it was not true for all lows, most searched for the embedded letter by proceeding from left-to-right in each row and then down the rows until the letter was located. This manner of search was performed either with a pencil or with one of their fingers. In performing the search in this letter-by-letter or serial approach, subjects obviously took longer in locating the target.

The conclusion from the Wallace and Patterson study seems to be that highs and lows process information in different manners. While both categories of subjects do accurately perform the search, highs appear to be efficient visual searchers while lows appear to be inefficient. Given the nature of the letter-search task, an error rate was nonexistent.

To determine if search strategies and error rate might be influenced if subjects had to seek out more ambiguous, multiple targets, Priebe and Wallace (1986) had subjects find objects embedded within pictorial scenes. A series of cartoon-like drawings from various issues of *Highlights for Children Magazine* were used as stimuli. Within each drawing, various objects are hidden and the task is to locate them. While these drawings are intended for children, many are sufficiently challenging even for adults.

Before being presented with a pictorial scene, each subject was given a list of objects which were embedded. An average of 11 objects were so embedded in each of a series of scenes. Subjects were then handed a pencil and were asked to find the embedded objects and to trace around them when located. As in the Wallace and Patterson study, the experimenter was concerned not only with the ability of subjects to find embedded stimuli, but also with the processes involved in finding the stimuli.

As in the Wallace and Patterson study, highs and lows exhibited different strategies in performing the visual search. Highs generally examined the list of objects-to-be-found for about 20 sec and then proceeded to find the objects. Rarely did they refer back to the list to see what objects still needed to be located. In essence, it appeared that they were storing the list in memory and then relying on this stored list from which to complete the search.

Lows generally performed the search in a different manner. First, they spent little time studying the list of objects-to-be-found. Rather, having spent on the average of 7 sec on the list, they proceeded to use it as a checklist. They would determine an object-to-be-located, find it in the pictorial scene, and then return to the list to check it off. They then proceeded to the next object and so on. While many of these subjects did proceed to find objects in the order specified on the list, this was not always the case. As ascertained in a postexperimental interview, some subjects seemed to search in a random order as a function of which objects appeared to be easiest to find. In examining the performance of both groups of subjects, it was found that lows made more incorrect identifications within the pictorial scenes. They would often identify an object as being the one they were to find when in fact their response was in error. In terms of number of correct objects found, the difference between the two groups was not statistically significant, although in later studies (Wallace, 1989, 1990a), highs did find more objects correctly while still making fewer misidentifications.

While it appears that highs are more efficient visual searchers than lows, there may also be other processes that influence performance. To continue the search for cognitive correlates of hypnotic susceptibility, Crawford (1981) studied the relationship between performance on various gestalt closure tasks involving fragmented stimuli and hypnotic susceptibility level. When subjects are presented with fragmented stimuli, the general tendency is to organize the fragments according to the laws of Gestalt psychology. As an example, if dots are presented in a circular form, subjects generally respond according to the law of closure and report the totality of the dots as forming a circle. To examine gestalt closure, Crawford used a closure speed test and the Harshman (1974) and Street (1931) figures. She reported that hypnotic susceptibility level was positively correlated to performance. The better performance of highs was theorized to be the result of their ability to more easily shift into a passive, holistic, associational mode of information processing when appropriate.

In a related study, Crawford and Allen (1983) examined performance on a variety of visual memory discrimination tasks that required detecting differences between successively presented pairs in which one member of the pair was slightly altered. As in the Crawford (1981) study, highs consistently showed enhanced performance. However, in this study, highs demonstrated superiority only during hypnosis and not during the waking state. In addition, it was reported that highs showed enhanced imagery vividness as measured by the Vividness of Visual Imagery Questionnaire or VVIQ (Marks, 1973).

Two cognitive strategies appeared to mediate visual memory performance. Crawford and Allen described the first as a detail strategy that involved the memorization and rehearsal of individual details for the task. The second, described by Crawford (1981), was referred to as a holistic strategy that involved examining and remembering the whole picture with accompanying imagery. Both highs and lows reported similar, predominately detail-oriented strategies during the waking state. During hypnosis, however, highs shifted to a significantly more holistic strategy.

Although hypnotic susceptibility level appears to be a discriminant in many of the aforementioned perception and cognition studies, it is possible that the imaging ability of subjects or their imagery vividness may also account for some of the variance. As was previously mentioned, Crawford (1981) reported a positive relationship between imagery vividness and hypnotic susceptibility. Others have also reported such a positive relationship (e.g., Hilgard, 1979; Nadon, Laurence, and Perry, 1987; Sutcliffe, Perry, and Sheehan, 1970), although the relationship has not always been linear nor consistent (see Morgan and Lam, 1969; Perry, 1973), except that low hypnotizability is reported to almost always be associated with poor imaging ability (Perry, 1973; Sutcliffe et al., 1970).

If there is a positive relationship between imaging ability and hypnotic susceptibility, then one would expect to find that subjects who are judged to be vivid imagers would perform in a manner similar to that described for high hypnotic subjects. And as will be discussed later, this is generally the case. However, prior to doing this relationship, let us examine methods by which imaging ability can be assessed.

IMAGING ABILITY

The study of imagery in psychology has come a long way since the early work of Perky (1910) where perception was compared with the image of imagination. And in a manner similar to the previous discussion of the measurement of hypnotic susceptibility, a major advance in the study of imagery has been the development of imagery tests involving imagery ratings. These tests include the Sheehan (1967) QMI or Vividness of Imagery Scale, the Gordon (1949) Test of Visual Imagery Control, and the Marks (1973) VVIQ. Each of these tests has been used in assessing the imaging ability of subjects in a number of different experiments. From a perusal of the various citations of the use of these tests, the VVIQ has become the most popular. And while there are critics who argue that it is neither a reliable nor a valid test (Chara, 1989), there are many investigators who have found it to be quite reliable as well as valid in assessing imaging ability (see Marks, 1989).

Using the VVIQ as a method for assessing imaging ability, Wallace and his colleagues have conducted a number of experiments to determine if imaging ability can predict performance in a cognition or perception task. In essence, if hypnotic susceptibility and imaging ability are related variables, then those tasks that have been shown to discriminate in terms of performance as a function of hypnotic susceptibility should likewise be discriminable in terms of imaging ability.

Since visual search strategies were found to differ as a function of hypnotic susceptibility level (Priebe and Wallace, 1986; Wallace and Patterson, 1984) and since hypnotic susceptibility and imaging ability have been reported by many to be related variables, it was predicted that vivid imagers should show superior performance in a visual search task compared to poor imagers. In essence, if in the Priebe and Wallace study subjects were storing lists of objects in memory and forming images of such to use in performing a visual search, then vivid imagers should be more adept at this compared with poor imagers.

To examine this possibility, the same stimuli and stimuli lists used by Priebe and Wallace were used by Wallace (1988) on vivid and poor imagers. And as expected, vivid imagers performed differently compared to poor imagers. Like subjects in the Priebe and Wallace study who were judged to be high in hypnotic susceptibility, vivid imagers also exhibited a different search strategy compared to poor imagers.

Vivid imagers spent a significantly longer period of time, an average of 22 sec, examining the list of objects that were embedded within a particular pictorial scene. This was contrasted to an average of 8 sec for poor imagers to examine the stimulus list. And like high hypnotics, vivid imagers did not tend to use the stimulus list as a checklist as did the poor imagers. Rather, they examined the list, stored the information in memory, and then searched for embedded objects by relying on images stored in memory. In essence, when comparing the performance of high hypnotics in the Priebe and Wallace study with vivid imagers in the Wallace study, the differences were not statistically different.

In addition to the results reported by Wallace on vivid and poor imagers in a pictorial visual search, differences have been reported between vivid and poor imagers on other tasks where imagery might be utilized as part of a task strategy. For example, differences have been found between the two groups of imagers in their ability to perform in a proofreading task (Wallace, in review).

Six passages were prepared from articles that appeared in issues of *Time Magazine* or the Cleveland *Plain Dealer* newspaper. Each passage contained between 250 and 275 words and was typed (double-spaced) on a single page. The content of topics spanned the range from serious news items such as the 1984 war in Lebanon to more casual items such as the history of astronomy.

Each passage contained 26 misspelled words. As in the procedure of an earlier experiment by Haber and Schindler (1981), all misspellings were created by substituting one incorrect letter for a correct one in such a way as to produce a nonexistent English word. For 13 of the misspellings in each passage, the substituted incorrect letter was in the same shape category as the correct letter. For the remainder, the substitute incorrect letter was in a different shape category. Also, within each passage, 13 of the misspelled words were function words (e.g., the) and 13 were content words (e.g., star). As much as was possible, both types of words were matched for length (most misspelled words were three or four letters in length). Also, the incorrect letter was always positioned in the middle, the position reported by Haber and Schindler to produce the most failures to detect a misspelling. Although in words with misspellings the mode number of letters was three or four, some longer words were misspelled in each passage so that subjects would not adopt a search strategy of looking only for three- or four-letter words.

After proofreading the various scripts, each subject was interviewed to ascertain what strategies had been used in the search for misspelled words. Also, words that subjects failed to pinpoint as being misspelled were orally presented to determine if subjects knew the correct spelling. In all instances, subjects could correctly spell the misspelled words. They simply missed locating them.

Results indicated that vivid imagers were more adept at finding misspelled words compared to poor imagers. However, this appeared to be the case only for words where the substitute letter that produced a misspelling was similar in shape to the one removed. This was likely the case because misspellings created by the use of different-shaped letters draw more visual attention than misspellings produced from the replacement of one letter with another same-shaped letter. As a result, when the misspelling draws this additional attention, it does not seem to matter whether a subject is a vivid or poor imager. Both groups respond in a comparable fashion. However, poor imagers exhibit a 22 percent greater error rate in failing to find misspellings consistent of words with similar-shaped letter substitutions. When averaged over the two types of words, vivid imagers do perform more accurately in a proofreading task.

With vivid imagers appearing to be as efficient as high hypnotic subjects in processing information, one could draw the conclusion that high hypnotics and vivid imagers may be one in the same. That is, subjects who are vivid imagers may be high hypnotics and vice-versa. As was previously discussed, there have been a number of investigators who have reported a positive correlation between imaging ability and hypnotic susceptibility. However, the correlation was never reported as being perfect. As a result, it was necessary to conduct experiments to determine to what degree hypnotic susceptibility and imaging ability jointly and separately play a role in information processing.

HYPNOTIC SUSCEPTIBILITY AND IMAGING ABILITY INTERACTIONS

Recently, Wallace (1990b) examined the relationship between hypnotic susceptibility level and imaging ability. Specifically, he attempted to replicate the Crawford (1981) finding that high hypnotics are more adept than low hypnotics at performing gestalt closures. This was attempted despite the fact that Popham and Bowers (1987) failed to replicate the relationship reported by Crawford.

Since Popham and Bowers failed to replicate Crawford, it was reasoned that one possible difference between the two studies was that Crawford examined the issue of imaging ability as it related to hypnotic susceptibility while Popham and Bowers did not. The implication of this is that Crawford may have discovered an interaction between hypnotic susceptibility level and imaging ability. Thus, Crawford may have found that high hypnotics perform better in a gestalt closure not because of their hypnotic susceptibility per se, but also because they were also vivid imagers and made use of their imaging abilities in a cognitive task. As a result, the variance accounted for by Crawford in terms of hypnotic susceptibility might further be partitioned into an imagery component.

Two experiments were conducted by Wallace. In the first, he repeated the conditions used by Crawford; subjects were administered the Closure Speed Test (Thurstone and Jeffrey, 1966) and the Street (1931) Test. In the second, he presented fragmented stimuli to subjects as an intense light pulse to the retina of an eye which when perceived, appeared as an afterimage. In addition, four groups of subjects were tested in each experiment as constituted by a matrix of hypnotic susceptibility level (high or low) by imaging ability (vivid or poor).

While it has been reported that low hypnotizability is almost always associated with poor imaging ability (Perry, 1973; Sutcliffe et al., 1970), Wallace was able to find subjects to complete all four cells of the 2x2 matrix. Thus, vivid imagers were found amongst high and low hypnotics. Similarly, poor imagers were found amongst the two hypnotic groups.

From a group of 411 individuals who participated in two mass-testing sessions, the total number who met the criteria for the experiments were as follows: 50 (or 12.2 percent) were classified as being high hypnotics as well as vivid imagers, 28 (or 6.8 percent) were high hypnotic and poor imagers, 27 (or 6.6 percent) were low hypnotics and vivid imagers, and 39 (or 9.5 percent) were low hypnotics and poor imagers. Thus, despite previous reports, there are individuals who comprise the four combinations of hypnotic susceptibility by imaging ability.

When subjects were administered the Closure Speed Test and the Street Test, those who were both high in hypnotic susceptibility and vivid in imaging ability clearly showed the best performance. Of the 24 correct closures on the former test, subjects who were high hypnotics as well as vivid imagers averaged 15.3 correct. This average was significantly different from that obtained by the other three groups. In addition, the performance of subjects who were both poor imagers and high in hypnotic susceptibility (an average of 10.4 correct) was not significantly different from the performance of those who were both poor imagers and low in hypnotic susceptibility (an average of 9.7 correct).

With respect to responses on the Street Test with a maximum of 14 correct identifications, again those who were both high in hypnotic susceptibility and vivid in imaging ability performed best (an average of 10.9 correct identifications) and this performance was significantly different than that obtained from the other three groups. Also, as in the previous experiment, subjects classified as poor imagers and high in hypnotic susceptibility did not demonstrate significantly better performance (an average of 8 correct identifications) than did subjects classified as being both poor imagers and low in hypnotic susceptibility (an average of 7.8 correct identifications).

In the experiment where subjects were required to report on their perception of a fragmented stimulus as an afterimage, again subjects judged high in hypnotic susceptibility as well as vivid in imaging ability were clearly superior to the other three groups. Of the 10 possible correct responses, the high hypnotic/vivid imager group averaged 9 correct. This was significantly greater than that achieved by any of the other three groups. Also, as in the Closure Speed Test and in the Street Test, subjects classified as being poor imagers and high in hypnotic susceptibility did not demonstrate significantly better performance (an average of 7.2 correct identifications) than subjects classified as being poor imagers and low in hypnotic susceptibility (an average of 7.1 correct identifications).

In addition to being superior in identifying fragmented stimuli as afterimages, high hypnotic/vivid imager subjects reported perceiving the longest enduring afterimage (an average of 66.7 sec). This duration was significantly longer compared to that reported by the other three groups. Also, subjects classified as being poor imagers but high in hypnotic susceptibility did not report a longer enduring afterimage (an average of 55.0 sec) than did those classified as being poor imagers but low in hypnotic susceptibility (an average of 54.1 sec).

The afterimage duration results replicate a previous study by Wallace, Garrett, and Anstadt (1974) where a less complex afterimage was reported as enduring longest by subjects classified as high in hypnotic susceptibility. These investigators did not evaluate imaging ability of their subjects.

An explanation for why an afterimage endures longest for subjects classified as being both high hypnotics and vivid imagers may relate to their ability to utilize their attentional processes. Since it is unlikely that high hypnotic/vivid imager subjects have different retinal functioning and biochemical reactions when a light impinges on the photoreceptors compared to other subjects, the most likely explanation is that these individuals attend to the stimulus in a more concentrative manner compared to other subjects. This attentional component permits them to focus in on the relevant stimulus and for a longer period. The result is a report of a longer enduring afterimage.

Based on these findings, it appears that it is not necessarily hypnotic susceptibility that produces superior performance in a gestalt closure task. Rather, to some extent, subjects' making use of their vivid imaging abilities contributes to their superior performance. The cause of such performance cannot be hypnotic susceptibility level, per se, because subjects who scored high in hypnotic susceptibility and were also poor imagers did not perform any better on either of the two gestalt tasks than did those who scored low in hypnotic susceptibility and were also poor imagers.

Two studies by Wallace (1988, 1990b) also add support to this conclusion. Subjects who were classified as low in hypnotic susceptibility were trained to improve their perceptual and cognitive performance by using the strategies employed by high, hypnotic subjects. On the basis of a number of earlier studies (e.g., Wallace et al., 1976; Wallace and Patterson, 1984), it was found that subjects who performed best in a number of cognitive performance tasks did so because they used strategies that helped them maximize their performance.

In the Wallace (1990b) study, subjects who performed best initially were those who scored high in hypnotic susceptibility. With training, however, low hypnotics were found to be capable of improving their performance to a level indistinguishable from their counterparts. In a related study (Wallace, 1988), subjects classified as vivid imagers initially performed better on various cognitive tasks than did those classified as being poor imagers. Also, with training in the use of the efficient strategies employed by vivid imagers, poor imagers improved their performance to a level indistinguishable from vivid imagers. A post hoc analysis of the Wallace (1990b) data indicated that the majority of high hypnotics were also initially (before training) high imagers. Thus, it appears that imaging ability may be an important factor in contributing to the initial exhibition of efficient cognitive strategies.

AN IMAGERY PARADOX

While it has been demonstrated that vivid imagery is a trainable skill (Wallace, 1988), an imagery paradox exists. Ahsen (1985, 1986, 1987) has questioned the assumption that if one is judged to be a vivid imager on a standardized test for assessing such (i.e., the VVIQ), that this individual upon retest will still score in the range considered vivid in imagery. In fact, Ahsen has found evidence that imagery as assessed on a standard questionnaire is not necessarily as reliable nor as stable a trait as has been predicted. Thus, Ahsen (1985) has defined what might be called an unvividness paradox. In a series of experiments he found that subjects who are initially judged to be vivid imagers may on occasion not be vivid or may be what he labeled unvivid.

One reason for the apparent unstable aspect to imagery may be that cognitive strategies play a role in determining when and if imagery is to be vivid. That is, in one situation, a subject may be judged to be a vivid imager because he/she has developed an appropriate strategy for dealing with the production and/or utilization of an image. In another situation the same subject may not have developed the appropriate strategy. As a result, this person demonstrates what would be considered to be vague or unvivid imagery. This might occur despite the fact that the individual may have scored high on an imagery questionnaire.

Recently, Wallace and Kokoszka (1990) discovered another possible reason for the unvividness paradox, the presence of a ultradian cycle related to imaging ability. A number of studies have demonstrated the existence of ultradian cycles or rhythms that seem to have an average duration of approximately 90 min (Kleitman, 1983). These cycles have been noted for many physiological responses such as gastric motility (Hiatt and Kripke, 1975), eating, drinking, and smoking (Friedman and Fisher, 1967), urinary flow (Lavie and Kripke, 1981), and the ability to fall asleep throughout the day (Lavie and Scherson, 1981).

Ultradian cycles have also been shown to exist for such diverse behavioral activities as vigilance (Okara, Matousek, Nueth, and Petersen, 1981; Orr, Hoffman, and Hegge, 1974), response to apparent motion such as beta movement (Lavie and Sutter, 1973), perception of spiral aftereffects (Lavie, Lord, and Frank, 1974; Lavie, Levy, and Coolidge, 1975), and reports of fantasy (Kripke and Sonnenschein, 1978).

Not all research has demonstrated the existence of 90-min cycles. Some have reported shorter cycles (30- to 60-min), for example, in human respiration (Horne and Whitehead, 1976). Others have reported longer cycles (up to 6.5 hrs in duration) in alpha brain-wave activity associated with variations in mood (Tsuki, Fukuda, Okuno, and Kobayashi, 1981).

If ultradian rhythms exist for a variety of physiological and behavioral responses, Wallace and Kokoszka speculated that such a rhythm may explain variations in imagery vividness on test-retest situations for, an example, the VVIQ. If such exists, one reason some individuals demonstrate vivid imaging ability at one time and poor ability at another time is because in the former, subjects are being tested during a valley in the cycle. If a spontaneous cycle in arousal during the waking state does exist with regard to imaging ability, then variations in such ability across times-of-testing can be expected.

To examine this possibility, Wallace and Kokoszka administered to a group of 60 individuals the VVIQ six times over a period of 3 hrs. Following each administration, completed tests were collected to prevent subjects from comparing responses on subsequent administrations. Between administrations the experimenter discussed current events with the participants. To determine if cyclicity was present in the performance of subjects during the various administrations, the highest and lowest scores per subject were compared. Of the total 60 subjects, 52 exhibited cyclicity. The most common cycle, represented by the performance of 42 subjects, was 90 min. This corresponds to the most common ultradian period reported by other investigators for behavioral phenomena (Kleitman, 1983). However, 8 subjects exhibited a 60-min cycle and 2 exhibited a 120-min cycle. For individuals exhibiting cyclicity, the difference between their highest and lowest VVIQ score was significant.

As expected, variability in imaging ability appears to be present during a series of administrations of the VVIQ. Clearly, the majority of subjects exhibited both vivid and poor imaging ability as a function of time-of-administration. While this lends further support to Ahsen's (1985) unvividness paradox, it also helps to some extent to explain why the unvividness paradox appears to exist.

It thus appears that imaging ability may be regulated, to some extent, by the existence of an ultradian rhythm, perhaps one concerned with or related to level of attention or arousal. This contention is supported by Kripke and Sonnenschein (1978) who reported the presence of EEG alpha waves during daydream activity, characterized by vivid sensory imagery. And such activity appeared to occur in 90-min periods that were correlated with continuous alpha activity.

While the Wallace and Kokoszka study did not assess EEG activity during administration of the VVIQ, it is possible that such activity might be correlated with peaks and valleys in imaging ability. If imaging ability is most keen while a subject is relaxed (where alpha activity might be present), this might encourage imaging activity that might not be present while a subject is fully aroused or, at least, not sufficiently relaxed. For example, it has been documented that attempts to hypnotize individuals are very difficult if the subject is incapable of creating images during the induction procedure (Hoyt, Nadon, Register, Chorny, Fleeson, Grigorian, Otto, and Kihlstrom, 1989; Kahn, Fromm, Lombard, and Sossi, 1989). Thus, high scores on the VVIQ might be associated with periods of relaxation. This is the time when subjects might be most capable of utilizing imagery, at least the type assessed by the VVIQ. When subjects are excited or not relaxed, imaging ability as assessed by the VVIQ may not be as keen.

If imaging ability runs in a cyclical fashion, the possibility may exist that this may impact on performance on tasks where imaging ability is a criterion for subject selection. For example, a study previously discussed by Wallace (1988) reported that subjects classified as vivid imagers (on the VVIQ) were more adept at finding embedded objects within a series of pictorial scenes compared to individuals classified as being poor imagers. Perhaps if subjects who were classified as vivid imagers were to be tested during a valley in their ultradian cycle for imaging ability, their performance would approximate that of the poor imager. Similarly, if poor imagers were tested during a peak in their ultradian cycle, their performance might approximate that of the vivid imager.

To determine if peaks and valleys in a possible, imagery-related, ultradian cycle affect the performance of subjects in a cognitive task, Wallace, Kokoszka, and Turosky (1990) repeated the Wallace (1988) study. And as in the Wallace and Kokoszka study, subjects were administered the VVIQ over a number of sessions. The first administration established a baseline of imaging ability. The VVIQ was then repeated continuously every half hour until a 15-point increase or decrease in performance was noted. This was approximately the range of performance between the average high and low score of subjects in the Wallace and Kokoszka study.

When a change in performance had been observed, an experimenter who was blind with respect to the subject's imaging ability, presented subjects with a list of words that represented what was embedded within a specific pictorial scene. Subjects were asked to examine such a list prior to each pictorial presentation. No time limit was set for this period but in no instance did a subject take longer than 28 sec to perform the examination. When subjects indicated that this had been accomplished, the first picture from a set of 3 was presented.

Subjects were then instructed to examine the cartoon-like drawing and to locate all the embedded objects by circling them with a pencil. They were told that they would have a maximum of six minutes in which to find the objects, and they should try and locate them before the elapsed time. As in the Wallace (1988) study, timing began when the subjects were presented with each picture; timing ended when the subjects indicated that they had found all the hidden objects or the six-min period had elapsed.

After finding the embedded objects, the subjects were administered additional forms of the VVIQ. This continued every half hour until, as before, subjects demonstrated a 15-point increase or decrease in their imaging ability. When such a change was noted, the subjects were administered a second set of stimuli they had not previously encountered.

When comparing performance as a function of changes in imaging ability, those originally classified as vivid or as poor imagers did not show an improvement nor a decline in correctly finding more embedded objects as their score changed with peaks and valleys in their possible, imagery-related ultradian rhythm. This was also the case with respect to incorrect identifications. Also, when originally-classified, poor imagers demonstrated vivid imaging ability on a subsequent administration of the VVIQ, their vivid VVIQ score was not significantly different from that originally obtained by those classified as vivid imagers. This was also true when originally-classified vivid imagers produced a poor VVIQ score. However, because VVIQ scores were variable across administrations, additional evidence is provided to support Ahsen's (1985, 1986, 1987) unvividness paradox. That is, vivid imagers can sometimes demonstrate poor imaging ability and poor imagers can demonstrate vivid imaging ability.

Incidentally, of the subjects in the aforementioned study, all but one demonstrated an ultradian rhythm. Of the remaining 23 subjects, 21 exhibited a 90-min rhythm, 1 exhibited a 60-min rhythm, and 1 produced a 120-min rhythm.

Despite the fact that imaging ability is vulnerable to change as a function of time-of-administration, it does not appear that this change significantly influences performance on a task that has been shown to be affected by subjects' imaging ability level. Thus, although ultradian cyclicity has been shown to exist for both vivid and poor imagers, it does not appear that such rhythms influence performance in a cognitive and/or perception task, at least not one involving the detection of embedded objects within pictorial scenes. It was reassuring to find that the best predictor of performance in the aforementioned task was the subject's original VVIQ score as obtained in a mass testing. In fact, 21 of the 24 subjects exhibited their best or poorest VVIQ score in the first administration. For these individuals, their ultradian rhythm appeared to have begun with this administration.

EXPERIMENTAL CONCLUSIONS

With many studies having been conducted in the areas of hypnotic susceptibility and imaging ability, it is safe to conclude that these variables do influence performance in a number of perception and cognition tasks. A number of investigators have shown that hypnotic susceptibility, per se, is a potent factor. Similarly, other investigators have demonstrated that imaging ability, per se, is a strong factor. And related to these findings, it has also been demonstrated that both factors may interact in determining performance in a cognition or perception task. The commonalty that appears to tie these variables is that they involve a cognitive style whereby subjects utilize an efficient strategy in the performance of a task. This is especially the case where the task involves a form of attending, whether it be selective or focused (see Crawford, 1981; Crawford and Allen, 1983; Wallace, 1979; Wallace, Knight, and Garrett, 1976; Wallace and Patterson, 1984).

So where do we go from here? Future studies should examine the processes that underlie the attainment of efficient, cognitive strategies by individuals classified as high hypnotics and/or vivid imagers. Why is it that these individuals possess an attribute or skill that is only present to a much lesser degree in most subjects? One possibility is that this skill was taught to them, either in a formal sense (school) or in an informal sense (they picked it up as part of their life experiences). As an example, perhaps when they were taught arithmetic in school, they were taught a style that differed from that of other individuals.

There is some evidence to suggest that this may be the case, to some degree. Wallace and Patterson (1984) asked high and low hypnotics to perform addition problems that involved a carry function. Thus, when they added numbers such as 34 + 87, they would have to add the 4 + 7 and produce an 11. The one from the 11 then had to be carried to the left column of the remaining numbers and added to it to obtain the sum. Interestingly, when low hypnotics were presented with such addition problems, they performed the task in a manner that often resulted in them having to write the carry number (1) above the left column of numbers to be added. Seldom did one observe such behavior in subjects judged to be high hypnotics. As such, high hypnotics carried the number 1 as an image or memory to produce the sum. Low hypnotics, at least in this experiment, seldom did this. It is as if they could not store an image of a carry number or, perhaps more realistically, they did not utilize a cognitive style or strategy that involved doing this. In other words, they were either not taught to carry a number in memory or they just never did it that way.

If low hypnotics and/or poor imagers are simply inefficient in the processing of information, this might have implications for a variety of behaviors in the real world. It has already been demonstrated that these individuals can be taught efficient strategies for information processing (Wallace, 1988, 1990a). Thus, might these laboratory studies have value for natural situations? Let me speculate on this.

POTENTIAL APPLICATIONS OF AN EFFICIENT COGNITIVE STYLE

If the previously-discussed, cognitive style was learned, does this imply that those who learned it are more intelligent? More creative? Better employees at certain types of jobs? Unfortunately, little light can be shed on these questions. To date, studies have not been conducted on these problems. However, let us examine a possible problem that might benefit from future investigations concerned with hypnotic susceptibility, imaging ability, and information processing.

Many elementary school students are often described by their teachers as lazy. That is, they seem to always be daydreaming in class or at least, not sufficiently paying attention to what is going on in the classroom. Further, they often do not turn in their homework. And when it is turned in, it appears that the students did not put forth a great effort. Often, they seem to be doing only the minimum to pass the assignment.

In this situation, the teacher's evaluation may be correct, to some extent. The student is lazy. But why is this happening? One possibility is that the student does not have the necessary cognitive style to remain sufficiently attentive in the classroom. The student may be intelligent, and perhaps even creative, but she/he does not know how to utilize their ability. They may watch, as an example, students doing addition problems in a time test very quickly. However, they just cannot do it that quickly. They struggle and struggle and just do not seem to finish as many problems as their classmates. Their work may be just as accurate as their classmates, but they seem to work more slowly, less efficiently. Sometimes in frustration, they almost appear to be giving up since they do not think they can compete with their classmates. If this happens, we may see the beginnings of the problem student.

Some teachers, unfortunately, misinterpret the behavior of these students. They may write them off as being lazy, not working to their potential. But what if these students were to be taught the efficient cognitive style of their classmates? What if the teacher were to find the so-called brightest, fastest students in the class and teach the rest of the class the techniques used by these students in the performance of classroom activity and subsequent homework assignments? It has been demonstrated that inefficient information processors can be taught to be more efficient. Why cannot this be extended from the laboratory to the classroom? And if it is, might it result in students who otherwise might be written off as becoming better in the classroom? From the quantity of data that now exists concerning how individuals who are high hypnotics and/or vivid imagers perform in a cognitive task, this is the type of problem that deserves attention. And hopefully future research will move beyond the laboratory to determine to what extent inefficient information processors can be taught to be more efficient.

REFERENCES

Ahsen, A. (1985). Unvividness paradox. *Journal of Mental Imagery, 9,* 1-18.

Ahsen, A. (1986). Prologue to unvividness paradox. *Journal of Mental Imagery, 10,* 1-8

Ahsen, A. (1987). Epilogue to unvividness paradox. *Journal of Mental Imagery, 11,* 13-60.

Barber, T. X., and Glass, L. B. (1962). Significant factors in hypnotic behavior. *Journal of Abnormal and Social Psychology, 64,* 222-228.

Chara, P. J., Jr. (1989). A questionable questionnaire: A rejoinder to Marks. *Perceptual and Motor Skills, 68,* 159-162.

Crawford, H. J. (1981). Hypnotic susceptibility as related to gestalt closure tasks. *Journal of Personality and Social Psychology, 40,* 376-383.

Crawford, H. J., & Allen, S. N. (1983). Enhanced visual memory during hypnosis as mediated by hypnotic responsiveness and cognitive strategies. *Journal of Experimental Psychology: General, 112,* 662-685.

Friedman, S., & Fisher, C. (1967). On the presence of a rhythmic, diurnal, oral instinctual drive cycle in man. *Journal of the American Psychoanalytic Association, 15,* 317-351.

Gordon, R. (1949). An investigation into some of the factors that favour the formation of stereotyped images. *British Journal of Psychology, 39,* 156-167.

Graham, C., & Evans, F. J. (1977). Hypnotizability and the development of waking attention. *Journal of Abnormal Psychology, 86,* 631-638.

Haber, R. N., & Hershenson, M. (1980). *The psychology of visual perception.* New York: Holt, Rinehart, and Winston.

Haber, R. N., & Schindler, R. M. (1981). Error in proofreading: Evidence of syntactic control of letter processing? *Journal of Experimental Psychology: Human Perception and Performance, 7,* 373-379.

Harshman, R. (1974). *Harshman figures.* Unpublished test (available from Department of Psychology, University of Western Ontario, London, Ontario, Canada)

Hiatt, J. F., & Kripke, D. F. (1975). Ultradian rhythms in waking gastric activity. *Psychosomatic Medicine, 37,* 320-325.

Hilgard, J. R. (1979). *Personality and hypnosis* (Second Edition). Chicago: University of Chicago Press.

Horne, J., & Whitehead, M. (1976). Ultradian and other rhythms in human respiration. *Experientia, 32,* 1165-1167.

Hoyt, I. P., Nadon, R., Register, P. A., Chorny, J., Fleeson, W., Grigorian, E. M., Otto, L., & Kihlstrom, J. F. (1989). Daydreaming, absorption and hypnotizability. *International Journal of Clinical and Experimental Hypnosis, 37,* 332-342.

Kahn, S. P., Fromm, E., Lombard, L. S., & Sossi, M. (1989). The relation of self-reports of hypnotic depth in self-hypnosis to hypnotizability and imagery production. *International Journal of Clinical and Experimental Hypnosis, 37,* 290-304.

Kleitman, N. (1983). Basic rest-activity cycle: 22 years later. *Sleep, 5,* 311-317.

Karlin, R. A. (1979). Hypnotizability and attention. *Journal of Abnormal Psychology, 88,* 92-95.

Kripke, D. F., & Sonnenschein, D. (1978). A biologic rhythm in waking fantasy. In K. S. Pope & J. L. Singer (Eds.), *The stream of consciousness.* New York: Plenum, 321-334.

Lavie, P., & Kripke, D. F. (1981). Ultradian circa 1 1/2 hour rhythms: A multioscillatory system. *Life Sciences, 29,* 2445-2454.

Lavie, P., Levy, C. M., & Coolidge, F. L. (1975). Ultradian rhythms in the perception of the spiral after-effect. *Physiological Psychology, 3,* 144-146.

Lavie, P., Lord, J. W., & Frank, R. A. (1974). Basic rest-activity cycles in the perception of the spiral after-effect: A sensitive detector of a basic biological rhythm. *Behavioral Biology, 11,* 373-379.

Lavie, P., & Scherson, A. (1981). Ultrashort sleep-waking schedule. I. Evidence of ultradian rhythmicity in "sleepability". *Electroencephalography and Clinical Neurophysiology, 52,* 163-174.

Lavie, P., & Sutter, D. (1973). Differential responding to the beta movement after waking from REM and NONREM sleep. *American Journal of Psychology, 88,* 595-604.

Marks, D. F. (1973). Visual imagery differences in the recall of pictures. *British Journal of Psychology, 64,* 17-24.

Marks, D. F. (1989). Construct validity of the Vividness of Visual Imagery Questionnaire. *Perceptual and Motor Skills, 69,* 459-465.

Miller, R. J. (1975). Response to the Ponzo illusion as a reflection of hypnotic susceptibility. *International Journal of Clinical and Experimental Hypnosis, 23,* 148-157.

Mitchell, M. B. (1970). Hypnotic susceptibility and response to distraction. *American Journal of Clinical Hypnosis, 13,* 35-45.

Morgan, A. H., & Lam, D. (1969). *The relationship of the Betts Vividness of Imagery Questionnaire and hypnotic susceptibility: Failure to replicate* (Research Memorandum No. 103). Stanford, CA: Hawthorne House.

Nadon, R., Laurence, J-R., & Perry, C. (1987). Multiple predictors of hypnotic susceptibility. *Journal of Personality and Social Psychology, 53,* 948-960.

Okawa, M., Matousek, M., Nueth, A. L., & Petersen, I. (1981). Changes of daytime vigilance in normal humans. *Electroencephalography and Clinical Neurophysiology, 52,* S17.

Orr, W. C., Hoffman, H. J., & Hegge, F. W. (1974). Ultradian rhythms in extended performance. *Aerospace Medicine, 45,* 995-1000.

Perky, C. (1910). An experimental study of imagination. *American Journal of Psychology, 21,* 422-452.

Perry, C. (1973). Imagery, fantasy, and hypnotic susceptibility. *Journal of Personality and Social Psychology, 26,* 217-221.

Popham, C. E., & Bowers, K. S. (1987, October). *A nonreplication of the effects of hypnotizability and hypnosis on holistic processing.* Paper presented at the annual meeting of the Society for Clinical and Experimental Hypnosis, Los Angeles.

Priebe, F. A., & Wallace, B. (1986). Hypnotic susceptibility, imaging ability and the detection of embedded objects. *International Journal of Clinical and Experimental Hypnosis, 34,* 320-329.

Register, P. A., and Kihlstrom, J. F. (1986). Finding the hypnotic virtuoso. *International Journal of Clinical and Experimental Hypnosis, 34,* 84-97.

Sheehan, P. W. (1967). A shortened form of Betts' Questionnaire Upon Mental Imagery. *Journal of Clinical Psychology, 23,* 386-389.

Shor, R. E., & Orne, E. C. (1962). *Harvard Group Scale of Hypnotic Susceptibility, Form A.* Palo Alto, CA: Consulting Psychologists Press.

Street, R. F. (1931). *A gestalt completion test* (Contributions to Education No. 481). New York: Columbia University Teachers College.

Sutcliffe, J. P., Perry, C. W., & Sheehan, P. W. (1970). Relation of some aspects of imagery and fantasy to hypnotic susceptibility. *Journal of Abnormal Psychology, 76,* 279-287.

Thurstone, L. L., & Jeffrey, T. E. (1966). *Closure Speed Test administration manual.* Chicago: Industrial Relations Center, University of Chicago.

Treisman, A., & Geffen, G. (1967). Selective attention: Perception or response? *Quarterly Journal of Experimental Psychology, 19,* 1-18.

Tsuki, Y., Fukuda, H., Okuno, H., & Kobayashi, T. (1981). Diurnal rhythm of alpha wave activity. *Electroencephalography and Clinical Neurophysiology, 52,* S43.

Van Nuys, D. (1973). Meditation, attention, and hypnotic susceptibility: A correlational study. *International Journal of Clinical and Experimental Hypnosis, 21,* 59-69.

Wallace, B. (1979). Hypnotic susceptibility and the perception of afterimages and dot stimuli. *American Journal of Psychology, 92,* 681-691.

Wallace, B. (1986, November). *Modification of cognitive search strategies.* Paper read at the annual meeting of the Psychonomic Society, New Orleans.

Wallace, B. (1987). Hypnotic susceptibility and proofreading accuracy. *American Journal of Psychology, 100,* 289-294.

Wallace, B. (1988). Imaging ability, visual search strategies, and the unvividness paradox. *Journal of Mental Imagery, 12,* 173-184.

Wallace, B. (1989). Improving cognitive search skills in resistant hypnotic subjects. *Journal of General Psychology, 116,* 351-358.

Wallace, B. (1990a). Hypnotic susceptibility and the modification of cognitive search strategies. *International Journal of Clinical and Experimental Hypnosis, 38,* 60-69.

Wallace, B. (1990b). Imagery vividness, hypnotic susceptibility, and the perception of fragmented stimuli. *Journal of Personality and Social Psychology, 58,* 354-359.

Wallace, B., & Fisher, L. E. (1991). *Consciousness and behavior* (Third Edition). Boston: Allyn and Bacon.

Wallace, B., Garrett, J. B., & Anstadt, S. P. (1974). Hypnotic susceptibility, suggestion, and reports of autokinetic movement. *American Journal of Psychology, 87,* 117-123.

Wallace, B., Knight, T.A., & Garrett, J. B. (1976). Hypnotic susceptibility and frequency reports to illusory stimuli. *Journal of Abnormal Psychology, 85,* 558-563.

Wallace, B., and Kokoszka, A. (1990, May). *Ultradian rhythms and imaging ability.* Paper read at the meetings of the Midwestern Psychological Association, Chicago.

Wallace, B., Kokoszka, A., & Turosky, D. (1990). *Ultradian rhythms and imaging ability.* Unpublished manuscript.

Wallace, B., & Patterson, S. L. (1984). Hypnotic susceptibility and performance on various attention-specific cognitive tasks. *Journal of Personality and Social Psychology, 47,* 175-181.

Weitzenhoffer, A. M., & Hilgard, E. R. (1959). *Stanford Hypnotic Susceptibility Scale, Forms A and B.* Palo Alto, CA: Consulting Psychologists Press.

Weitzenhoffer, A. M., & Hilgard, E. R. (1962). *Stanford Hypnotic Susceptibility Scale, Form C.* Palo Alto, CA: Consulting Psychologists Press.

DEEP TRANCE SUBJECTS: A SCHEMA OF TWO DISTINCT SUBGROUPS

Deirdre Barrett, Ph.D.

Harvard Medical School
Behavioral Medicine Unit
1493 Cambridge Street
Cambridge, MA 02139

This chapter will review previous research on characteristics of deep trance subjects with special attention to the trait of fantasy proneness. Then a study will be presented which distinguishes two types of deep trance subjects. One fits the characterization of fantasy proneness and the other is distinguished by dissociative phenomena.

INTRODUCTION

As Spanos and Barber pointed out in their 1974 article on hypnotic susceptibility, research in this area has been converging on the propensity to become absorbed in fantasy or imaginative activity as the personality characteristic most associated with deep trance subjects.

Josephine Hilgard (1970, 1979) found the childhood histories of her deep trance subjects were more likely than less hypnotizable subjects' to involve imaginary playmates, parental encouragement of fantasy play, and reading of much fiction. A significant number of high susceptibles also remembered being punished harshly and using their well-developed fantasy ability to tune out the punishment while it was occurring or to engage in self-soothing later. As adults, the high susceptibles were more likely than others to be avid consumers of drama, film, and fiction, to daydream more, and to be more creative.

Tellegan and Atkinson (1974) found hypnotic susceptibility to correlate with their scale of absorption in imaginative activity, containing questions about vividness of imagery, intensity of emotional involvement in fantasy, tendency to tune out external stimuli when imaging, and experiences of synesthesia. Absorption has also been found by multiple regression analysis to account for factors such as positive attitudes toward hypnosis, which in turn have been linked to hypnotic susceptibility (Spanos & McPeake, 1975).

Wilson and Barber (1981, 1983) studied 27 women, representing approximately the 4% most hypnotically responsive, and reported that all but one of them were distinguished by a constellation of fantasy-related characteristics: 1) They spent much of their waking time engaged in fantasy; the majority said they fantasized at least 90% of their waking time simultaneous with carrying on real life activities. 2) They reported their imagery to be every bit as vivid as their perceptions of reality; sixty-five percent said this was the case with their eyes open; thirty-five percent had to close their eyes for the visual component of their imagery to look completely real. 3) They experienced physiologic responses to their images such as requiring a blanket to watch Dr. Zhivago on TV in a warm room, vomiting when they (mistakenly) thought they had eaten spoiled food, and being able to reach orgasms in response to fantasy with no physical stimulation. The majority of their female subjects had experienced physiological symptoms of false pregnancy at least once when they had reason to suspect they might be pregnant. 4) They had unusually early ages for their first memory, many dating back to infancy. Only one of Wilson and Barber's high hypnotizable subjects did not display this constellation of fantasy-related characteristics, and only a small minority of their low and medium susceptible subjects displayed any of them.

Their study used both traditional and nontraditional scales (Barber & Wilson, 1978/79) in selecting those they judged to be the best hypnotic subjects including the rather ideosyncratic variable of the ability to go into a trance instantly or quickly as one of their criteria. This is not a criteria for any of the most widely used scales of hypnotic susceptibility, which typically give the subjects about fifteen minutes of induction before beginning the specific suggestions whose responses will be scored for hypnotizability.

Lynn and Rhue (1986) developed a "fantasy-proneness" scale based closely on the characteristics Wilson and Barber had described. They found that 80% of fantasy-prone subjects scored as highly hypnotizable while a little over 1/3 of the non-fantasizers did so. Lynn and Rhue (1988) and Huff and Council (1987) found that high and medium fantasizers did not differ on hypnotic responsiveness while low fantasizers were less hypnotically susceptible. Spanos (1989) found an even lower degree of correlation between fantasy proneness and hypnotic susceptibility.

Several dreamlike qualities have been suggested to be more characteristic of daydreams in high hypnotizable subjects than of those in low hypnotizables. Barrett (1990) found highly hypnotizablesubjects to be likelier than medium hypnotizables to have daydreams containing magical or surreal content, abrupt transitions of scenes, a sense of awaking with a start at their conclusion, and occasional amnesia for content.

In characterizing frequent nightmare sufferers, Hartmann (1984) has described them as having "thinner boundaries" in many senses including those between sleeping and waking. He reported that the concept "daymare" was a meaningful one to nightmare sufferers only; they reported that their fantasies could take on very terrifying turns of content and be difficult for them to terminate. Frequency of nightmares has been found to correlate with hypnotic depth (Belicki & Belicki, 1984), as has Hartmann's measure for thinness of boundaries (Barrett, 1989).

Other categories of dreams that have been found to correlate significantly with hypnotizability include dreams which the dreamers believed to be precognitive and dreams in which the dreamer seems to be out of his or her body (Zamore and Barrett, 1989). The same study found Tellegen's Absorption Scale to correlate positively with dream recall, ability to dream on a chosen topic, reports of conflict resolution in dreams, creative ideas occurring in dreams, amount of color in dreams, pleasantness of dreams, bizarreness of dreams, flying dreams and precognitive dreams.

METHOD

The present study set about to examine to what extent other highly hypnotizable people resembled Wilson and Barber's fantasizers and what traits might characterize deep trance subjects who were not extreme fantasizers. As being able to enter a trance instantly was the most unusual of Barber and Wilson's criteria, it was hypothesized that this might distinguish fantasizers from other deep trance subjects. In addition to exploring the replicability of Wilson and Barber's findings about fantasy activity among high hypnotizables, other points of interest were characteristics of hypnotic experience and how these interact with a person's waking fantasy style.

For this study, thirty-four extremely hypnotizable subjects were selected from among approximately 1200 undergraduate subject volunteers who had been hypnotized in the course of other research projects and demonstrations in classroom and dormitory settings over a seven year period. They were selected using two standard scales: The Harvard Group Scale of Hypnotic Susceptibility, Form A (Shor and Orne, 1962) and The Stanford Scale of Hypnotic Susceptibility, Form C (Weitzenhoffer and Hilgard, 1962). All subjects scored either 11 or 12 on both scales. This constituted a very similar criterion for hypnotic susceptibility to Wilson and Barber's with the exception of not requiring instant or rapid hypnotic induction.

Subjects were hypnotized a total of three to four times, with zero to one of these experiences being solely for the present experiment, depending on what the protocol in the screening project had been. Their hypnotic experiences included both ones in which an amnesia suggestion and removal cue were given and ones in which they were not, age regression suggestions, a hypnotic hallucination of a candle which they were asked to blow out, a post-hypnotic hallucination of a person they knew arriving at the experimental room to talk with them, and an attempted instant re-hypnosis followed by several measures of trance depth.

They were interviewed from two and a half to four hours and were asked about the fantasy-related phenomena which Wilson & Barber and J. Hilgard reported. They were also asked about the "dreamlike" qualities of surrealism, abrupt transitions within daydreams, startling out of them, and occasional amnesia for content that Barrett (1979, 1990a) has described. They were asked about the "daymare" phenomena that Hartmann (1984) found among nightmare sufferers. They were also asked about how real and/or involuntary the hypnotic phenomena they experienced felt and about how much hypnosis was like other experiences.

All subjects, either in their preliminary screening or specifically for the present experiment, also completed the Tellegen and Atkinson (1974) Absorption Scale and responded to the Field Inventory Scale of Hypnotic Depth (Field, 1965) in terms of their HGSHS-A experience. Field's scale consists of true-false items that assess subjective response to hypnosis and has a subgroup of six items that reflect the degree to which hypnosis is different from other experiences.

FANTASIZER GROUP

The first subgroup of deep trance subjects was selected by their ability to enter trance instantly, since Wilson and Barber had used this as a criteria for the group they characterized. These 19 people, 7 male and 12 female, also had a number of other characteristics which distinguished them from subjects who did not achieve their deep trances immediately. Most of these characteristics clustered around vividness of fantasy processes, so they are referred to for the rest of this discussion by Wilson and Barber's term "fantasizers".

Vivid Imagery and Fantasies

Fantasizers scored extremely high on Tellegen and Atkinson's Absorption Scale: 32-37 of 37 items, with a mean of 34. During their interviews, they described five related characteristics of fantasy-proneness that Wilson and Barber found most characteristic of their group: extensive history of childhood fantasy play, majority of adult time devoted to fantasizing, hallucinatory vividness to their imagery, physiological effects from their imaging, and a variety of "psychic" experiences.

They all described rich fantasy life as children. They had at least one, most many, imaginary companions. These included a real playmate who had moved out of state, a princess, an entire herd of wild horses, and space aliens among others. The fantasizers greatly enjoyed stories, movies, and drama; they tended to prolong their experience of these by incorporating them into their fantasy lives, providing another source of imaginary companions. For example one subject described that, after seeing the movie Camelot, he had spent two years engaging daily in an elaborate scenario in which he was the son of Arthur and Guinivere and commanded the King's court. Periodically he would appoint new knights of his own invention to the roundtable. His real-life brother was cast in the role of Mordred, but all the other characters were either from the film, or completely from his own imagination. The fantasizers described these imaginary companions as every bit as vivid as real persons. In addition to ongoing fantasies, these subjects described a wide variety of brief fantasy as children, such as watching a friend blow soap bubbles and imagining one was a bubble or seeing a tulip and suddenly developing a fantasy about a being a fairy that lived inside it. Seventeen of them found this changing of realities at will so compelling that before encountering its formal philosophical discussions they had formulated their own versions of the famous musing of Chuang-tzu: "One night, I dreamed I was a butterfly, fluttering here and there, content with my lot. Suddenly I awoke and I was Chuang-tzu again. Who am I in reality: A butterfly dreaming that I am Chuang-tzu, or Chuang-tzu dreaming that I was a butterfly?" (trans. 1970)

Parents of fifteen of the fantasizers were remembered as explicitly encouraging their fantasy. For example, on a rainy day when one boy was bored, his mother would begin play suggestions with "You could pretend to be..." Another said her parents' formula response to her requests for expensive toys was "You could take this...(household object) and with a little imagination it would look just like...(that $200 whatever-Susie- just-got). And you know this worked for me--although Susie couldn't always see it." One mother very specifically trained hypnotic ability by reading trance inductions exercises about age regression, being an animal, speeding up time, etc. to her son from the book Mind Games (Masters & Houston, 1972)

Their adult fantasy continued to occupy the majority of their waking hours. They all fantasized throughout the performance of routine tasks and during any unoccupied time. Six of them said they did not "fantasize" or "daydream" when dealing with the most demanding tasks, but still continued to have vivid images in response to any sensory words or geometric tasks that occurred . The other thirteen said they continued to have elaborate ongoing fantasy scenarios. Some experienced them superimposed and intertwined with the ongoing tasks: "I'm listening to my boss's directions carefully, but I'm seeing the Saturday Night live character 'Mockman' next to him mocking all his gestures". Others experienced the fantasies as simultaneous or separate, happening "on a side stage", as one subject described it: "somehow I'm seeing the real world and experiencing my fantasy one at the same time."

Fantasizers also continued to have momentary vivid fantasies inspired by ongoing events. One young man had come to the interview directly from an archery class where he described that as he shot arrows at a target and watched others do so, he would briefly experience himself as the arrow being hurled by the force of the string through the air and felt himself piercing the fiberboard target. Another described that while passing up chocolate cake at lunch because of a diet, she momentarily "became" a microbe burrowing through the cake, tasting and smelling it as she devoured it, and feeling it squish around her body. She reported experiencing a sense of satiation with this fantasy indulgence.

All of these subjects described some of the dreamlike, surreal content, sudden transitions, and surprise that two earlier studies have reported for deep trance subjects' daydreams (Barrett, 1979, 1990a). When asked whether they "startled" out of daydreams which they could not recall, four said they experienced this occasionally although usually they had a "tip of the tongue" feeling about the fantasy and its memory would "come back" to them shortly. Seven of them reported that they occasionally had frightening content that seemed not to be under their control as in the "daymares" reported by Hartmann's nightmare sufferers.

Like Wilson & Barber's subjects they experienced physical effects from their imagery. Seven of the twelve female fantasizers had experienced false pregnancy symptoms. Even more of Wilson's subjects had experienced some such symptoms and full-blown cases (so to speak) presenting for treatment have been linked to high hypnotic susceptiblility (Barrett,1989). All of the fantasizers, male and female, described sometimes experiencing physical sensations to visual stimuli such as shivering when seeing a painting of the Alps, feeling hot, dry and impulsively getting something to drink in response to looking at desert photos, and getting nauseated from motion sickness at a film set on a tossing submarine. Ten of them said they tried to avoid either fictional depictions or real newsreel footage of violence and injuries because they experienced pain akin to real injuries. For four of them, this might precipitate ill feelings for hours or days. One such subject who had long-ago learned to avoid television news, described several weeks previously that she had been watching a nationally televised swim meet in which a diver had unexpectedly been injured. As she described the scene, she clutched herself tightly, grimaced as if in pain, tears came to her eyes, and she described this as minimal compared to her reaction when watching the scene which had left her shaken and physically aching for hours.

Fourteen of the fantasizers could experience orgasm through fantasy in the absence of any physical stimulation and all of them reported frequent, vivid and varied sexual fantasies. Although most of them tended to have fairly active and varied sex lives, all of them had fantasies of many more variations than they actually engaged in. Seventeen of this group were exclusively heterosexual and two males were predominantly homosexual with a bit of heterosexual experience. However all of the women and two of the heterosexual men mentioned homosexual fantasies. Other fantasy partners included animals, children, statues, and a variety of suggestively shaped inanimate objects.

Wilson and Barber reported that their subjects often obtained greater enjoyment from their fantasized sex than their actual sexual relationships. When our group was queried, they said this was not a meaningful comparison as their two categories of sexual experience were fantasy only vs. fantasy superimposed on real activity, of which the latter was often preferred. Real partners were heard to utter imaginary sexy comments, were dressed in hallucinatory erotic attire, had movie star's faces (and occasionally other parts) superimposed onto theirs, were joined by additional imaginary partners, and were transformed into science-fiction creatures and circus animals. Only two subjects (one male, one female) said they tried not to fantasize during real sex and both of these said they often failed.

Fantasizers all had some experiences which they considered "psychic": 14 had premonitions about events that were going to happen, 12 said that they could sometimes sense what significant others were thinking or feeling at a distance, 9 had dreams which came true, 13 had out of body experiences, and 8 had seen ghosts. Fifteen firmly believed these experiences were real paranormal phenomena and the remaining four said they were undecided about their reality.

Early Memories and Parental Discipline

The earliest memories of the fantasizers were all identified as being before the age of three, and before the age of two for eleven subjects. For the purposes of this study, subjectively believed age and detail of first memories were compared. This study was not set up to definitively check whether the ages were accurate, or whether indeed the memory was directly recalled rather than fantasized from stories told by parents. For randomly selected college students, the average age of subjectively recalled first memory is about three and a half and two to six is the usual range (Barrett 1980, 1983). The youngest memory that had a specific time estimate was of age eight months. This subject remembered two scenes: one in which he was being carried by his father down a hospital corridor and another in which he was lying on his back with one green-gowned man prodding his stomach while another pressed a plastic mask over the patient's nose and mouth. He remembered excruciating pain in both scenes. He was quite convinced that these were memories of an appendectomy he had undergone at eight months, and that he had remembered details of this which surprised his parents the first time they discussed it with him.

More typically, the incidents were too minor to be remembered by parents or to be tied to an exact date but sounded like those of a preverbal or early verbal child. For example one that the subject estimated as before age two: "I remember being in my crib which was pushed against a wall with a window above it. I was looking up at the window and it must have been raining outside because water drops were running down the outside of it. I was fascinated because I'd never noticed the window doing this before. This was a stage when I would point at things and ask 'whah?' and my mother would say the name for it. I pointed at the water drops and said 'whah?' and my mother said 'window'. I already knew this word so I frustratedly pointed again at the glass with the drops on the outside and repeated 'whah?'. I guess she thought I meant the pane of glass itself-or maybe she even said "rain" and I misunderstood-- because what I heard her say was 'pain'. I thought I recognized this as the word for when I hurt myself and I realized that the drops were like the tears that ran down my face at those times. I watched amazed that the window could cry with pain like me. I think it was a long time before I corrected this impression and came to connect the drops with the 'rain' that fell when I was outside and that could also run down the window's 'pane'.

Several of this group's earliest memories were of surreal events, most likely memories of fantasies or dreams such as this one: "I remember waking up in the middle of the night. In the air over me there were these big neon letters of the alphabet, maybe eight inches tall dancing around. They looked so wonderful. I recognized an 'A' and a 'D' because I knew the first few letters, but most of them were shapes I didn't know from later in the alphabet. They seemed to be floating into my room from the hall. I got out of bed and went into the hall where there were more neon letters in a line coming from my parents' room. I followed the line into my parents' bedroom. They were sound asleep, not knowing anything was going on. The letters were appearing from the bathroom off their room, so I went in there and traced them to the shower. They were coming out of the drain on the floor; one by one they would pop up out of the drain and dance out of the room. I watched them there for a while and then I went back to my room and watched them in bed until I fell asleep again. I remember thinking I must tell my parents about this in the morning, but I don't know if I did. I must have been about to turn three because I could say the alphabet by three years old."

When asked about how their parents had disciplined them and about any possible abuse, eleven of the subjects said that their parents had disciplined them solely by some combination of two strategies: 1) rewards or withholding of rewards and 2) reasoning with them, often emphasizing empathy: "One time I'd gotten in a fight at nursery school with another little girl because there was this doll there that was her favorite or regular toy to play with. I'd gotten it first that day; she tried to take it away from me and I pushed her down. The teacher called my mother and told her about it. Mother told me I should think about what she had felt like when she fell down, and it became like I really was her hitting the floor, scraping one knee, and crying. I could also feel her desperation and thinking it really was her doll (even though it was the school's); she had named it and everything. After that I wouldn't have done that again."

Eight of this group reported discipline that they experienced as harsh including frequent spankings, being locked in their rooms for extended periods, and verbal belittling. They typically used fantasy and imaginary companions to restore self esteem after these incidents. Wilson and Barber reported that their subjects' fantasies in these situations did not revolve around retaliation except indirectly toward other objects. In the present sample, more than half of these fantasies were of retaliation against parents, albeit tempered by leniency on the part of the offended child. One child fantasied producing electric shocks to repel spankings. More typically some other powerful being intervened against the parent sometimes because of punishing the child, sometimes for some other reason. Parents were kidnapped by aliens, chained in King Arthur's dungeon, arrested by the police, or sent back to grade school. In most cases however the next step was that the child intervened on the parents' behalf and the parents were released feeling repentant and/or indebted.

None of the nineteen fantasizers reported any severe beatings or sexual abuse by immediate family or caretakers. Two female subjects in this group did report abusive sexual behavior on the part of other adults, in one case a social acquaintance of the family, in the other a stranger. In asking about discipline and potential abuse, a characteristic of this group was that they all answered immediately and in detail. As with their other early memories, there were no "don't remember" responses and no hesitancy in talking about even the unpleasant memories.

Fantasizers' Experience of Hypnosis

Despite being such deep trance subjects, these 19 people scored only just above average (mean=18) on the Field Inventory and very low on the subgroup of Field items which reported surprise at hypnotic phenomena. Nine of the 19 described hypnosis as not different than what they experienced in their waking fantasy activity and the remaining ten found hypnosis mildly different by being somewhat more intense in some aspect but still similar to their other imagery experiences. These differences included hypnotic imagery being more consistently hallucinatory for six subjects, and two saying they felt much more subjective time had gone by in hypnosis than it would if they were fantasizing for a similar amount of real time. One drama major said "Hypnosis is a lot like what I do with method acting only you can get more into it. When I'm doing an acting exercise, I can only get so far into the experience because some part of me has to keep watching that I don't become the character so much that I'd just walk out of the class if he was mad, but with the hypnosis you don't have to watch that sort of thing at all. During the age regression I could leave my adult self behind completely."

These subjects were all quite aware that what they experienced during hypnosis were phenomena they produced themselves. None of them conceptualized it at all in terms of something the hypnotist was doing to them. "Hypnosis was a lot like what I do when I'm daydreaming or experiencing something from the past except it's even easier because your voice conjures up the images automatically," said one subject. The fantasizers generally seemed proud of their ability at hypnosis. All of them enjoyed the hypnotic experiences, although several remarked that the lengthy interviews about fantasy and memory were more personally significant to them. "Seeing the things you described in hypnosis is nice but pretty much like my daydreaming all the time, but talking about what my daydreams are like and how big a part of my life they are isn't something I've ever gotten to do before in this much detail."

Fantasizers experienced hypnotic amnesia only when it was specifically suggested--and not always absolutely then. Six of the eight fantasizers scoring 11 rather than 12 on the HGSHS-A had the amnesia suggestion as their only failed item. Some had partial recall although they had formally passed it. Others described that it seemed not as completely real an effect as the other hypnotic phenomena, citing working to keep items out of consciousness or being very aware they could counter the suggestion if they chose.

The fantasizers were also likely to know hypnotic hallucinations were not real without needing to be told this. When asked how they were sure they knew there had not been a real candle lit in the room for instance, fourteen of them cited some cognitive strategy which they had long practiced for differentiating the hallucinations of their waking fantasies from reality. Nine of them also usually retained the knowledge that the hypnotist had given verbal suggestions to hallucinate what they then experienced which made the deduction simple. In response to the HGSHS-A suggestion about hallucinating a fly during his first group induction, one subject had the following experience: "When you told us there was a fly buzzing around us, one appeared circling my head. Then I realized you had suggested it to everyone, and I saw and heard fifty of them circling around each student in unison. At the same time the rock group Kansas' song *The Gnat Attack* began to play as if there was a stereo in the room. I thought all this was delightful and very funny. As soon as you said we could shoo the flies away, the music stopped too."

This group showed a moderate degree of muscular relaxation during hypnosis akin to what an average person might look like awake but at rest. There was not a dramatic loss of muscle tone, all of them remained seated in the chair without problem and most shifted position occasionally during the trance. They moved easily when asked to do so for candle-blowing and for tasks while age regressed. When asked to, they also talked readily in trance, some of them with a bit softer or more monotone voice than awake, but no one in this group was difficult to understand. All subjects in this subgroup awoke from the trance immediately alert. Some began talking about their trance experience before the experimenter asked any questions. The most immediate response upon awakening from hypnosis for the fantasizers was a big smile.

DISSOCIATION GROUP

The other subgroup of fifteen subjects was selected for scoring as very highly hypnotizable on standard measures of hypnosis (scores of 11 or 12 on the HGSHS-A and SSHS-C) but not meeting Wilson and Barber's additional criteria of being able to enter a trance instantly. They scored about average (range 16-33, mean=26) on the Absorption Scale and did not display many of Wilson and Barber's fantasizers' characteristics.

In fact, the most distinctive quality to this subgroup's descriptions of fantasizing was the amnesia that had been noted for some subjects in a previous study (Barrett, 1989). The majority of them said their fantasizing was often characterized by inability to remember some or all of the content. Six of them said the only reason they knew they must daydream was that they were often startled to be spoken to, or otherwise have their attention summoned to the real world, with a sense that their mind had been occupied elsewhere. The reports of this group were quite dissimilar to most characterizations of "fantasy proneness" and "high absorption". They had so much more in common with the dissociative phenomena emphasized in Ernest Hilgard's (1977) neodissociation theory of hypnotic susceptibility that this subgroup is referred to to as the "dissociaters" for the remainder of this discussion.

Imagery and Fantasies

The fantasies which the dissociaters did recall from both childhood and the present were more mundane than the other subgroup's. They tended to be pleasant, realistic scenarios about events they would like to happen in their near future. None of them said these fantasies were as real in their sensory imagery as their perception of reality. Dissociaters were somewhat more like the fantasizers in how they reacted to external drama. They described that as both children and adults, they could become so absorbed in books, films, plays, and stories being told to them that they could lose track of time, surroundings, or their usual sense of identity. Their lack of equal vividness in self-directed fantasy seemed to stem partly from an external locus of control. It just did not seem to them that vivid images could be their own production and so they tended to experience them mainly in response to others' lead as in hypnosis or in listening to stories. Sometimes this absorption in external stimuli was intertwined with amnestic phenomena; several subjects commented that they thought they got very caught up in horror movies, but then could not remember their content shortly afterwards.

One of the most dramatic incidents of amnesia was recounted in answer to a routine inquiry of one of the dissociaters as to whether she had ever been hypnotized before. She answered "maybe" and described the following experience: "One time, my boyfriend and I were watching a police show on TV. There was this scene where they were going to use hypnosis with a witness. The detective began to swing a watch and tell the witness that he was going to go deep asleep. I don't remember anything after that until I started awake and said 'what happened?' about twenty minutes later. My boyfriend says the show continued with questions during the hypnosis, several scenes of what other characters were doing, a commercial break, and then came back to the scene where the detective was waking the witness up. But I don't remember any of that. I guess I was hypnotized by the watch."

Other amnestic experiences seemed to be triggered by more personal associations. One suggestion subjects were given in hypnosis was that they would see a book "with something important for you in it. You may take it down from the bookshelf and open it." One woman reported the book she saw was *Sybil*. She had opened it in the trance but could not recall anything she had read then. She also said that in reality, she had bought the book two years before and was sure she had read it but could not remember anything about it. When asked if she could produce even a sentence about the main subject of the the book, she insisted she had no idea. An obvious diagnostic question loomed. However when asked about specific multiple personality symptoms (as were all of the subjects showing pronounced dissociation) it was clear she did not have Sybil's malady. The only signs she and five others reported were "blackouts" which however only lasted hours at most. Neither she nor any others in this group had ever been told they behaved oddly or called themselves anything else during these times. She said she was by others' reports either inactive or acting normally during those times. She had never had longer blackouts, never found clothes she did not remember buying in her closet, and never met anyone who knew her by another name. She recalled some abuse in childhood and suspected much more than she directly recalled; she was currently in therapy partly to uncover this material. So it seemed that the childhood abuse and her related psychotherapy was probably the basis for the book *Sybil* coming up as such a strong personal association.

The way in which dissociaters appeared most like the fantasizers was in the frequency of their dramatic psychophysiological reactions. Five of the ten women had experienced symptoms of false pregnancy. They reported getting cold watching arctic scenes and becoming nauseated aftereating supposedly spoiled food that they later learned was fine. One developed a rash after being told by a prankster friend that a harmless vine she had handled was poisen ivy. Three of them also reported feeling pain when witnessing others' traumas. This might have been true of more of them, as six remarked that they often could not remember moments around witnessing injuries. After a swine flu vacination, one subject had a hysterical conversion-like episode of ascending paralysis that mimicked Guilliane-Barre syndrome, but which had remitted after a few minutes of reassurance from her physician about safety of the vaccine.

None of this group said they achieved orgasms solely from fantasy. All of them reported sexual fantasies but six subjects remarked that they sometimes couldn't remember them afterward. The interview did not specifically ask for examples of sexual fantasies. The fantasizer subgroup, as already described, volunteered voluminous content in the course of answering questions about frequency and vividness of these fantasies. The dissociaters rarely volunteered much detail so less characterization was possible of their sexual fantasy content. Most of the ones that were mentioned were mundane. The few who volunteered details consistently seemed to do so in the context of wanting reassurance about their normality. One subject was worried that she fantasized about anyone besides her boyfriend, and a male was bothered by thoughts of his girlfriend's attractive mother. A woman who in her early teens had been a victim of sexual abuse, now, in her early twenties, found herself fantasizing about the abuse in an arousing way during masturbation and intercourse. She seemed reassured to hear that that was not unheard of among rape and abuse victims and that it did not invalidate her perception that the sexual contact had been predominantly frightening and abusive at the time it occurred. Childhood sexual abuse may have been a common event for this group, as will be discussed in the next section.

Fewer subjects in this subgroup believed they had psychic experiences, and for nine of the eleven who did so, these experiences were confinedsolely to altered states of consciousness: dreams most commonly for seven of them, automatic writing for two, and trance-like seance phenomena for two. One subject reported that the spirit of her father who had died when she was nine regularly appeared to her in dreams dressed in the uniform in which he was buried and gave her advice on current problems. During hypnosis, when she was told that she could open her eyes and "see someone that you know and like" seated across from her, she had opened her eyes and seen her father. She felt certain that her nocturnal visitations were real but was not certain whether the hypnotic hallucination was her father's spirit or not.

Early Memories, Discipline and Abuse

The earliest memories of the dissociaters were later than average (mean=5 and for six subjects between ages 6 and 8) This was opposite the trend for the fantasizers. When asked about parental discipline and possible abuse, four of these subjects remembered abusive behavior. For three of them this involved physical violence and for two of them it involved sexual abuse. In addition to these four with direct memories, two subjects said they did not remember but had been told that they had been battered as children (in one case an older sibling remembered witnessing this, in another case a social worker had monitored the parents following a teacher's report of abuse). One additional subject in this group described a severe history of early childhood multiple fractures and burns for which his parents presented improbable explanations. Another subject experienced nausea and vomiting whenever anyone touched a certain portion of her thigh. Six of the remaining seven subjects reported some signs such as nightmares of beatings, dreams of injured children, or lack of recollections before the ages of 7 or 8 that have been associated with an increased likelihood of childhood abuse (Barrett and Fine, 1980).

In addition to this hint that between six and fourteen of the dissociaters had been abused by parents, three of them reported other major traumas in childhood, in one case a very painful and extended medical condition, and for two the death of a parent when they were under ten.

This subgroup scored very high on the Field questionnaire, mean = 33, usually answering 'true' to all six items which express surprise and amazement at hypnotic phenomena. They were muchlikelier to conceptualize hypnotic phenomena as due to some amazing talent of the hypnotist rather than as produced by themselves. They were resistant to hearing that it was something within their control, and in some sense this may really be less true for this group, for them it is less consciously controlled. Six of them asked many questions seeking reassurance that their hypnotic susceptibilty was normal. Two described hypnosis as partially unpleasant, not in terms of any specific content being negative but they did not like the concept that they were hallucinating. All described hypnosis as the more striking and interesting part of the experimental process; much of the interview about fantasy and imagery was not of great personal relevance.

These subjects frequently experienced spontaneous amnesia for hypnotic events. Amnesia was consistent and total for them whenever it was suggested, and it sometimes persisted even once removal cues had been given. Half of them experienced some degree of spontaneous amnesia for trance events when it had not been suggested.

Dissociaters were often surprised at some of their hypnotic experiences, especially hypnotic hallucinations. They were much likelier than fantasizers to believe their hypnotic hallucinations were real until told otherwise. The few who realized they were not real, distinguished them on the basis of their implausibility rather than by any other method for telling hallucinations from reality. They almost never remembered the verbal suggestions for the hallucinations, and when they did, still ignored the association with their perceptions. One subject remained convinced that, coincidentally at the moment that I suggested the HGSHS-A fly hallucination to a roomful of subjects, a real fly happened to begin to buzz around him.

The dissociaters exhibited an extreme loss of muscle tone during trance, often slumping; two needed to be propped up so that they did not fall out of their chairs. When asked to move or speak during the trance, their voices and movements were markedly subdued; four were partially inaudible. Six reported that their trance had to lighten for them to be able to move or speak at all.

When they were instructed to awaken, they would usually open their eyes, but most blinked and looked confused at first. Four asked disoriented questions such as "what happened?" or "Where was I?" They appeared to need almost to struggle to talk, and were slow to begin to answer questions. All of these behaviors were transient and all subjects were fully alert within a couple minutes.

DISCUSSION

In summary, this study found two distinct subgroups of high hypnotizable subjects. The "fantasizers" strongly resembled Wilson and Barber's subjects. They scored extremely high on absorption and low on a subgroup of Field Inventory items which reported surprise at hypnotic phenomena. They reported many deep trance-like experiences in their waking life, had an unusually early age for first memories, responded extremely rapidly to hypnotic inductions, and did not experience hypnotic amnesia unless it was specifically suggested. They consistently enjoyed their hypnotic experiences but did not view them as something drastically different from their waking fantasy and imagery.

The dissociative subgroup scored near average on absorption and very high on the Field Inventory items indicating surprise at hypnotic phenomena. They did not report many trance-like experiences in their waking life except "startling" out of daydream states for which they then had amnesia. They did not respond rapidly to hypnotic inductions, although they could eventually attain a trance depth equal to the fantasizers. They tended to have a late age for their first memory and many showed some evidence of a history of childhood abuse. They frequently experienced spontaneous amnesia for hypnotic events. Dissociaters were very surprised at some of their hypnotic experiences; a few were anxious about them and required reassurance that phenomena such as hypnotic hallucinations were not pathological.

The original criteria for distinguishing between the two groups was being able to achieve a deep trance instantly vs. needing time to make the transition. However another dichotomy that divides the same subject groups is the characterization of having very vivid fantasies ongoing the majority of the time vs. having a fantasy life characterized most conspicuously by dissociative phenomena. While not directly identifying dissociaters as the alternate category, previous studies emphasizing vivid fantasy as the major characteristic of many deep trance subjects, have all observed that some deep trance subjects do not fit these characterizations. Josephine Hilgard observed, "Evidence builds from a number of directions in regard to the role of imaginative involvement in hypnotizability. However, we must not forget that the relationship is far from perfect." (1979, p. 494) In statistical studies Lynn and Rhue (1988), Huff and Council (1987), and Spanos (1989) all found that although the correlation between hypnotizability and fantasy-proneness was consistently positive and significant, it was not linear. Low fantasizers are less hypnotically susceptible while high and medium fantasizers differ little on hypnotic responsiveness.

Even Wilson & Barber reported one dramatic exception in their second study (1983) of a highly hypnotizable subject who did not display any of their fantasizer characteristics. They did not describe the subject in enough detail to tell if perhaps this person was a dissociater who could atypically achieve that dissociated state instantly. If Wilson and Barber had not used "rapid or instant" response to hypnosis as a criteria, it seems likely that they would have found more exceptions to their characterizations of fantasy-proneness.

A patient of Morton Schatzman's whom he has described in detail in *The Story of Ruth* (Schatzman, 1980) was cited by Wilson and Barber as resembling their subjects because of her frequent and vivid hallucinations in the absence of psychosis. However in light of the distinctions in the present study, she might have more in common with the dissociaters. At least before therapy, she was not aware of her own imagery ability. She learned to control it mostly with verbal hypnotic-like suggestions and did this mainly in the presence of her therapist. She also had a history of severe violent and sexual abuse in childhood and was initially amnestic for much of her early years like the present study's dissociaters. Although in therapy she eventually gained detail for childhood memories equal to that of the fantasizers, she achieved this through very dissociative means: "Ruth said that now that she could summon an apparition of herself she would never have trouble remembering anything about herself. On that occasion the apparition had told her, 'Get to know yourself. Ask me questions.'" (p. 181)

The dissociative characteristics of hypnosis have been acknowledged at least since Puysegur (1837) focused on 'somnambulistic' behavior and amnesia as the distinguishing features of hypnotic trance. That some of the most hypnotizable persons have a variety of other dissociative phenomena was well documented in Breuer snf Freud's (1893) *Studies in Hysteria*. Ernest Hilgard (1973) has refined some of these observations in his "neodissociation" theory of hypnosis. His "hidden observer" experiments (1979) demonstrate that hypnotized subjects, while consciously oblivious to pain or noise, may process these stimuli in a dissociated manner. He also reported that the same people who would manifest a "hidden observer" for hypnosis, described analogous phenomena when awake. One subject reported answering questions without awareness of speaking; another could be reading in the room next to a soft conversation and later have knowledge of the content of the conversation without having even realized he could hear it. Some of these observations about the intimate link of dissocation and hypnosis seem to have gotten temporarily overlooked in the enthusiasm over the discovery of the more consciously controlled imagery experiences of the fantasizers. Interest in dissociation and especially its relation to trauma are presently experiencing a resurgence of interest.

In Frankel's recent review (1990) of the relation of hypnosis and dissociation, he questions the standard model of these traits as distributed on a continum. He suggests instead that Weitzenhoffer's (1989) view that the phenomemna of deep hypnosis are discontinuous with moderate hypnotic achievements may also be the appropriate model for dissociative phenomena. The two types of trance subjects described in the present study do not follow a normal distribution in relation to each other either. They appear to be more of a dichotomy, or at least a bimodal distribution.

Perhaps the most interesting question about this apparant dichotomy is whether the predominance and vividness of fantasy are really absent in the dissociaters, or whether this is an illusory difference stemming from their propensity for amnesia. In other words, do they have sparse fantasies in addition to their dissociative phenomena or do they have vivid fantasies for which they are amnestic in the same way they sometimes block out hypnotic experiences, memories of their early years, and unpleasant perceptions in their present?

Some of the evidence, such as their reports of frequently startling out of daydreams, suggests that the amount of time spent in fantasizing may be greater than they are consciously aware. Their dramatic physiological reactions to imagery and their sometimes vivid imagery in reaction to externally absorbing stimuli also support the idea that their imagery life may have a similarity to that of fantasizers that amnesia masks in terms of self-directed daydreams. Or, as mentioned earlier, they may have some of the same imagery ability which they do not utilize as much due to a more external locus of control. However, it appears that the difference in fantasy reports is at least partly due to their really not having as vivid or extensive fantasies: the dissociaters amnestic periods don't seem to equal the amount of time fantasizers are daydreaming.

Discussing the findings on their fantasizers, Wilson and Barber wrote: "We realized that the major reason why some individuals are excellent subjects is that they live in a fantasy world of their own creation that is very much like the world the hypnotist asks them to 'go into'" (1983, p. 375). It appears that the dissociaters are another group who have the ability to go in to this world but who do not dwell there as steadily as the fantasizers and do not have easy access to memory of their experiences there.

REFERENCES

Barber, T. X. and Wilson, S. C. (1978). The Barber Suggestibility Scale and the Creative Imagination Scale: Experimental and Clinical Applications. *American Journal of Clinical Hypnosis,* 21, 84-108.

Barrett, D. L. (1979). The Hypnotic Dream: Its Content in Comparison to Nocturnal Dreams and Waking Fantasy. *Journal of Abnormal Psychology,* 88, 584-591.

Barrett, D. L. (1980). The First Memory as a Predictor of Personality Traits. *Journal of Individual Psychology,* 36, 136-149.

Barrett, D. L. (1983). Early Recollections as Predictors of Self-Disclosure and Interpersonal Style. *Journal of Individual Psychology,* 39, 92-98.

Barrett, D. L. (1988). Trance-related Pseudocyesis in a Male. *International Journal of Clinical and Experimental Hypnosis,* 36, 256-261.

Barrett, D. L. (1989/March). *'Thick' vs. 'Thin' Boundaries: A Concept Related to Hypnotic Susceptibility.* Paper presented at Eastern Psychological Association Meeting, Boston, MA.

Barrett, D. L. (1990). *Daydreams of Deep Trance Subjects: They Strikingly Resemble Nocturnal Dreams.* Manuscript under editorial review.

Barrett, D. L. & Fine, H. J. (1980). A Child was Being Beaten: The Therapy of Battered Children as Adults. *Psychotherapy: Theory, Practice, and Research,* 17, 285-293.

Belicki K. & Belicki D. (1984). Predisposition for nightmares: A study of hypnotic ability, vividness of imagery and absorption. *Journal of Clinical Psychology,* 42, 714-718.

Breuer, J. & Freud, S. (1937). *Studies in Hysteria* (Trans. by J. Strachey). New York: Basic Books.

Chuang-tsu (trans. 1970). *Madly Singing in the Mountains.* London: Arthur Waley.

Field, P. (1965). An Inventory Scale of Hypnotic Depth. *International Journal of Clinical and Experimental Hypnosis,* 13, 238-249.

Frankel, F. (1990). Hypnotizability and Dissociation. *American Journal of Psychiatry,* 147, p. 823-829.

Hartmann, E. H. (1984). *The Nightmare: The Psychology and Biology of Terrifying Dreams.* New York: Basic Books.

Hilgard, E. R. (1977). *Divided Consciousness: Multiple Controls in Human Thought and Action.* New York: John Wiley and Sons.

Hilgard, E. R. (1979). Divided Consciousness in Hypnosis: The Implications of the Hidden Observer. In E. Fromm and R. E. Shor (Eds.), *Hypnosis: Developments in Research and New Perspectives,* 2nd Edit. Hawthorne, NY: Aldine.

Hilgard, J. (1970). *Personality and Hypnosis: A Study of Imaginative Involvement* . Chicago: University of Chicago Press.

Hilgard, J. (1979). Imaginative and sensory-affective involvements: in everyday life and in hypnosis. In E. Fromm and R. E. Shor (Eds.), *Hypnosis: Developments in Research and New Perspectives,* 2nd Edit. Hawthorne, NY: Aldine.

Huff, K. and Council, J. (1987). *Fantasy proneness and psychological coping.* Paper presented at the meeting of the American Psychological Association, New York.

Lynn, S. J. and Rhue, J. W. (1986). The fantasy prone person: Hypnosis, imagination, and creativity. *Journal of Personality and Social Psychology,* 51, 404-408.

Lynn, S. J. & Rhue, J. W. (1988). Fantasy proneness: Hypnosis, developmental antecedents, and psychopathology. *American Psychologistt,* 43, 35-44.

Masters, R. & Houston, J. (1972). *Mind Games: The Guide to Exploring Inner Space.* New York: Viking Press.

Puysegur, A. M. Marquis de. (1837). *An Essay of Instruction on Animal Magnetism* (Trans. by J. King). New York: J.C. Kelley.

Schatzman, M. (1980). *The Story of Ruth*. New York: Putnam.

Shor, R.E. & Orne, E. C. (1962). *The Harvard Group Scale of Hypnotic Susceptibility, Form A.* Palo Alto, CA: Consulting Psychologists Press.

Spanos, N. P. (1989/June). *Imagery and Hypnosis: Some Recent Developments*. Paper presented at the Third World Conference on Imagery, Washington, D.C.

Spanos, N. P. & Barber, T. X. (1974). Toward a Convergence in Hypnosis Research. *American Psychologist*, 29, 500-511.

Spanos , N. P. & McPeake, J. D. (1975). The Effects of Involvement in Everyday Imaginative Activities and Attitudes Toward Hypnosis on Hypnotic Susceptibility. *Journal of Personality and Social Psychology*, 31, 247-252.

Spiegel, H. (1974). The grade 5 syndrome: The highly hypnotizable person. *International Journal of Clinical and Experimental Hypnosis,* 22, 303-319.

Tellegan, A. & Atkinson (1974). Openness to Absorbing and Self-Altering Experiences ("Absorption"), a Trait Related to Hypnotic Susceptibility. *Journal of Abnormal Psychology,* 194, 83, 268-277.

Weitzenhoffer, A. (1989). *The Practice of Hypnotism Vols. I & II.* New York: John Wiley & Sons.

Weitzenhoffer, A. and Hilgard, E. (1962). *Stanford Scale of Hypnotic Susceptibility, Form C.* Palo Alto, CA: Consulting Psychologists Press.

Wilson, S. C. & Barber, T. X. (1981). Vivid Fantasy and Hallucinatory Abilities in the Life Histories of Excellent Hypnotic Subjects ("Somnambules"): A Preliminary Report. In Eric Klinger (Ed.), *Imagery: Volume 2: Concepts, Results, and Applications.* NY: Plenum Press.

Wilson, S. C. & Barber, T. X. (1983). The Fantasy-Prone Personality; Implications for understanding imagery, hypnosis, and parapsychological phenomena. In A. A. Sheikh (Ed.), *Imagery: Current Theory, Research, and Application* (pp.340-390). New York: Wiley.

Zamore, N. and Barrett, D. L. (1989). Hypnotic Susceptibility and Dream Characteristics. *Psychiatric Journal of the University of Ottawa,* 14, 572-574.

ADULTS WHO HAD IMAGINARY PLAYMATES AS CHILDREN

John F. Connolly, M.A.

The Imaginary Companion Project
P.O. Box 18143
Rochester, NY 14618

Imagine that you have a personal relationship with a being that you know is not real in the same way that you are. This being, which you are able to describe and interact with easily, could be like a friend, a protector, a teacher, a confidant, or a trouble maker. You are able to hear its words or thoughts with your mind. Your experience is vivid and real and often meaningful, but no one else can see or hear or interact with it the way that you do. If you were to seek out a deeper understanding of such a relationship it would be quickly evident that the orientation of your advisor would define the nature of your experience. In religious circles you would talk about angels, spirits, and the experience of prayer. In metaphysical or parapsychological circles you would talk about spirits, ghosts, fairies, channeling, reincarnation, aliens, mediums, and your higher self. In artistic circles you would talk about the autonomy of the character in your novel or the finding of your voice. In psychotherapeutic circles, you would talk about hallucinations, introjects, archetypes, and the techniques of active imagination, gestalt therapy, psychoimagination, and hypnosis. In healing and personal growth circles you would talk about your inner child, creative visualization, dialogue methods, focusing, psycho-synthesis and intensive journal writing. In social circles you probably wouldn't talk about it at all.

The focus of this paper is to talk about the naturally occurring phenomenon of imaginary playmates. Of specific interest are adults who had an imaginary playmate (IP) when they were children. If they "experienced" a relationship with a being that they knew was not physically real, then what implications might this have for their later development? Is there a difference between those that had IP's and those that did not, in vividness of imagery, creativity, suggestibility, or belief in other non-physical realities?

This paper will review what is known about IP's and what is known about their adult cohorts. We will also discuss the goals of the Imaginary Companion Project which was initiated to collect and to preserve the often fascinating childhood stories about IP's that have survived the ravages of time, memory, and experience.

OVERVIEW AND HISTORY

Most of the literature has focused on IP's as a time-limited adaptation or coping mechanism for environmental and developmental stress. Depending on the orientation of the author, the role and function of the IP has been assigned varying degrees of pathology or creativity.

Mary Watkins (1986), in her book *Invisible Guests: The Development of Imaginal Dialogues,* identifies imaginary playmates as just one example of a wide variety of human experiences in which there is a dialogue between an individual and an imaginary character or being. In her analysis she weaves together the full experience of inner dialogues and takes the reader outside the limitations of studied psychology to draw on the depths of knowledge available in the fields of literature, mythology and religion. In these fields imaginal dialogues are of central rather than peripheral signficance. She argues that while childhood imaginal dialogues do change with age, it does not necessarily follow that they are simply converted into conversation with "real" others or transformed into private and abstract thought. As a developmental psychologist and practicing clinician she argues tenaciously and eloquently:

> Here we will steal over the fences that have traditionally segregated private speech, play, imaginary companions, fantasy, prayer, religious experiences, the writing of novels, the reading of literature and thought itself...It is not enough that these experiences suffuse the intimacy of our talk and thought. They need a conceptual space as well, where they can exist with integrity: a place where their 'development' is not reduced to a change from their presence in childhood to their absence in adulthood. They need speace in theory so we can ask, 'Given their presence, their diversity, enduringness and multiformity, what might their development ential?' Only when we have accepted their continued presence can we move closer both to describing the variations in their structures and to wondering at the multiplicity of their possible function. (Watkins, 1986, p. 4).

One premise of her work is that contemporary psychological theory has taken a myopic view of imaginal dialogues and that by doing so has impaired its ability to see the phenomenon in its broader context. She argues that there is a continuum upon which the function of imaginal dialogue exists. It exists in its own right rather than merely as a subset or appendage of another developmental issue.

Initially, psychiatry and psychology viewed IP's to be signs of disturbance pathology or regressive development. When the primary charge of a profession is to heal the pain and distress of psychic disturbances and when there is only a limited amount of agreement on definitions, diagnosis and treatment, it would only seem reasonable that those schooled in a medical model of disease would focus on the pathological aspects of a phenomenon such as IP's.

Consider an orientation that regularly found itself exploring the uncharted territories of hallucinations, amnesia, dissociation, multiple personality disorder, depersonalization, possessions, defensive structures, and manifestations of organic lesions. Because of the similarity in the phenomena, it would be quite reasonable to view IP as an example of something gone wrong or least having the potential to do so. In psychoanalytical parlance an IP is referred to as an introject. An introject is:

> An unconscious symbolic internal psychic representation of a hated or loved external object whose goal is the establishment of the closeness and constant presence of the object. It is considered an immature defense mechanism. In the case of a loved object, anxiety consequent to separation or tensions arising out of ambivalence toward the object is diminished. In the case of a feared or hated object, internalization of its malicious or aggressive chracteristics serves to avoid anxiety by symbolically putting those characteristics under one's own control" (Kaplan, 1985, p. 498).

Rucker (1981) sees IP's as a temporary resting place for afffects and impulses that the child could not otherwise tolerate. Since they usually appear during the Oedipal stage - a time when aggression toward the mother is most threatening to psychological stability and self-esteem, IP's have also been referred to as:

"aids in impulse control" (Fraiberg, 1959),
"developmental buffers" (Nagera, 1969),
"instruments of the forces that oppose change..from individuals who are dominated by
    infantile fixations and prefer fantasy to external object relations" (Schaefer, 1968),
"manifestations of personality difficulties such as dominance, fear, over sensitivity,
    irresponsibility, and sex role dissatisfaction" (Svendsen, 1934), and
"possible precursor of later borderline pathology" (Myers, 1976).

As Levenson (1986) points out, the majority of analytical theorists do not necessarily see IP's as a sign of severe pathology. In fact, many think it can be viewed as a creative way to handle the stress and anxiety of age-appropriate developmental tasks. However, the experience of a childhood IP is not seen to be related to later vivid imaginal experiences. The focus of these theories concerns itself more with the disappearance of the phenomenon as an indicator of healthy adjustment than with the potentials that IP's have for future development.

RESEARCH COMPOSITES

When children with IP's are subjected to empirical investigation and compared to control groups of children with no reported IP's, composite pictures begin to take form. The children are at least three years old and usually not older than ten. They are of equal or higher intelligence, more linguistically advanced, better able to concentrate and more interested in interacting with adults. They are self-initiators, more self-reliant, less frequently bored, more socially cooperative, less aggressive, less impulsive, smile more frequently, watch less T.V. and show no difference in behavioral or emotional problems. Depending on how IP is defined, these children are joined by anywhere from 15 to 50 percent of their peers.

As for the playmates, there are often two or more per child with boys having males and girls having either or both. They are most likely to be around during quiet times and almost always leave when "real" friends are present. For younger children they are more likely to be animals and change to human-like for older children. Most have commonplace or composite names but many have unusual and creative ones of unknown origin. They are perceived with visual and auditory senses and between a third and a half require physical space while at the same time they are described as not real. Eighty percent of their interactions are playful affectionate and friendly and are conducted in a happy mood. Twenty percet are hostile and argumentative and reflect an agnry mood. (Ames & Learned, 1946; Curtis, 1979; Caldeira, 1978; Hurlock & Burnstein, 1932; Levenson, 1985; Manosevitz, 1973 & 1977; Rucker, 1979; Schaefer, 1969; Singer, 1967, 1973, 1983; Turner, 1972.)

PSYCHOLOGICAL INTERACTIONS

When the phenomenon of IP's is based on empirical findings, rather than theoretical speculation, a different picture emerges than is theorized from the traditional analytical perspective. When the interaction between the child and the IP is examined (Levenson, 1985) about 20% of such encounters are of an angry or argumentative nature. It is this same 20% of children who are more likely to have argumentative and uncooperative interactions with their peers. These are the types of behavior that most often elicit the involvement of a parent, an authority figure, or a mental health professional. Therefore, it is likely that the reputation of IP's as scapegoats for the expression of hostile impulses would have arisen from this skewed sample selection. Even the linkage between aggression and IP's for this subgroup is open to question. Singer (1979) found that while positive affect and IP's were closely tied with each other, the occurrence of anger and aggression was best predicted by a third factor: the type and the amount of television viewing. Levenson (1986) discovered that 80% of the interactions between children and their IP's were friendly, and playful and conducted in a positive affective state. This, along with Singers (1979) findings that these children are seen as happier, more socially cooperative, with more advanced linguistic skills, and more intense concentration ability challenges psychological theory to explore a phenomenon that appears to be merging as a developmental plus. In fact, as Singer (1979) and Bettelheim (1977) point out, the development and effective practice of imaginative ability is crucial for healthy adjustment. The individual who lacks this capacity is the one who elicits the most alarm. It is this person that is more likely to be impulsive, have greater academic and interpersonal difficulties and present major obstacles for therapeutic intervention. Singer succinctly states;

It does seem possible to conclude, that as early as ages 3 and 4, we can identify children who just seem happier than others and are also more cooperative and helpful with others. Can imagination be the underlying factor? It think it is. . . (Singer, 1979, p. 208)

ADULTS WHO HAD IP'S AS CHILDREN

There has been a minimal amount of research regarding adults who had IP's as children. What is known is hampered by different definitions, reliance on long term memory recall, and faulty experimental design. There are only two published studies on the subject (Hurlock & Bumstein, 1932, and Schaefer, 1969) and both used high school students as subjects. Neither study gave a definition of IP's. Hurlock & Burnstein (1932) found that almost half of the males (48%) and a quarter of the females (25%) who had IP's carried their playmates into adolescence. They also reported no evidence of hateful interactions and found that 80% of encounters with IP's were of a kind, pleasant, or loving nature. This corresponds with the findings of Levenson (1985) that show a similar percentage of positive interaction. Schaefer (1969) in his survey of high school students enrolled in an art school found a significantly higher level of creativity for those students who reported having had IP's when they were children. Attempting to see if this correlation existed with children at the time that they still had their fantasy friends, Manosevitz (1977) discovered no difference in creativity measures between those children who had IP's and those that did not. This adds some doubt to the idea that later creativity differences are predicted by having had a childhood IP.

Barber and Glass (1962) in an investigation of the correlates of hypnotic suggestibility found consistent predictors in the fantasy activities of book reading, daydreaming, and the occurrence of IP's. This lends support to the notion that the specific underlying imaginative activity involved in the creation of IP's does not cease with the quieting of playmate activity but finds its expression in related processes. If hypnotic suggestibility can be predicted by the occurrence of IP's, then what other phenomena, beliefs, or behaviors might emerge as we examine them more closely.

NEW FINDINGS

In a recent unpublished study carried out by the author, a number of variables were examined for adults who had IP's and compared to those that did not have them. Sixty-nine community college students completed a six page questionnaire and a vividness of imagery scale (Sheehan, 1967). Twenty-four subjects (34%) reported having had an IP as a child. Forty-five students (66%) said they did not. Preliminary results examined the effect of IP's on the dependent variables of academic grades, vividness of imagery and beliefs in other non-physical realities. All these variables were predicted to be higher for subjects who had IP's. Predicted results, in the expected direction were found only with academic performance. There was a clear effect of having an IP on grades in school, t (67) = 2.66 p. <01. This indicates that those subjects who had IP's reported significantly higher grades than those who did not. This corresponds with earlier investigations (Singer, 1979) that reported advanced linguistic development for children who had IP's. This support is based on a premise that students with advanced linguistic skills would be more likely to have higher academic achievement in an education system that generally relies so heavily on language.

Significance was also found in three of seven subscales on the Betts mental imaging scale (Sheehan, 1967). However, the difference was in the oppositie direction that was thought likely. Auditory (t (67) = 2.08, p. <.05), gustatory (t (67) = 3.64, p. <.001) and organic (t (67) = 2.07, p. <.05) vividness all were signficantly lower for subjects who had IP's than those who did not. There was no difference for visual, tactual, kinesthetic, or olfactory vividness between the two groups. The reasons for the significantly lower auditory, gustatory, and organic vividness scores is unclear and worthy of further investigation. Given that subjects with IP's might be more prone to experience other forms of non-physical realities, the question of belief in spiritis, demons, ESP, and UFOs was posed. The effect of having an IP on this variable was non-significant at the .05 level. On the speculation that there might be some difference in philosophy or social orientation, political leanings were also examined. There was no difference between subjects who had IP's and those that did not on this variable.

While questionnaires and surveys of childhood images will provide important information, analysis and conclusions will be subject to doubt because of their reliance on the occurrence of long term memory. Certainly, the most effective way to study the influence of IP's on later development would be a longitudinal investigation. Short of that, a number of strategies that could add to the information base on IP's would be: an agreed upon definition of what an IP is, a call for the incorporation of an IP question on a wide range of measurement instruments, and the collection of stories about IP's for qualitative analysis. As to the question of defining IP's, a slight variation of the Manosevitz (1973) definition would provide the basis for identifying not only IP's but also other types of imaginary beings. A suggested definition would be:

an imaginary companion is a very vivid, invisible imaginary character (person, animal or object) with which a child interacts during his play and daily activity.

IMAGINARY COMPANION PROJECT

In 1988, in an effort to more thoroughly examine IP phenomena, the author established the Imaginary Companion Project. The goals of this project are to investigate the nature and function of IP's, their relationships to other imaginal experiences such as inspiration, prayer, creativity, angels, and psycho-therapy, to name a few, and finally to collect stories of individual experiences. It is these stories that have yielded some of the most fascinating information. Something gets lost in the translation of a vivid imaginal experience into a quantifiable series of numbers, tables and levels of signficance. One is reminded of the saying, "It is only the fool that seeks to understand the beauty of a rose by taking it apart petal by petal."

In order to collect additional stories, a cooperative venture was undertaken with author and free lance writer Betty Utterback. An ad was placed in a writers' magazine soliciting stories from adults who had IP's when they were children. The following stories were chosen to highlight the qualities of these unique experiences.

A Friend, Companion, Teacher

I'd like to tell you about Dodie. I don't remember exactly when Dodie came to live with me, or how she got her name. I'm sure she told me what it was. Your psychologist friend will point out that she filled a vast, hollow place for a child growing up alone on a farm in Northern Ohio. Perhaps that was her only purpose. Perhaps.

Since reading your notice, I've tried to remember if she took the blame for my misbehavior, as many imaginary playmates do. My mother could give a truer answer, but I don't think so. If she did, I've forgotten.

She was my playmate, my companion, always cheerful, ever cooperative, ever present, just for me. I remember telling my mother about things she said or things we did, but I can't remember being scolded for any of those things. Nor did we set a place for her at the table, although she ate with us. She had her own imaginary plate and chair just like mine.

I had a rope swing hanging from a wild cherry tree, and it was one of our favorite places to play. Dodie and I would swing to other worlds. One of our favorite places was a large palace where we lived as princesses. Sometimes she was the princess, and I was her favorite maid. Other times we were sisters. She was always older because she knew more and was braver.

We also liked to play in the woods on my parents' farm. It wasn't a large woods, and it was pastured, so the weeds were kept down and it was a good place to play, but the trees made shadowy corners that frightened me.

At the edge of the clearing stood an old Sycamore tree. It had a low, inviting branch, but its bark was patch and multicolored. I was afraid of it. I'd seen a high school play with a "python," a fake snake made from cloth with patches painted on it. The tree reminded me of the snake, and I called it "the python tree." Dodie wasn't afraid of it. She climbed it to show me it wouldn't hurt me. Then she coaxed me into climbing it too -- not up high where I could fall and be hurt, just the low branch where we could snuggle in and talk.

I don't remember much about how she looked, except that she had gorgeous brown eyes. I do remember her eyes. If I see eyes like that now, I call the person an "old soul."

The day I started to school, Dodie missed the bus. I didn't realize it until we were pulling away from my house and it was too late.

The next morning she was sick, and a few days later, she died. I held a big funeral and buried her in the in the lot behind the barn. Then I forgot about her. Life goes on.

She's still there, I suppose, forty-odd years later, in an imaginary grave with an imaginary tombstone. Maybe the next time I go home, I'll take flowers -- imaginary ones, of course.

I remember Dodie's companionship most, but I've come to understand she was also my teacher. She taught me that you have to reach out. You have to stretch to grow and to achieve. That's not easy for me. I'm far too timid. Many times I've had to force myself to reach.

A few years ago, I'm not sure when I became aware of it, I realized that every time I take a deep breath and step into the unknown, an image flashes through the back of my mind. It's an image of the most beautiful brown eyes you've ever seen, clear and sparkling, the kind you fall into, the kind of eyes that belong to an old soul.

Dodie? I don't know. Maybe. Or maybe an image constructed by my subconscious to encourage me. I suspect we give other people far too much credit for teaching us -- and our own higher selves far too little.   (LC)

Scapegoat - Pathology

I had a "friend" named Billy Ray with whom I shared all my secrets from three to age seven. No one knew about him. He made me feel safe while he was around. At night we would talk over the day's events. He even made suggestions which I sometimes followed.

The problem came at age seven when I felt I no longer needed him. He didn't go away. He became another personality and I created unconsciously another personality at age eight to protect me from Billy Ray. His name is Harry.

I am currently under treatment for multiple personalities. It's a long story beginning with the emergence of Bill Ray into the open in 1975. My life became hell after that. I have been hospitalized 18 times, attempted suicide 14 times. On the suicide I just found out while at this hospital the reason I could never commit suicide was because one of the other personalities would call for help. I have been in and out of psychotherapy for 14 years. But it's only the last 27 months here that I've made any progress.

I don't know if any of this will help you, but if you want more information, please feel free to write, my charge is murder committed by Bill Ray not by me.   (WR)

A Disturbing Thought

I have a twelve year old cousin who had an imaginary friend when he was smaller. It drove his father crazy. One day his dad had had enough of it and asked him where BoBo (his friend) was, and when he pointed it out, my uncle stomped down as hard as he could and smashed BoBo into the ground. My cousin turned pale and wouldn't talk for the rest of the day. That is how he lost his imaginary friend.   (KA)

A Mentor

In respect to solely my own experience and knowledge, an imaginary friend has always been a vital part of my life. As a writer and thinker, I've always cultivated and developed an inner voice which has been various people I respect or admire. Since childhood I've been a loner and introverted and this imaginary friend has helped me to depend on my thoughts and personality as well as building my own self-esteem. Through this imaginary friend I've developed a positive attitude towards my own abilities, expectations, goals and demeanor. Through childhood, adolescence, young adulthood and manhood I've attributed this inner voice to a figure of fame or person I respected and wanted to be like. This helped me to learn and grow without dissipating or diluting my own true personality. Now, at the age of 35, I depend less on transferring the inner voice to another entity and realize that the inner voice or imaginary friend is and was always myself at a later age or stage in my life.   (AD)

An Uncovering Tool

I have a somewhat interesting experience with that. Not only did I have an imaginary playmate but I had several. And more interesting than just the playmates was the way in which I communicated with them.

I'm not sure how I got started doing this, but as far as I can remember and speculate, what must have happened is I got my "tool" for Christmas or a birthday and just immediately began using it as a security medium.

What the "tool" was, was a leather cowboy holster. And what I used to do was put the gun part of the holster in one of my hands and shake it while I talked to it pretending it was one of several of a cast of characters. I remember how it used to feel so good in my hand to hold that leather and pretend it was anyone I could imagine.

I had this quirk unti I was about 9 or 10 years old. It caused me a lot of embarrassment as a child and I was always looking for a "safe" place to carry on.

As a matter of fact, the embarrassment is what led to my extermination of the whole deal. I just up and tossed the thing in a garbage can one day, and that was that. (JL)

The project continues to collect stories of imaginary playmates and invites people to request a questionnaire, and to send their stories to The Imaginary Companion Project, PO Box 18143, Rochester, NY 14618-18143.

REFERENCES

Achterberg, J. (1985). *Imagery in Healing: Shamanism and Modern Medicine*. Boston: Shambhala Publications, Inc.

Ames, L. & Learned, J. (1946). Imaginary companions and related phenomena. *Journal of Genetic Psychology, 69*, 147-167.

Barber, T. X., & Glass, L. B.(1962). Significant Factors in Hypnotic Behavior.*Journal of Abnormal and Social Psychology, 64*, 222.228.

Bettelheim, B. (1977). *The Uses of Enchantment: The Meaning and Importance of Fairy Tales*. New York: Random House.

Burnham, S. (1990). *A Book of Angels*. New York: Ballantine Books.

Caldeira, J. (1978). *Imaginary Playmates: Some Relationships to Preschoolers' Spontaneous Play and Television Viewing*. Paper presented at meeting of Eastern Psychological Association.

Curtis, J. T. (1979). *Personality characteristics of children with imaginary companions*. Unpublished Doctoral Dissertation, University of Texas.

Delaney, M. M. (1973). *Of Irish Ways*. Minneapolis: Dillion Press, Inc.

Dengrove, E. (ed.) (1976). *Hypnosis and Behavior Therapy*. Springfield, IL: Charles C. Thomas.

Friaberg, S. (1959). *The Magic Years*. New York: Scribner.

Fromm, E., & Shor, R. E. (eds.)(1979). *Hypnosis: Developments in Research and New Perspectives*. New York: Aldine Publishing Co.

Gawain, S. (1978). *Creative Visualization*. New York: Bantam Books.

Graves, A. P. (1983). *The Irish Fairy Book*. New York: Arlington House.

Grof, S. (1988). *The Adventure of Self-Discovery*. Albany, NY: State University of New York Press.

Hurlock, E. G. & Buranstein, W. (1932). The imaginary playmate: A questionnaire study. *Journal of Genetic Psychology, 41*, 380-392.

Jaynes, J. (1976). *The Origin of Consciousness in the Breakdown of the Bicameral Mind*. Boston: Houghton Miffling Co.

Jung, C. G. (1979). *Word and Image*. Princeton, NJ: Princeton University Press.

Kaplan, H. (ed). (1985). *Comprehensive Textbook of Psychiatry IV*. Baltimore, MD: Williams and Wilkins.

Levenson, N. (1981). *An Examination of Pre-conditions for the Emergency of the Imaginary Companion*. Unpublished Doctoral Dissertation, Adelphi University.

Manosevitz, M., Prentice, N. M., & Wilson, F. (1973). Individual and Family correlates of imaginary companions in preschool children. *Developmental Psychology, 8*, 72-79.

Manosevitz, M., Fling, S., & Prentice, N. (1977). Imaginary companions in young children: relationships with intelligence, creativity, and waiting ability. *Journal of Child Psychology and Psychiatry, 18*, 73-78.

Merton, T. (1972). *New Seeds of Contemplation*. New York: New Directions Publishing Corp.

Missildine, W. H. (1982). *Your Inner Child of the Past*. New York: Simon and Schuster, Inc.

Myers, M. (1976). Imaginary companions, fantasy twins, mirror dreams, and depersonalization. *Psychoanalytic Quarterly, 45,* 503-523.

Negera, N. (1981). Capacities for integration, oedipal, ambivalence, and imaginary compansions. *The American Journal of Psychoanalysis, 41,* No. 2, 129-137.

Ornstein, R. E. (1974). *The Nature of Human Consciousness: A Book of Readings.* New York: Viking Press.

Piaget, J., & Inhelder, B. (1971). *Mental Imagery in the Child.* New York: Basic Books.

Rucker, N. (1981). Capacities for integration, oedipal, ambivalence, and imaginary companions. *American Journal of Psychoanalysis, 41,* No. 2, 129-137.

Schaefer, C. E. (1969). Imaginary companions and creative adolescents.*Developmental Psychology, 1,* 747-749.

Sheehan, P.W. (1976).A shortened Form of Betts' Questionnaire Upon Mental Imagery. *Journal of Clinical Psychology,* 23, 386-389.

Shleman, B. L. (1976). *Healing Prayer.* Notre Dame, IN: Ave Maria Press.

Shorr, J. E. (1973). *Psychotherapy Through Imagery.* New York: Thieme-Stratton Inc.

Singer, J. L. (1974). *Imagery and Daydream Methods in Psychotherapy and Behavior Modification.* New York: Harcourt Brace Javonovich.

Singer, J. L. (1979). *Proceedings, International Year of the Child.* New Haven, CT: Yale University Press.

Singer, J. L. (1973). *The child's world of make-believe: experimental studies of imaginative play.* New York: Academic Press.

Singer, J. L. (1976). Imaginative play in early childhood: some experimental approaches. In A. Davids (Ed.), *Childs personality and psychopathology.* New York: Wiley.

Singer, J. L., & Singer, D. (1981). *Television, imaginatio, and aggression: a study of preschoolers .* Hillsdale, NJ: Erlbaum.

Svendsen, M. (1934). Children's imaginary companions. *Archives of Neurology and Psychiatry, 32,* 985-999.

Tart, Charles (ed.) (1969). *Altered States of Consciousness.* New York: John Wiley.

Taylor, T. L. (1989). *Messengers of Light: The Angels' Guide to Spiritual Growth.* Tiburon, CA: J. J. Kramer Inc.

Turner, J. D. (1972). *An investigation of the role the imaginary companion plays in the social development of the child.* Unpublished Doctoral Disseration, Miami University.

Veltri, J. A. (1981). *Orientations, Volume II.* Guelph, Ontario: Loyola House.,

Watkins, M. (1986). *Invisible Guests.* Hillsdale, NJ: Erlbaum

Watkins, M. (1984). *Waking Dreams.* Dallas, TX: Spring Publications.

IMAGINED INTERACTIONS, IMAGERY, AND MINDFULNESS/MINDLESSNESS

James M. Honeycutt, Ph.D.

Center of Imagined Interaction Research
Department of Speech Communication
Louisiana State University
Baton Rouge, LA 70803

People sometimes have imagined interactions in which they imagine talking with someone. For example, before entering a job interview, the interviewee may rehearse in his/her mind what the interviewer might ask and how the self will respond. After an argument with a romantic partner, the self may replay the encounter and feel despair at not having said various things that are currently in one's mind. In the first scenario, a proactive imagined interaction has occurred while a retroactive imagined interaction has occurred in the second. It is also possible that the retroactive encounter in the second scenario acts as preinteraction stimulus for the next encounter with the romantic partner. Thus, the conflict picks up where it left off. These examples reflect what has previously been referred to as imagined interactions (Honeycutt, 1990; Honeycutt, Edwards, and Zagacki, 1989-90; Honeycutt, Zagacki, and Edwards,1989).

Imagined interactions (IIs) may keep the conflict alive in the absence of actual interaction. They may serve a variety of functions including the transference of emotions and generating self-confidence (Honeycutt et al., 1989). IIs may be accompanied by various feelings ranging from anger to joy. This paper will review the theoretical foundation of the II construct and discuss this in terms of the transference phenomenon as demonstrated in research findings on emotional reactions to the elicitation of IIs. In addition, some links to mindlessness and overlearned schemata are discussed.

We have previously defined IIs as attempts to simulate real-life conversations with significant others (Honeycutt et al., 1989; 1989-90; 1990). Mead (1934) describes internal conversations in terms of self-concept development in which individuals assume the perspective of others in order to understand the self. We respond to ourselves by taking the role of others, imagining how they might respond to one's messages within particular situations, and thus one can test and imagine the consequences of alternative messages prior to communication (Edwards, Honeycutt, and Zagacki, 1988; Honeycutt, 1990; Zagacki, Edwards, and Honeycutt, 1988).

Rosenblatt and Meyer (1986) discuss IIs occurring between clients and therapists in terms of transferring unwanted feelings and attributes to the therapist. This may allow the client to put the therapist in an empathic frame of mind permitting the client to feel understood (Steiner, 1976). The transference phenomenon is known in the psychoanalytic literature for the expression of emotions at a target who is not physically present. Transference is a pervasive phenomenon occurring in a variety of situations in common, everyday experience to the extent that individuals bring hidden agendas to their interactions. Singer (1987) has used a cognitive-affective perspective to explain transference. His model assumes that people draw on scripts in transference as they act out internal fantasies. This may occur when having an II as persons may replay previous encounters with others.

Mental Imagery, Edited by R.G. Kunzendorf
Plenum Press, New York, 1990

IIs may be viewed as a type of instrumental thought process as well as a type of simulation heuristic. For example, Klinger (1978; 1981) has distinguished ongoing thought between operant thought processes and respondent thought processes. Operant thought is concerned with problem solution, or analysis of an issue confronting one, and is active rather than passive. It is volitional as it is checked against new information concerning its effectiveness in moving toward a resolution. Operant thought involves a higher level of mental activity.

Klinger's (1981) notion of respondent thought involves all other thought and is nonvolitional. Most of what we consider daydreams, dreams, and fantasies are respondent thought. IIs are not simply instances of self-talk. Rather, IIs are a "type of social cognition in which communicators experience cognitive representations of conversation with accompanying verbal and nonverbal features" (Honeycutt et al., 1989, p. 170). IIs that are used for message planning and that serve a rehearsal function seem to reflect the operant thought process. A critical function of many IIs is rehearsal for anticipated interaction.

Individuals may draw upon procedural records (Greene, 1984) and envision interactive strategies for goal accomplishment. In such instances, the II may be experienced in the form of what Abelson (1976) originally referred to as "vignettes." These are representations of events of short duration similar to a panel in a cartoon strip where a visual image is accompanied by a verbal caption. Like a cartoon reader, an individual having an imagined interaction is afforded the luxury of moving back and forth over the panel, even "rewriting" the strip if appropriate. The analogy to cartoon strips is important to understanding imagined interactions. For like these strips, imagined interactions may be visual and verbal. Moreover, interactants may possess, like cartoon characters, much power over the imagined conversation (e.g., topic changes, anticipating the other's response, time-travel, pause, and so on) not afforded real-life interactants.

Berger (in press) discusses how previous encounters can be used as a basis for the planning of future actions. Previous actions may be modified depending on what the outcome was in order to facilitate a successful future outcome. Persons may replay previous encounters and modify the interaction in order to anticipate the other's responses to the changes. Thus, imagined interactions, like vignettes, may provide information for actors to utilize during real conversation. This information-production and rehearsal function of cognition seems similar to what Greene (1984) attends to in his early discussion of procedural records. He has argued that much cognitive research assumes that cognitive systems have developed to facilitate action (see also Norman, 1980), and that the functions of cognitive systems are best understood in terms of their implications for action. As a kind of cognitive information bank, a procedural record specifies certain communicative actions associated with particular interaction goals. They provide functional information about interaction goals and related behaviors. We have proposed that, as individuals engage in imagined interactions, procedural records are activated (and perhaps reconstituted) which may inform behavior related to specific situational exigencies (Honeycutt et al, 1989). An example of this is how individuals may choose various message strategies in order to influence another.

O'Keefe (1988; 1990) has argued that individuals may construct different messages for situations in which there is the need to influence or control others. She discusses this in terms of regulative messages where the individual is seeking to accomplish goals. There are three types of message designs discussed by O'Keefe that may be imagined during a proactive II.

An expressive message design is one where the individuals unload their emotions and thoughts onto the recipients. Thus, there should be a great deal of positive or negative emotional affect associated with the II if an expressive design is being imaged. The conventional message is rule-governed, in which individuals follow socially-governed norms (e.g., be polite) as a means to an end. The highest level of message is rhetorical, in which the self is uniquely negotiated in situations. It is person-oriented and characterized by harmony or desire for consensus (O'Keefe, 1988).

Conventional messages are produced more than expressive and rhetorical messages. In addition, females produce more rhetorical messages than males (O'Keefe, 1988). Our own research has revealed that women report having more IIs than men as well as pleasant ones (Edwards, Honeycutt, and Zagacki, 1989). It may be that the greater II activity of women produces the procedural record for which rules are produced.

Uniform messages characterize many everyday interactions (e.g., conversation among friends) but most notably where there is no interpersonal conflict. According to O'Keefe, situations which require goal achievement reflect different message logics and presumably different messages. She speculates that individuals pick message types first (e.g., expressive, etc.) and then think about using them. By having IIs, individuals may envision various messages, speculate on another's reactions, and replay the II much as the cartoon reader who goes back and rereads the script while possibly anticipating what will occur in the next series of vignettes. Given the rehearsal function of IIs, non-uniform message designs may be reflected in IIs that occur prior to anticipated encounters.

Differences Between IIs and Fantasy

Fantasies are a type of respondent thought (Klinger, 1981). Previously, my colleagues and I have attempted to distinguish IIs from fantasy (Honeycutt et al., 1989). Caughey (1984) discusses fantasy as a type of daydreaming in terms of a sequence of mental images that occur when attention drifts from focused rational thought. On the other hand, IIs simulate conversational encounters that individuals expect to experience or have experienced during their lives. Some of these encounters may never transpire or they may be quite different from what was envisioned. Yet, communication fantasies involve highly improbable or even impossible communication encounters. Thus, talking with deceased others or celebrities are fantastical and rarely serve as the basis for real communication exchanges (Edwards et al., 1988).

Previous studies of II partners reveal that many of the IIs occur with romantic partners (33%), friends (16%), family members (12%), individuals in authority (9.4%), work associates (8%), ex-relational partners (6%), and prospective partners (4%) (Edwards et al., 1988; Honeycutt et al., 1989-90; Zagacki et al., 1988).

Imagery Mode of IIs

IIs occur in different imagery modes. They may utilize visual or verbal imagery as well as a combination of these modes. In forming an image of the scene of an II, individuals may visualize the other and self with functions varying with the type of imagery. For example, pleasant IIs have been associated with mixed imagery compared to verbal imaging (Zagacki et al., 1988). Furthermore, some individuals may have omniscient or direct images. The omniscient perspective is where individuals see themselves along with others such as watching ourselves on videotape.

The direct perspective is where individuals see only other interactants much as they would during real encounters. An example of this is reported by Berger (in press) in a series of planning studies in which individuals comprised plans for achieving particular types of social goals. The data revealed that individuals who were thinking of plans for asking someone for a date, or planning for meeting a potential new roommate in order to get the other to like the self, recalled previous episodes in similar situations in which they had done this. The role of the individual in the recalled episodes was a central figure seeking to achieve the goal rather than as a detached observer of the scene.

Another imaging consideration concerns the distinction between immediate and reflective operations of IIs. Individuals are capable of shifting from the immediate mode in which they experience directly an II, to a reflective mode where they move out of the II in order to deliberate over the II happenings and then move back into the immediate mode. This may be associated with rehearsal and message planning as contingency plans are envisioned. Singer (1985) indicates how thoughts may be modified and acted upon by further thoughts in much the same way that experience is modified by new information from the environment. These "further thoughts" may be an instance of the reflective operation of IIs.

CHARACTERISTICS AND MEASUREMENT OF IIs

A number of characteristics and functions of IIs have been identified in previous studies. A multidimensional instrument ("Survey of Imagined Interaction" SII) has been used to measure how often individuals have IIs, topics, whom they are with, how discrepant or similar they are to real conversations, how detailed they are and the functions they serve (Edwards et al., 1988; Honeycutt et al., 1989; 1989-90; Zagacki et al., 1988). The SII begins by describing IIs as "those mental interactions we have with others who are not physically present" and goes on to describe some potential characteristics of II such as being ambiguous or detailed and how they may address a number of topics or examine one topic exclusively. The interactions may be one-sided where the person imagining the discussion does most of the talking, or they may be more interactive where both persons take an active part in the conversation.

The SII measures various characteristics of IIs. The first dimension reflects "discrepancy" between imagined and real conversations. We have found loneliness is associated with having discrepant and vague IIs (Honeycutt et al., 1989-90). The second factor reflects reports of how pleasant feelings may be associated with IIs. Some are pleasant while others are conflictual and elicit negative affect. The third general feature assessed by the SII is "activity". IIs may occur with relative frequency and regularity in a variety of contexts and situations. Still others, may have recurrent IIs with the same individuals.

Two other characteristics related to II activity are "proactivity" and "retroactivity." IIs may occur before or after actual encounters. These characteristics are not necessarily independent. Earlier analysis has revealed that the correlations between these two characteristics is moderate (r = .34). In addition, retroactivity (r =.65) and proactivity (r = .47) have demonstrated strong relationships with activity (Honeycutt et al., 1989-90). These correlations reinforce a general "activity" simplex identified by Edwards et al. (1988) using correlagram analysis. Thus, some IIs may have simultaneous features in which they occur after an encounter and previous to the next anticipated encounter. Caughey (1984) discusses how inner dialogue can help one to recreate previous encounters in order to determine if different courses of action could have resulted in other outcomes.

After an argument with one's relational partner, X may recreate in his/her mind what was said while being in the immediate mode discussed earlier. Furthermore, negative affect may be experienced. It may be that when switching to a reflective II mode, X may feel distress or anger over the encounter and envision what he or she will say next time they talk with Y. Thus, a retroactive II is experienced, yet it may be immediately linked with a proactive II (e.g., "Last time, I bit my lip. Next time, I see him/her, I am going to say exactly how I feel."). Given that IIs tend to occur with significant others, it may be that many of them are linked and occur between encounters reviewing and previewing conversations. Further analyses is needed to specify the degree to which activity, retroactivity, and proactivity are isomorphic or different characteristics of IIs. However, subsequent confirmatory factor analysis of the SII characteristics on other datasets indicates that proactivity, and activity may reflect a general "activity" dimension while the other characteristics are independent. [A confirmatory factor analysis of the SII dimensions in other datasets (e.g., Honeycutt, 1989b) using Package 1.0 (Hamilton & Hunter, 1988) has confirmed cohesive factors reflecting general II features for the following dimensions: activity (.79), retroactivity (.79), discrepancy (.87), pleasant (.84), proactivity (.69), specificity (.68), variety (.65), self-dominance (.76), self-understanding function (.72), rehearsal (.76), catharsis (.60).]

Another characteristic that we have assessed reflects the degree of self-talk or dominance in the II. Individuals may see themselves as being relatively dominant in the II while the other listens. Analyses of sample protocols reveals that the self utters more lines of dialogue and words than the other (Edwards et al., 1988). This helps the individual plan messages and thus self-talk is important. It is also related to a cathartic function in which individuals may have IIs in order to release tension.

"Specificity" is another characteristic reflected on the SII scale. Some individuals report having very detailed and specific images of the scene of an II. They may be able to imagine the context or the environment in which an II encounter is imagined. On the other hand, others report only vague images about the scene of the II or what is said. They may simply report having them but are unable to provide little details.

Another characteristic reflected in the SII is "variety." This represents the diversity of II topics and partners. Some individuals have IIs with a variety of others while others have recurring IIs with the same individuals over selected topics. For example, college students who have IIs with parents are more likely to discuss finances and school than they are with romantic partners. The topics are more diversified when having IIs with relational partners. A pilot analysis of IIs in the elderly has revealed such topics dealing with family matters, health, money, current events, and religion (Honeycutt, 1989a).

Aside from rehearsal, other functions of IIs include catharsis, self-understanding, and psychological relationship maintenance. IIs can function to create catharsis for the individual by relieving tension and reducing uncertainty about another's actions. Self-understanding can be enhanced through clarifying thoughts. Caughey (1984) has discussed how inner dialogue may help individuals to retain a sense of values and purpose.

IIs may function to maintain relationships. Knapp (1984) originally posited increased use of covert dialogue as relationships began to come apart. Partners in these kinds of situations are marking time until the relationship ends or they may remain in this state of stagnation. During this stage, overt dialogue is at a standstill because partners feel they 'know' how an anticipated interaction will go because of previous repetitive interaction experiences going nowhere. Since they 'know' how it will go, it is not necessary to say anything. However, we have found that IIs occur very early in relationships. In addition, positive emotions may be attributed to the excitement that accompanies relational initiation and growth (Honeycutt et al., 1989). For example, individuals may imagine pleasant activities with relational partners, such as engaging in small talk, planning dates, and discussing shared interests. [It is noted that Caughey (1984) discusses cases in which individuals fantasize that they are involved with a celebrity and live in their own private world. This is different insofar as the individuals have never actually had a relationship with the celebrity.]

When assuming a functional approach to analyzing IIs, there is an implicit belief that there may be therapeutic benefits at some level whether it be increased self-awareness, tension-relief, or feeling pleasant thoughts about the II. Support for this assumption is available in a study by Schultz (1978) investigating the use of imagery to alleviate depression. He studied four imagery conditions across 60 depressed, male psychiatric patients. One condition labelled the "aggressive imagery procedure" had depressed males recalling someone saying something which angered the self. In the "socially gratifying imagery" condition, the individual was instructed to recall someone saying something which was very pleasing. The "positive imagery" condition had the patient recall a place he used to visit in order to relax. Finally, the "free imagery" condition had patients reporting all images, thoughts, fantasies, and ideas which occurred to him without trying to direct his thoughts.

Ratings of depressive feelings taken 10 minutes after the imagery induction revealed that the first two conditions produced lower levels of depression than the less socially oriented conditions. I would argue that the aggressive and socially gratifying inductions forced the patient to have retroactive IIs that were negative and pleasant, respectively. Schultz also reports that in comparing the socially gratifying and positive imagery conditions, depression was lowered after the socially gratifying induction. Whatever the case, IIs may elicit different kinds of emotional affect and through transference linger on for some time.

IIs AND MINDFULNESS

Langer, Blank, and Chanowitz (1978) have demonstrated how individuals may process information mindlessly, by not carefully attending to information in their immediate environment. There is an absence of flexible cognitive processing. Mindlessness occurs when the individual relies on old, established ways of thinking. For example, a person may have a schema about abortion and mindlessly attend to arguments made by pro-life or pro-choice sides because of previous exposure to the arguments. In this regard, Roloff (1989) indicates how schemata lend themselves toward stability and resistance to change. Thus, mindlessness is a type of perception that is rigid to the extent that individuals rely on previous distinctions (Langer, Chanowitz, and Blank, 1985). On the other hand, mindfulness implies creative thought and attention to information. Mindful individuals are presumed to make distinctions and create categories.

Langer (1989) reviews a number of studies which reveal that we cling to preformulated categories and conceptions rather than thinking conditionally. For example, if we are told that an object is an X and the need arises whereby the object could be used in other ways (e.g., it could be a Y or Z, A, etc...), individuals who are thinking categorically are less likely to generate alternative uses for the object compared to individuals who are told that the object could be an X. Categorical thinking enhances mindlessness while conditional thought facilitates mindful processing.

The question has arisen as to the prevalence of mindlessness and mindfulness. Folkes (1985) has argued that the extent of mindlessness that is found in the research of Langer and her associates (1978) is overestimated. Folkes found in a series of four studies that reactions to verbal requests to intrude on a person's use of a copying machine were mindfully processed when an uncontrollable reason (e.g., because I feel really sick) rather than a controllable reason (e.g., because I don't want to wait) was given for intrusion. Langer and her associates (1978) argued that redundant information (e.g., Excuse me, I have 5 (20) pages. May I use the Xerox machine because I have to make copies?) elicited more compliance than when a simple request was made. Within this debate, Langer and her colleagues (1985) have indicated that it is necessary to understand how mindlessness occurs and when mindfulness is likely to be operating.

Langer (1978) lists a number of situations when thought is enhanced. Individuals are likely to be mindful or engaging in thought when encountering novel situations for which no script can be utilized. IIs may play a role here by envisioning contingency plans for actions in which the confidence that a given plan will be instantiated is low. Langer also posits that thought is more likely when experiencing positive or negative affect that is discrepant with the consequence of previous enactments of the behavior. It would be interesting to investigate the affect associated with retroactive IIs after real encounters had occurred.

Langer and Piper (1987) also argue that conditional thought enhances mindfulness. Mindfulness is conceived in terms of being process-oriented while mindlessness is concerned with outcome by using well-learned categories which enable an individual to easily classify behavior and information (Langer, 1989). These types of information processing are not necessarily incompatible. Langer and Piper (1987) view mindlessness resulting from mindfulness in which "one mindfully creates categories and then is able to mindlessly use them" (p.281).

Mindlessness results from a premature cognitive commitment in which our conceptions lead us to shut down the epistemic search for alternative categories, courses of action, etc... According to Langer (1989):

> Throughout our lives, an outcome orientation in social situations can induce mindlessness. If we think we know how to handle a situation, we don't feel a need to pay attention. If we respond to the situation as very familiar (a result, for example, of overlearning), we notice only the minimal cues necessary to carry out the proper scenario" (p. 34).

A process orientation directs attention toward steps that may be necessary to accomplish an outcome. The process orientation reflects, "How do I do it" rather than "Can I do it?" (Langer, 1989, p. 34).

How does mindfulness lead to the formation of categories which may lead to subsequent cognitive commitments when a similar scenario is next encountered with mindlessness being reflected in subsequent encounters? One way this can be done in the social arena is by having IIs in which relevant procedural records can be activated. For example, having a retroactive II after a given encounter has occurred puts one in a mindful state while replaying the encounter. Further, the individual may think of contingency plans while imaging what another individual might say in the future. Thus, an II that is concurrently retro and proactive can be used to plan for contingencies. The critical point is that IIs are somewhat mindful, particularly when used for rehearsing messages.

One way to test this would involve assessing the IIs of individuals at a job fair who are undergoing various employment interviews. There may be a curvilinear relationship between interview experiences (number of interviews) and II interview-activity. Presumably, persons with no interviews have fewer procedural records to activate and may have less IIs. After having been through a few interviews, proactive and retroactive IIs may be linked as the previous interviews are reflected or ruminated upon while preparing for ensuing interviews. On the other hand, after having been in a number of interviews, the person may believe he/she has a sufficient memory structure for anticipating what will happen in the next interview. Thus, mindlessness sets in. IIs are seen as a type of cognitive activity that is relatively mindful. We may go back and reexperience the II like the cartoon reader who rereads the script. This conceptualization of IIs as mindful sets up the idea that overlearned schema are reflective of mindlessness which is preceded by mindful states. Hence, IIs can play a role in the development of memory structures. As previously indicated, overlearned structures or schemata may be viewed as states of mindlessness. It would not be necessary to set up contingency plans for that which has been experienced repeatedly and is expected again.

Singer (1985) argues that overlearned schemas, prototypes, scripts, personal constructs, and transferences are reflected in everyday life through thought processes outside of conscious awareness. This may be in the form of fleeting thoughts, fantasies, and daydreams. Daydreaming may be one way we sustain interest and arousal in boring or redundant situations with the prospect that, because the situations are so redundant or overlearned, we will not miss too much of what is happening. Klinger (1987) has reported that 100% of lifeguards and 79% of truck drivers report vivid daydreams at times. Besides daydreaming, they spend half their work time planning ahead or reviewing past events. This may be related to pro and retroactive IIs. IIs viewed as mindful activity with the elicitation of relevant procedural records may create the conditions for "mindlessness" (e.g., greeting ritual at the airport for someone not seen in a long while, "Hi, how are you doing? Fine."). If this were the case, we would expect more proactive IIs before novel situations.

126

An intriguing study in this area would involve assessing the IIs of individuals at a job fair who are undergoing various employment interviews. I would posit a curvilinear relationship between interview experiences (number of interviews) and II interview-activity. Presumably, persons with no interviews have fewer procedural records to activate and may have less IIs. After having been through a few interviews, proactive and retroactive IIs may be linked as the previous interviews are reflected or ruminated upon while preparing for ensuing interviews. On the other hand, after having been in a number of interviews, the person may believe he/she has a sufficient memory structure for anticipating what will happen in the next interview.

IIs are seen as a type of cognitive activity that is relatively mindful. We may go back and reexperience the II like the cartoon reader who rereads the script. This conceptualization of IIs as mindful sets up the idea that overlearned schema are reflective of mindlessness which is preceded by mindful states. Hence, IIs can play a role in the development of memory structures. Overlearned structures or schemata may be viewed as states of mindlessness. It would not be necessary to set up contingency plans for that which has been experienced repeatedly and is expected again. Langer (1978) lists a number of situations when thought is enhanced. Individuals are likely to be mindful or engaging in thought when encountering novel situations for which no script can be utilized. IIs may play a role here by envisioning contingency plans for actions in which the confidence that a given plan will be instantiated is low. Langer also posits that thought is more likely when experiencing positive or negative affect that is discrepant with the consequence of previous enactments of the behavior. It would be interesting to investigate the affect associated with retroactive IIs after real encounters had occurred.

Our research is taking a functional approach to the analysis of IIs. This approach has allowed us to create a typology of functions. We are interested in determining if the specific functions we have identified so far are generalizable across a variety of situations, tasks, and/or relationships.

REFERENCES

Abelson, R. P. (1976). Script processing in attitude formation and decision-making. In *Cognition and Social Behavior,* J. S. Carroll and J. W. Payne (eds.). Hillsdale, NJ: Erlbaum.

Berger, C. R. (in press). A plan-based approach to strategic communication. In *Cognitive Bases of Interpersonal Communication,* D. E. Hewes (ed.). Hillsdale, NJ: Erlbaum.

Caughey, J. L. (1984). *Imaginary Social Worlds.* Lincoln, NE: University of Nebraska Press.

Daly, J. A., Vangelisti, A., and Daughton, S. M. (1987). The nature and correlates of conversational sensitivity. *Human Communication Research,* 14, 167-202.

Edwards, R., Honeycutt, J. M., and Zagacki, K. S. (1988). Imagined interaction as an element of social cognition, *Western Journal of Speech Communication,* 52, 23-45.

Edwards, R., Honeycutt, J. M., and Zagacki, K. S. (1989). Gender differences in imagined interactions. *Sex Roles,* 21, 259-268.

Fiske, S. T. and Taylor, S. E. (1984). *Social Cognition.* Reading, MA: Addison-Wesley.

Folkes, V. S. (1985). Mindlessness or mindfulness: A partial replication and extension of Langer, Blank, and Chanowitz. *Journal of Personality and Social Psychology,* 48, 600-604.

Greene, J. O. (1984). A cognitive approach to human communication: An action-assembly theory. *Communication Monographs,* 51, 289-306.

Hamilton, M. & Hunter, J. (1988). *PACKET 1.0, A multiple groups confirmatory factor analysis routine for microcomputers.* Storrs, CT: University of Connecticutt.

Honeycutt, J. M. (1989a). A pilot analysis of imagined interaction accounts in the elderly. In *Louisiana: Health and the elderly,* R. Marks and J. Padgett (eds). New Orleans, LA: Pan American Life Center.

Honeycutt, J. M. (1989b). *Transferrence in everyday life: Imagined interactions, message planning, and emotional affect.* Seminar paper presented at the annual Speech Communication Association Conference, San Francisco, November.

Honeycutt, J. M. (1990). A functional analysis of imagined interaction activity in everyday life. In *Imagery: Current Perspectives,* J. E. Shorr, P. Robin, J. A. Connelia, and M. Wolpin (eds.). New York: Plenum.

Honeycutt, J. M., Zagacki, K. S., and Edwards, R., 1989, Intrapersonal communication and imagined interactions. In *Readings in Intrapersonal Communication,* C. Roberts and K. Watson (eds.). Scottsdale, AZ: Gorsuch Scarisbrick Publishers.

Honeycutt, J. M., Edwards, R., and Zagacki, K. S. (1989-1990). Using imagined interaction features to predict measures of self-awareness: Loneliness, locus of control, self-dominance, and emotional intensity. *Imagination, Cognition, and Personality*, 9, 17-31.

Kihlstrom, J. F. and Cantor, N. (1984). Mental representations of self. In *Advances in Experimental Social Psychology*, Vol., 17, L. Berkowtiz (ed.). New York: Academic Press.

Klinger, E. (1978). Modes of normal conscious flow. In *The Stream of Consciousness: Scientific Investigations into the Flow of Human Experience*, K. S. Pope and J. L. Singer (eds.). New York: Plenum.

Klinger, E. (1981). The central place of imagery in human functioning. In *Imagery: Concepts, Results, and Application*, Vol. 2, E. Klinger (ed.). New York: Plenum.

Klinger, E. (1987). *What people think about and when they think it*. Paper presented at the annual American Psychological Association Conference, New York.

Klos, D. S. and Singer, J. L. (1981). Determinants of the adolescent's ongoing thought following simulated parental confrontations. *Journal of Personality and Social Psychology*, 41, 975-987.

Langer, E. J. (1978). Rethinking the role of thought in social interaction. In *New Directions in Attribution Research*, Vol. 2, J. H. Harvey, W. Ickes, and R. F. Kidd (eds.). Hilldfslr, NJ: Erlbaum.

Langer, E. J. (1989). Mindfulness. Reading, MA: Addison-Wesley.

Langer, E. J., Blank, A., and Chanowitz, B. (1978). The mindlessness of ostensibly thoughtful action: The role of placebic information in interpersonal interaction. *Journal of Personality and Social Psychology*, 36, 635-642.

Langer, E. J., Chanowitz, B., and Blank, A. (1985). Mindlessness-mindfulness in perspective: A reply to Valerie Folkes. *Journal of Personality and Social Psychology*, 48, 605-607.

Langer, E. J., and Piper, A. I. (1987). The prevention of mindlessness. *Journal of Personality and Social Psychology*, 53, 280-287.

Mead, G. H. (1934). *Mind, Self and Society*. Chicago: University of Chicago Press.

Norman, D. A. (1980). Copycat science or does the mind really work by table look-up? In *Perception and production of fluent speech*, R. A. Cole (ed.). Hillsdale, NJ: Erlbaum.

O'Keefe, B. J. (1988). The logic of message design: Individual differences in reasoning about communication. *Communication Monographs*, 55, 80-103.

O'Keefe, B. J. (1990). The logic of regulative communication: Understanding the rationality of message designs. In *Seeking compliance: The production of interpersonal influence messages*, J. P. Dillard (ed.). Scottsdale, AZ: Gorsuch Scarisbrick Publishers.

Roloff, M. E. (1989). Issue schema and mindless processing of persuasive messages: Much ado about nothing? In *Intrapersonal Communication Processes*, C. V. Roberts and K. W. Watson (eds.). Scottsdale, AZ: Gorsuch Scarisbrick Publishers.

Rosenblatt, P. and Meyer, C. (1986). Imagined interactions and the family. *Family Relations*, 35, 319-324.

Schank, R. C. (1982). *Dynamic Memory*. New York: Cambridge University Press.

Schultz, K. D. (1978). Imagery and the control of depression. In *The Power of Human Imagination*, J. L. Singer and K. S. Pope (eds.). New York: Plenum.

Sherman, S. J. and Corty, E. (1984). Cognitive heuristics. In *Handbook of Social Cognition*, Vol. 1, R. S. Wyer, Jr. and T. K. Srull (eds.). Hillsdale, NJ: Erlbaum.

Singer, J. L. (1985). *Private experience and public action: The study of ongoing thought*. Paper read at the Henry A. Murray Lecture, Symposium on Personality, Michigan State University, East Lansing Michigan.

Singer, J. L. (1987). Reinterpreting the transference. In *Reasoning, Inference and Judgement in Clinical Psychology*, D. C. Turk and P. Salovey (eds.). New York: Free Press.

Zagacki, K. S., Edwards, R., and Honeycutt, J. M. (1988). *Imagined interactions, social cognition and intrapersonal communication: Elaboration of a theoretical construct*. Paper presented at the annual Speech Communication Association Convention, New Orleans, November.

AN INTRAPERSONAL PROCESS IN CROSS-CULTURAL ADAPTATION:

IMAGINED INTERACTIONS AMONG TEMPORARY SOJOURNERS

Dominique M. Gendrin, Ph.D.

Department of Communication and Theatre
McNeese State University
Lake Charles, LA 70609

The individual experience in cross-cultural adaptation has been studied by a variety of disciplines. Researchers in communication, social psychology, sociolinguistics, cultural anthropology, and psychiatry have attempted to explain the varying impact of cross-cultural adaptation on the individual. In an effort to integrate the various perspectives, Kim (1988) developed a theoretical framework from which to study the cross-cultural adaptation process. Adaptation is defined as "the internal transformation of an individual challenged by a new cultural environment in the direction of increasing fitness and compatibility in that environment" (Kim, 1988, p. 9). Underlying this definition of adaptation is the assumption that culture and cognition are inseparable.

Research in intercultural communication has highlighted the close interdependence among culture, communication, and individual social cognition. According to Forgas (1988), "Culture exists in the minds of individuals, and it is individual perceptions, interpretations, and representations of culture, which in their innumerable daily manifestations, help to maintain or change our stable sense of the relevant knowledge structures shared by individuals." (p. 188). This theorist argued that intercultural communication may be analyzed in terms of the cognitive representations of the individuals involved, and suggested that the consequences of conflicting cognitive representations in intercultural communication be investigated. Of recent interest in cognition studies, Imagined Interactions have been found to play a relevant role in the social and psychological life of the individual (see Honeycutt, 1990, for a review). Imagined interaction is defined as "a process of cognition whereby the actors imagine themselves in interaction with others" (Edwards, Honeycutt, & Zagacki, 1988, p. 24). Thus, the purpose of this investigation is to establish a link between Imagined Interaction and the process of cross-cultural adaptation. The paper is divided into three parts. First, Kim's (1988) theory of cross-cultural adaptation is reviewed from a systemic perspective, with an emphasis on intrapersonal processes. Second, the research and findings on Imagined Interaction as developed by Honeycutt and his colleagues are examined. Finally, the theoretical and practical implications of imagined interactions in the adaptation process of cultural strangers are explored.

CROSS-CULTURAL ADAPTATION

Kim (1988) proposed a theory of cross-cultural adaptation based on the General Systems perspective which views immigrants and sojourners as "open systems," interacting within a given cultural environment that is different from the home culture in which they were born and raised. The theory suggests that individuals respond to their environment in a way that will enable them to maintain an equilibrium in their internal structure. As open systems, individuals cope with drastic environmental changes with psychological stress, better known as "culture shock". According to Kim (1989) "the resulting stress, then, serves as the underlying psychological force that 'moves' individual systems to undergo *adaptation*, or the adaptive

Mental Imagery, Edited by R.G. Kunzendorf
Plenum Press, New York, 1990

transformation of internal conditions, which results in the system's *growth*." (p. 5). Therefore, the adaptation process takes place along a continuum of stress-adaptation-growth whereby individuals learn new patterns of the host culture (acculturation) while "unlearning" some of the old patterns of the native culture (deculturation). This "transformation" is said to be gradual and to lead to 'functional fitness' with the host environment. As these cultural strangers gradually decrease their intercultural stress and become functionally fit, psychological health is established.

This open systems perspective stresses the role of communication in the adaptive process. The individual is said to adapt to the host environment through various communication situations at the interpersonal level as well as through the mass media. Interpersonal communication activities involve interacting with host nationals as well as nationals of the same ethnic origin. The mass media also offer opportunities to cultural strangers to participate in the political, historical, and social life of the host culture.

While adaptation precludes active communicative interaction in the host environment, the underlying intrapersonal communication process of cultural strangers is a critical element of adaptation. According to Kim (1989), adapting to a culturally different environment means that individuals must have the internal capacity to construct messages that are appropriate to evolve in the host culture. In doing so, the cultural stranger achieves what she calls *host communication competence* or the ability to think, feel, and act in ways congruent to host nationals. One of the critical features of host communication competence is the skillful use of the dominant language of the host society. Not only does this ability to speak the host language enable the cultural stranger to be functional in that society, but it also enables him or her to think in a native way. Therefore, the acquisition of the host language becomes imperative to the adaptive process. The critical role of communication at the interpersonal as well as at the intrapersonal level is well established in the adaptation process of cultural strangers.

Kim's (1988) theoretical model for cross-cultural adaptation includes three additional dimensions which are as follows: 1) ethnic social communication which involves the proportion of ties with members of the same ethnic group and exposure to ethnic mass communication; 2) host environment receptivity, or the opportunity for strangers to participate in its social activities and the amount of pressure it exerts on strangers to conform to its patterns; and 3) individual predisposition which influences the amount of communication with the host environment, such as the cultural/racial background of cultural strangers and their personality attributes such as openness and resilience. The last dimension identifies adaptive outcomes of functional fitness, psychological health and intercultural identity.

TEMPORARY SOJOURNERS AND THE PSYCHOLOGICAL PROCESS OF ADAPTATION

The success of adaptation depends, in part, on the cultural strangers' motivation to adapt based on the degree of their permanence in the host environment. For instance, immigrants are more likely to commit themselves to participate fully in the host culture since there is little hope to return "home". Temporary sojourners are bound to return to their homeland and therefore are less committed to becoming full members of the host society. According to Furnham (1987), sojourners are characterized by the length and purpose of their stay. A sojourner tends to stay from six months to five years at a place with the intent to return "home." Foreign students, as representatives of sojourners, report living abroad to get a degree or professional training (Bochner, 1973; 1979; Bochner, Lin, & McLeod,1979; Klineberg & Hull, 1979). As sojourners enter a new or different culture, they necessarily go through an adaptation process known as acculturation. Acculturation is defined as "culture change that results from continuous, firsthand contact between two distinct cultural groups" (Redfield, Linton, & Herkovits, in Berry, Kim, & Boski, 1987, p. 64). The changes involved as a result of this cultural encounter are physical, biological, cultural, and psychological for the individual as well as for the cultural group. Sojourners can be further characterized by what is called integration. According to Berry (1984), integration involves having the individual establish relationships within the host culture while maintaining his or her cultural identity. Integration can be contrasted with assimilation which involves relinquishing one's cultural identity while maintaining relationships with other groups. In the case of temporary sojourners, it is assumed that they don't want to change their cultural identity while establishing significant relationships with other groups. Hence, it also is assumed that they strategize for positive encounters in order to function properly in their learning environment.

The psychological process of adaptation has been the focus of extensive research with an emphasis on the 'culture shock' that strangers go through when entering a new culture. (See

Furnham & Bochner, 1982; 1986; Taft, 1977; Torbion, 1982; for a review of literature on culture shock.) In her review on the psychological adaptation of sojourners, Furnham (1987) suggested that nearly all sojourners suffer from culture shock. Culture shock is generally viewed as "a stress reaction where salient psychological and physical rewards are generally uncertain and difficult to control or predict" (p. 46). Although culture shock often has been studied for its negative consequences, it also can be viewed as a creative force in the development and personal growth of the stranger.

Studies exploring the mental health of foreign students examined various factors affecting the success of their adaptation. For instance, the psychological stress of foreign students has been attributed to the cultural distance between their native culture and the host culture, their lack of social skills to make contact with host nationals, and their lack of prior experience in a foreign country (Furnham, 1987). Counseling studies identified problem areas of international students adjusting to their new life as follows: homesickness, obtaining housing, social relationships with members of the opposite sex (for those not married), English language usage, and finances (Stafford, Marian, & Shalter, in Wherly, 1986). Other studies concerned with the well-being of college students have identified indicators of adaptation and adjustment which include language skills, academic issues, cultural differences, racial discrimination, and social interaction with their hosts (Heikinheimo & Shute, 1986).

Successful adaptation to a culturally different environment has been linked to a variety of factors. For instance, Lee (1981) developed a profile of the foreign student who is most likely to succeed in an academic career in the United States: a Latin American or European graduate student who has good English skills, an American roommate, and a job waiting at home. Berry and Kim (1986) showed a positive relationship between sojourners' life satisfaction and their mental health as demonstrated by greater contact with the host society, greater knowledge of English, positive motivation, and academic satisfaction. Researchers agree that in order to maintain positive mental health, individuals need to be emotionally stable, establish meaningful interpersonal relationships, and experience satisfaction in various aspects of life (See Scott and Stumpf, 1984; Taft, 1986a, 1986b). Berry, Kim, & Boski (1987) stated that individuals make psychological attempts to "achieve a better fit (outcome) with other features of the system in which they carry out their life" (p. 63). Thus, sojourners may be best characterized as those individuals who will "fit" well enough to their environment so they can successfully achieve their temporary goals. Hence, an important issue to be addressed here is how temporary sojourners achieve better fitness and compatibility with their new environment at the intrapersonal level of adaptation. Temporary sojourners must test their perceptions, interpretations, and cognitive representations of their culture and the host culture. Sojourners must also review their own communication and that of others in order to adapt. Thus, it is argued that sojourners' Imagined Interactions play an important part in the intrapersonal process of cross-cultural adaptation. The following section presents a review of the research on Imagined Interactions.

IMAGINED INTERACTIONS

As suggested earlier, Imagined Interactions (IIs) are attempts to simulate real-life conversations with significant others (Edwards et al., 1988; Honeycutt, Edwards, & Zagacki, 1989-1990; Honeycutt, Zagacki, & Edwards, 1989). IIs are different from other cognitive processes in that they have all the features of real conversations (Edwards et al., 1988; Honeycutt et al., 1989a). Grounded in symbolic interactionism and script theory, these internal dialogues involve a process of social cognition which is directly related to the achievement of some intentional, social communicative goal. As such, they perform the important function of rehearsing for anticipated encounters (Edwards et al., 1988; Honeycutt, 1990). The individual's experience and knowledge are inscribed in various types of cognitive structures which are then activated in the form of procedural records in order to evaluate one's behaviors and goals in interaction. According to Honeycutt (1990), "it is possible that imagined interactions activate, and possibly constitute, procedural records for coping with specific interpersonal communication situations" (p. 17).

Extended research was conducted to identify and test the various characteristics and functions of IIs, using a multidimensional instrument ("Survey of Imagined Interaction" SII) [Honeycutt et al., 1989; Zagacki, Edwards, & Honeycutt, 1988]. The SII instrument yielded several dimensions of IIs. First the "discrepancy" dimension reflects the difference between imagined and real interactions. In looking at individual characteristics, lonely individuals were found to have more discrepant and vague IIs than non-lonely individuals. IIs are also characterized by their "pleasantness" and their "activity". The "activity" dimension was found to have a strong relationship with two other features of IIs, namely "proactivity" and "retroactivity" (Honeycutt et al., 1989-1990). These two features suggest that IIs may occur before or after real conversations. They may also occur consecutively to one another: "Given that IIs tend to occur with significant others, it may be that many of them are linked and occur between encounters reviewing and previewing conversations." (Honeycutt, 1989, p. 10). A degree of self-talk or dominance was observed also in IIs. The "dominance of self" dimension suggests not only that the actor talks more than the other, but also that this self-talk enhances self-understanding and can function as a catharsis (Edwards et al., 1988; Honeycutt, 1990; Honeycutt et al., 1989-1990; Honeycutt, Zagacki, & Edwards, 1989). IIs have been variously described as detailed or vague, thus illustrating the "specificity" of IIs. Finally, in line with the "variety" dimension of IIs, individuals can imagine conversations with various partners on diverse topics or converse over several topics with the same partner (Edwards et al., 1988). Honeycutt and his colleagues have taken a functional approach to the study of IIs, with the understanding that the individual can achieve greater self-understanding and maintain relationships. Hence, in addition to the rehearsal function of IIs, these internal dialogues serve as a form of catharsis, enhance self-understanding, and sustain psychological relational maintenance (Honeycutt et al., 1989).

TEMPORARY SOJOURNERS:
IMAGINED INTERACTIONS AND CROSS-CULTURAL ADAPTATION

Kim (1988) defined cross-cultural adaptation as a process of change that takes place intrapersonally as the individual comes into a prolonged first-hand contact with a new culture. Honeycutt, Zagacki and Edwards' (1988) review of the research on IIs emphasized the importance of IIs as an intrapersonal process and its relevance to relational development. Specifically, Honeycutt and his colleagues identified major research issues regarding the features of IIs: 1) the frequency of IIs among particular individuals (e.g., lonely vs. none-lonely individuals); 2) the central topics in IIs (e.g., dating, conflicts and problems in work situations); 3) types of relational partners (romantic partners, family members and friends); 4) the dominant role of the self in IIs; 5) the linguistic features of IIs, such as turn-taking, number of statements vs. questions; 6) the rehearsing and review functions of IIs; and 7) the strong emotional tone of IIs. A theoretical question to be addressed here concerns the features of IIs among temporary sojourners. Considering the cognitive relevance of IIs and its potential for the individual's mental health, as well as its relational significance for future interactions, it is assumed that IIs play an important role in the adaptive process of temporary sojourners.

Rehearsing and Review Functions of Sojourners' IIs

Honeycutt et al. (1989) proposed that IIs serve to plan and solve communication situations using cognitive scripts or procedural records. Engaging in IIs enables the individual to assemble information and develop or change behavioral scripts. This paper suggests a similar cognitive activity whereby temporary sojourners evaluate their experiences in the new culture and revise old scripts/or develop new ones that are culturally "fit". This cultural fitness, however, requires that the individual unlearn old cognitive scripts and assemble new ones. This process of change, in turn, may create great psychological stress until the individual has integrated culturally appropriate cognitive representations of his/her new social life. This cross-cultural transformation can be explained by the link between culture and cognition.

In an extensive research effort aimed at understanding encounters with people from cultures other than our own, Forgas (1988) developed a sociocognitive approach to intercultural communication in which he suggested that people develop cognitive representations about prototypical interaction situations. These recurring encounters constitute 'natural units' in the stream of behavior and are referred to as social episodes. The cognitive representations of social episodes are necessarily linked to particular cognitive structures, such as cognitive schemata and scripts or procedural records. Cognitive scripts serve as a basis for developing procedural records which dictate specific goal states and the behaviors needed to achieve them (Edwards et al., 1988). Thus, imagined interactions provide the means by which sojourners may access information and related outcomes contained in cognitive structures in order to make sense of their cross-cultural experience. However, the use of IIs may be made dysfunctional when sojourners have not yet developed the appropriate psychological, emotional, and physical responses to the new cultural milieu.

Forgas (1988) demonstrated how the perception of social episodes reflects cultural differences (Forgas & Bond, 1985; Hofstede, 1980). Thus, a stranger, in the initial stage of adaptation, is likely to rely on cognitive representations that are incongruent with the intercultural experience. Consequently, it can be inferred that the stranger will frequently engage in IIs in order to evaluate the intercultural situation and develop a behavioral script that will be cross-culturally effective. Edwards et al. (1988) reported more occurrences of IIs before actual encounters rather than after them. The rehearsal nature of imagined interaction enables individuals to plan for the verbal and nonverbal behaviors of anticipated encounters. This is confirmed by Berger and Calabrese's (1975) theory of uncertainty reduction which acknowledges the individual's ability to explain and predict accurately other peoples' behaviors. Berger (1979) further stated that individuals engage in proactive and retroactive explanations about the behaviors of others.

Gundykunst and Hammer (1987) and Gudykunst (1988) expanded the uncertainty reduction theory to partially explain intercultural adaptation. According to these theorists, sojourners, as they enter a host culture, are not cognitively sure how to behave, and thus experience greater uncertainty than members of the host culture. Furthermore, as temporary sojourners enter the host culture, they rely on an implicit theory of culture (their own) to guide their behavior and interpret the behavior of others. Hence, Gudykunst et al. (1987) made the assumption that the stranger's behavior takes place at relatively high levels of awareness. Therefore, it is reasonable to assume that sojourners would mentally rehearse future encounters with members of the host culture to reduce their uncertainty and facilitate their integration. It is also reasonable to infer that they would use past encounters as a basis to evaluate and develop behavioral scripts for more successful encounters. Consequently, IIs should function proactively and retroactively in the psychological adaptation of temporary sojourners.

Dominance of Self in Sojourners' IIs

Research on the functions of IIs indicated the dominant role of the self (Honeycutt, 1990; Honeycutt et al., 1989; Honeycutt et al., 1989-1990). In accordance with the fundamental attribution error, Edwards et al. (1988) reported that IIs generate more information about the self than about others. The fundamental attribution error illustrates the individual tendency to underestimate situational or external factors when observing the behaviors of others. Yet, when the same behavior is performed by the actor him/herself, attributions are external (Heider, 1944; Kelley & Michela, 1980; Nisbett & Ross, 1979; Ross, 1977). This attribution is not only intracultural, but also occurs at the intercultural level. Brislin (1981) suggested that when an individual observes another person's behavior, there is a strong tendency to downplay situational factors and interpret the behavior as a cultural trait. This is confirmed by Jaspar and Hewstone's (1982) notion that outgroup members' behaviors are perceived to be dispositional while ingroup members's behaviors are made situational. These cultural trait attributions should affect the way cultural strangers process information in an interpersonal situation. This phenomenon, in turn, should be reflected in sojourners'IIs.

Gudykunst and Hammer (1987) expanded the fundamental attribution error by assuming that "strangers" overestimate the influence of culture in explaining host national's behaviors, especially with respect to negative behaviors. In other words, strangers tend to attribute positive behavior of in-group members (other strangers) to dispositional factors and the positive behavior of out-group (members of host culture) members to situational factors. Conversely, negative behaviors by in-group members are attributed to situational factors, while negative behaviors of out-group members are attributed to dispositional factors (Hewstone in Gudykunst & Hammer, 1987). The latter findings support the role of IIs in engaging in self-talk to explain one's behavior and that of others in an intercultural context. As a consequence of this trait attribution process, sojourners' IIs may serve to reinforce negative stereotypes about host nationals while dismissing their negative behaviors as situational. This perceptual tendency could hinder the process of adaptation when sojourners have not yet acquired sufficient knowledge of their new cultural milieu.

Self-Awareness and Self-Understanding

In relation to self-dominance, it has been argued that IIs may help the self to sort out feelings and achieve greater understanding (Edwards et al., 1988; Honeycutt, 1990). Mead (1934) explained the development of self-concept through interactions with others: "The individual experiences himself as such, not directly, but only indirectly, from the particular standpoints of other individual members of the same social group" (pp. 138-140). Such interactional self-development raises the issue of self confirmation when interacting with individuals of different cultures. In evaluating the role of IIs in enhancing individual self-awareness, it is necessary to acknowledge a conceptual difference of self between cultures.

Gudykunst and Ting-Toomey's (1988) discussion of self-concept identified a distinction between individualistic and collectivistic cultures. A western conception of self is individualistic in that the self is viewed as being an entity unto itself and has an existence apart from the group to which the individual belongs. Thus, important goals for individuals to pursue in individualistic cultures include self-actualization and/or self-realization. This view contrasts with a non-western concept of self. In collectivistic cultures, individuals see themselves as interdependent with other human beings to the extent of denying their own self-importance. Consequently, the self in collectivistic cultures is relationally bound in order to promote the well-being of the group. This brief overview of self-concept in individualistic and collectivistic cultures suggests a degree of cultural variation which needs to be accounted for in examining the function of IIs in developing self-awareness among sojourners.

In view of these cultural differences, IIs may serve not so much to enhance a sense of self as an intra-psychic identity as to promote group membership and project or maintain a "social self" that is relationally bound. For instance, in her theory on culture and face work, Ting-Toomey (1988) argued that in collectivistic cultures, such as China, Korea, and Japan, the self serves to project an image of oneself in a relational situation and is defined conjointly by the participants in that situation. This self-projection constitutes what is called "facework." Although facework takes place in both individualistic and collectivistic cultures, western individuals are concerned with self-face maintenance or preserving the "I" identity while nonwestern individuals are concerned with both self-face and other-face maintenance in order to preserve relational harmony and avoid public shame and embarrassment. Thus, facework may become problematic in uncertainty situations such as intercultural encounters when the identity of the cultural stranger is called into question. Based on this conceptualization of face, and assuming that sojourners and host nationals do not share the same rules and moral codes governing the self, both parties will lose face. From the perspective of the sojourners, culturally individualistic individuals may see their identity threatened in an intercultural context and lose face while culturally collectivistic sojourners may suffer the embarrassment of losing face and shaming the other. It is possible, then, that sojourners engage in IIs to review those cross-cultural encounters and experience a degree of stress as the said encounter is incongruent with the self script. This is partially confirmed by Honeycutt et al.'s (1989-1990) finding that individuals may be less satisfied with their IIs when they occur retroactively since they cannot rewrite the script. This is especially the case when the reviewed encounter involves a conflict or a negative evaluation. Therefore, it could be argued that temporary sojourners experience unsatisfactory IIs after an actual encounter involving rejection or some negative evaluation of the self. It is possible to argue also that sojourners engage in IIs that would reconfirm a positive sense of self with its cultural boundaries by reviewing past encounters with significant others of the same culture. This is partially supported by Caughey's (1984) notion that inner conversations can serve to retain a sense of values. Such inner talk not only may function to maintain a sense of one's own "reality" but also serves to sort out one's emotions and feelings (Honeycutt, 1990). IIs may function to cope with unpleasant real-life situations and offer the sojourner the luxury of rewriting the script. Yet, to the extent that the new script does not reflect actual encounters, it may create greater psychological stress and hinder the process of adaptation. Honeycutt (1990) warns us against too much self-introspection at the expense of actual encounters. This would be especially true for the sojourner who may feel culturally isolated.

The Emotional Tone of Sojourners' IIs

Edwards et al. (1988) found that when individuals report an II concerning a relational partner, their emotions may be positive, negative, or mixed, depending on the stage of the relationship being imagined. For instance, positive emotions are more likely to be experienced when an individual is in the process of initiating and developing a new relationship (Honeycutt et al., 1988).

In view of sojourners's mental activities in their adaptive process, it is necessary to identify the emotions experienced during IIs. Because of the uncertainty experienced by sojourners in an intercultural context, it was suggested earlier that sojourners may rehearse actual encounters. Honeycutt (1989) argued that the emotional equality of IIs is goal-related: "IIs that serve a rehearsal function should be related to measures of emotional affect insofar as it can be argued that rehearsal is goal-directed and makes us attentive to cues that may produce incongruity between desires and expectancies." (p. 15). Thus, it may be assumed that positive emotions will be experienced when the sojourner anticipates an encounter with predictable outcomes. This could be the case when the relational partner is a co-national, or when the sojourner has achieved sufficient host communication competence to predict the responses of host nationals. Zagacki et al, (1988) showed how II emotional intensity was contingent upon the level of communication satisfaction experienced during IIs and specific feelings. For instance, positive emotions were associated with medium emotional intensity and high communication satisfaction. Sojourners knowing the host language and communication rules are likely to experience positive, satisfying IIs of medium intensity. Negative, unsatisfying, and strongly intense IIs may occur, however, when sojourners are unable to anticipate with certainty future interactions for lack of host communication competence. As sojourners acquire greater host communication competence, they may plan future encounters (proactivity) successfully and experience pleasant IIs in the process.

Relational Maintenance in Sojourners' IIs

In addition to the introspective function of IIs, this mental activity is said to enhance the development and maintenance of relationships. Individuals mentally replay relational episodes, reviewing past encounters and anticipating new ones, and speculating about possible outcomes. According to Honeycutt, Zagacki & Edwards (1990), individuals have IIs most frequently with intimate relational partners and about topics concerning relational matters.

Among the characteristics of these mental replays, an examination of the relationships represented in IIs from American students revealed the importance of significant others, namely: romantic partners, friends, family members, individuals in authority, individuals at work, ex-relational partners, and prospective partners (Edwards et al., 1988; Zagacki et al., forthcoming). Considering the differing social and emotional ties of temporary sojourners (e.g., foreign students) due to their presence in a culturally different setting, the relational partners represented in IIs should differ qualitatively and quantitatively from their American counterparts. Studies on friendship among international students identified specific patterns of social relationships. Foreign students tend to belong to three social networks with varying salience: (a) a primary network of co-nationals consisting of close-friends whose primary function is to provide opportunities for sojourners to rehearse and express their culture of origin; (b) a secondary network consisting of ties with significant host nationals, such as academics, landladies, student advisers and government officials whose function is instrumental in facilitating the academic and professional aspirations of sojourners; and (c) a third network of multinationals friends and acquaintances whose function is to provide recreational, non-cultural and non-task oriented activities (Bochner, McLeod, & Lin, 1977; Furnham & Alibhai, 1985). Therefore, one can anticipate that sojourners' IIs would involve co-nationals, host-nationals, and multinationals as relational partners, depending on the interactional goals reviewed or planned. Furthermore, Kim (1988) stressed the need for strangers to engage in social communication activities such as interpersonal activities in the host society. The interpersonal process involves making contacts with host nationals in order to become adjusted more quickly. Along with host interpersonal communication, temporary sojourners have access to individuals of the same national or ethnic origin. These ethnic groups enable the newcomer to find various forms of support during the initial phase of their adaptation. This intra-group relationship should recede as the sojourner becomes self-reliant in the new environment. An examination of the relational partners in sojourners' IIs could indicate the extent to which they can achieve communication competence in the host culture. One can anticipate that those individuals who have IIs with members of the host culture are more likely to adapt quickly than those who imagine conversing with ethnic nationals. The more resistant sojourners are to interacting with the host culture, the longer it will take them to acquire host communication competence and to adapt.

Apart from the relational partners imagined in interaction, an analysis of II topics stresses further this covert process of relational maintenance. Edwards et al. (1988) identified the following topics, in terms of importance: dating, relational conflict, school, work/job, family/home, money, friends, small talk, and ex-relationships. Of interest in the present investigation are the topics of sojourners' IIs. A theoretical question to be raised here is: To what extent are II topics of temporary sojourners about home-related events and to what extent are they related to current events in the host culture? It is reasonable to assume that sojourners may recall interpersonal situations that occurred in the home country with significant others, such as a quarrel with a friend, or a happy conversation with a relative. Studies on memory and emotions suggest that remembering an event depends on the similarity of a recaller's emotional state at the time of the event and the emotional state at the time of the recall (Bower, 1981). Specifically, individuals in a pleasant mood recall more pleasant events, and do it faster, than do individuals in an unpleasant mood. What people recall is enormously dependent on the mood at the time. Temporary sojourners are likely to mentally re-enact social events that took place in the home country especially at the initial stage of adaptation, when they have not yet taken an active part in the host culture. Thus, according to Bower's (1981) explanation, to the extent that they experience psychological stress in the host culture, sojourners may recall unpleasant conversations having taken place at "home". Lloyd and Lishman (1975) reported that among clinically depressed patients, the sadder ones could call up sad experiences more quickly than they could happy ones. Assuming that adaptation involves stress coupled with psychological and physical illness, IIs may involve topics related to negative life events associated with the adaptive process. Little research has been done in the area of sojourners' life events (Furnham, 1987). An analysis of II topics would shed some light on specific events experienced by sojourners. Yet, not all sojourners experience culture shock when first encountering another culture. Those individual embrace their intercultural experience as a positive challenge with little stress (Kim, 1988). It can be anticipated that these "satisfied" sojourners would have pleasant IIs when they recall conversations with significant others, having taken place in the home or the host country. As temporary sojourners acquire host communication competence over time, their IIs should involve more current relational events which will take on a specific emotional tone depending on the topic of conversation and the relational partner involved at the time.

CONCLUSION

This paper has attempted to address some of the theoretical and practical issues pertaining to the role of II in the process of cross-cultural adaptation. Several conclusions can be drawn from this analysis. First, it was established that II plays a fundamental role in the adaptation of temporary sojourners. Not only does it take place at the intrapersonal level of adaptation but it also functions to plan effectively for interpersonal communication activities. Second, IIs can facilitate as well as hinder the sojourners' adaptation process. To the extent that sojourners engage actively in the social communication activities provided by the host culture (interpersonal contacts and mass media), IIs function to review, rehearse, and plan ongoing encounters toward greater cultural fitness, and increasing mental health. Conversely, should sojourners delay the inevitable encounter with their host environment, IIs may become dysfunctional as they also can keep the cultural stranger in a mental state disconnected from the current situation. According to Kim (1988) the cultural stranger who adapts successfully to the host environment is one who is "fully engaged in the present moment with an inner posture of being ready to cease to 'fight' for or against the process of change, and [is] willing to 'let go' some of the existing inner conditions" (p. 172-173).

While the main functions of IIs in the adaptation of temporary sojourners are being examined empirically (in progress), other characteristics of IIs that are potent to the process of adaptation need to be researched. Of major interest in cross-cultural communication is the extent to which sojourners' IIs are in the native language, host language (e.g., English) or both. In view of the literature in sociolinguistics one should anticipate instances of code switching and/or diglossia. An examination of the language features of sojourners' IIs should further our understanding of the ways in which they achieve host communication competence.

REFERENCES

Berger, C. R. (1979). Beyond initial interactions. In H. Giles and R. St. Clair (Eds.), *Language and social psychology*. Oxford: Basil Blackwell.

Berger, C. R. and Calabrese, R. (1975). Some explorations in initial interactions and beyond: Toward a developmental theory of interpersonal communication. *Human Communication Research, 1*, 99-112.

Berry, J. W. (1984). Cultural relations in plural societies: Alternatives to segregation and their sociopsychological implications. In N. Millerand and M. Brewer (Eds.), *Groups in contact*. New York: Academic Press.

Berry, J. W. and Kim, U. (1986). Acculturation and mental health. In P. Dasen, J. W. Berry, and N. Sartorious (Eds.), *Health and cross-cultural   psychology: Towards applications.* London: Sage.

Berry, J. W., Kim, U., and Boski, P. (1987). Psychological acculturation of immigrants. In Y.Y. Kim and W. B. Gudykunst (Eds.), *Cross-cultural adaptation: Current approaches.* Beverly Hills: Sage Publications.

Bochner, S. (1973). *The mediating man: Cultural interchange and transnational education.* Honolulu: Culture Learning Institute.

Bochner, S. (1979). Cultural diversity: Implications for modernization and international education. In K. Kumar (Ed.), *Bonds without bondage.* Honolulu: University of Hawaii Press.

Bochner, S. (1981). *The mediating person: Bridges between cultures.* Cambridge, MA: Schenkman.

Bochner, S., Lin, A., and McLeod, B. (1979). Cross-cultural contact and the development of an international perspective. *Journal of Social Psychology, 107,* 29-41.

Bochner, S., Mcleod, B., and Lin, A. (1977). Friendship patterns of overseas students: A functional model. *International Journal of Psychology, 12,* 277-294.

Bower, G. H. (1981). Mood and memory. *American Psychologist, 36,* 129-148.

Brislin, R. (1981). *Cross-cultural encounters.* New York: Pergamon Press.

Caughey, J. L. (1984). *Imaginary social worlds.* Lincoln, NE: University of Nebraska Press.

Edwards, R., Honeycutt, J. M., and Zagacki, K. S. (1988). Imagined interaction as an element of social cognition. *Western Journal of Speech, 52,* 23-45.

Forgas, J. P. (1988). Episode representations in intercultural communication. In Y. Y. Kim and W. B. Gudykunst (Eds.), *Theories in intercultural communication.* Beverly Hills: Sage.

Forgas, J. P., & Bond, M. H. (1985). Cultural influences on the perception of interaction episodes. *Journal of Cross-Cultural Psychology, 11,* 75-88.

Furnham, A. (1987). The adjustment of sojourners. In Y.Y. Kim and W.B. Gudykunst (Eds.), *Cross-cultural adaptation: Current approaches.* Beverly Hills: Sage Publications.

Furnham, A. and Alibhai, N. (1985). The friendship networks of foreign students: A replication and extension of the functional model. *International Journal of Psychology, 20,* 709-722.

Furnham, A. and Bochner, S. (1982). The social psychology of cross-cultural relations. In S. Bochner (Ed.), *Cultures in contact: Studies in cross-cultural interaction.* Oxford: Pergamon Press.

Furnham, A. and Bochner, S. (1986). *Culture shock: Psychological reactions to unfamiliar environments.* London: Mathuen.

Gudykunst, W.B. (1988). Uncertainty and anxiety. In Y. Y. Kim and W. B. Gudykunst (Eds.), *Theories in intercultural communication.* Newbury Park, CA: Sage.

Gudykunst, W. B. and Hammer, M. R. (1987). Strangers and host: An uncertainty reduction based theory of intercultural adaptation. In Y.Y. Kim and W. B. Gudykunst, *Cross-cultural adaptation: Current approaches.* Beverly Hills, CA.: Sage.

Gudykunst, W. B. and Kim, Y. Y. (1984). *Communicating with strangers: An approach to intercultural communication.* New York: Random House.

Gudykunst, W. B. and Ting-Tommey, S. (1988). *Culture and interpersonal communication.* Beverly Hills, CA: Sage.

Heider, F. (1944). Social perception and phenomenal causality. *Psychological Review, 4,* 107-115.

Heikinheimo, P. S. and Shute, J. C. M. (1986). The adaptation of foreign students: Student views and institutional implications. *Journal of College Student Personnel,* 399-406.

Hofstede, G. (1980). *Culture's consequences: International differences in work-related values.* Beverly Hills, CA: Sage.

Honeycutt, J. M. (1989). *Transference in everyday life: Imagined interaction, message planning, and emotional effect.* Paper presented at the annual conference of the Speech Communication Association, San Francisco, CA.

Honeycutt, J. M. (1990). A functional analysis of imagined interaction activity in everyday life. In Joseph E. Shorr, Pennee Robin, Jack A. Connelia, & Milton Wolpin (Eds.), *Imagery: Current Perspectives* (pp.13-25). Baywood/Plenum Press.

Honeycutt, J. M., Edwards, R. and Zagacki, K. S. (1989-90). Using imagined interaction features to predict measures of self-awareness: Loneliness, locus of control, self-dominance, and emotional intensity. *Imagination, cognition, and personality ,* 9, 17-31.

Honeycutt, J. M., Zagacki, K. S., and Edwards, R. (1989). Intrapersonal communication, social cognition and imagined interactions. In C. Roberts, and K. Watson (Eds.), *Readings in intrapersonal communication*. Scottsdale, AZ: Gorsuch Scarisbrick Publishers.

Honeycutt, J. M., Zagacki, K. S., and Edwards, R. (1990). Imagined interaction and interpersonal communication. *Communication Reports*, 3, 1-8.

Jaspar, J. and Hewstone, M. (1982). Cross-cultural interaction, social attribution and intergroup relations. In S. Bochner (Ed.), *Cultures in contact*. New york: Pergamon Press.

Kelley, H. and Michela, J. (1980). Attribution theory and research. In M. Rosenzweig and L. Porter (Eds.), *Annual Review of Psychology*, 31, 457-501.

Kim, Y. Y. (1988). *Communication and cross-cultural adaptation: An integrative theory*. Clevedon, England: Multilingual Matters.

Kim, Y. Y. (1989, November). *Communication and Adaptation: The Case of Indochinese Refugees in the United States*. Paper presented at the annual conference of the Speech Communication Association, San Francisco, CA.

Klineberg, O. and Hull, W. (1979). *At a foreign university: An international study of adaptation and coping*. New York: Prager.

Lee, M. Y. (1981). *Needs of Foreign Students from Developing Nations at U.S. Colleges and Universities*. Washington, D.C.: National Association for Foreign Student Affairs.

Mead, G. H. (1934). *Mind, self, and society*. Chicago: University of Chicago Press.

Lloyd, G. G. and Lishman, W. A. (1975). Effect of depression on the speed of recall of pleasant and unpleasant experiences. *Psychological Medicine*, 5, 173-180.

Nisbett, R. and Ross, L. (1980). *Human inference: Strategies and shortcoming of social judgement*. Englewood Cliffs, NJ: Prentice Hall.

Ross, L. (1977). The intuitive psychologist and his shortcomings: Distortion in the attribution process. In L. Berkowitz (Ed.), *Advances in experimental psychology*, Vol. 10. New York: Academic Press.

Scott, W.A. and Stumpf, J. (1984). Personal satisfaction and role performance: Subjective and social aspects of adaptation. *Journal of Personality and Social Psychology*, 47, 812.

Taft, R. (1977). Coping with unfamiliar cultures. In N. Warren (Ed.), *Studies in cross-cultural psychology*, Vol. 10. London: Academic Press.

Taft, R. (1986a). The adaptation of recent Soviet immigrants in Australia. In I. Reyes-Lagunes and Y. H. Poortinga (Eds.), *From a different perspective: Studies of behaviors across cultures*. Lisse: Swets and Zeitlinger.

Taft, R. (1986b). The psychological study of the adjustment and adaptation of immigrants to Australia. In N. T. Feather (Ed.), *Survey of Australian psychology: Trend for research*. Sydney: Allen and Unwin.

Ting-Toomey, S. (1988). A face-negotiation theory. In Y. Kim and Gudykunst (Eds.), *Theories in intercultural communication*. Newbury Park, CA: Sage.

Torbion, I. (1982). *Living abroad: Personal adjustment and personnel policy in the overseas setting*. New York: John Wiley & Sons.

Wherly, B. (1986). Counseling international students: Issues, concerns, and programs. *International Journal for the Advancement of Counseling*, 11-22.

Zagacki, K. S., Edwards, R., and Honeycutt, J. M. (1988). *Imagined interaction, social cognition, and intrapersonal communication: Elaboration of a theoretical construct*. Paper presented on the Top Two Panel of the commission for the study of Intrapersonal Communication at the annual Speech Communication Conference, New Orleans, LA (November).

INFLUENCE OF IMAGINED INTERACTIONS ON COMMUNICATIVE OUTCOMES:
THE CASE OF FORENSIC COMPETITION

James M. Honeycutt, Ph.D., and J. Michael Gotcher, Ph.D.

Center of Imagined Interaction Research
Department of Speech Communication
Louisiana State University
Baton Rouge, LA 70803

Scholars have posited that the role of communication is to control the environment so as to realize physical, economic, or social rewards (Miller & Steinberg, 1975), the underlying assumption being that the message making process is not a random activity. Instead, in seeking to control the environment, communicators purposively weigh the perceived available message alternatives and select the one expected to produce the most favorable outcome. In other words, individuals use language to create and/or alter the world around them.

To facilitate the social construction of reality, individuals can mentally visualize the "reality" they desire and then attempt to bring that reality to fruition. For example, in an attempt to control the environment, mental imagery has been used by athletes to enhance performance. Sports psychologists have found it helpful for athletes to visualize themselves giving flawless performances before actual competition (May & Asken, 1987). Mental imagery after a successful performance has been valuable for athletes by enabling them to focus on exceptional aspects and record them for future performances (Orlick, 1980).

In the field of health, positive mental imagery has been correlated with improved prognosis (Siegel, 1988; Pettingale, Burgess, & Greer, 1988; Stavraky, Buck, Lott, & Worklin, 1968). Scholars in the field of psychoneuroimmunology have theorized that mental imagery can help patients destroy the disease from within (Cousins, 1988; Ornstein & Sobel, 1988). Bombeck (1989) posited that positive mental imagery has enabled children with cancer to live long and fruitful lives. Gotcher and Edwards (in press) reported how cancer patients used mental conversations to prepare for actual conversations with medical professionals. The mental conversations coupled with the actual conversations enhanced active coping processes of the cancer patients.

In order to control the environment through communication, communicators use language to construct reality through cognitive attitude structures (Fishbein & Ajzen, 1975) and cognitive scripts/schemas (Schank & Abelson, 1977). To explore the cognitive construction of reality, Honeycutt, Zagacki, and Edwards (1989; 1989-90) have examined mental imagery in an attempt to better understand social cognition and its relationship to message production, interpretation and storage. The goal of the research concerning mental imagery and language is to understand how individuals monitor, alter, and/or create actual communication interactions as a result of imagined encounters.

While ancedotal evidence abounds linking mental imagery to physical performance, little empirical evidence exists to substantiate the claim that mental imagery is used by communicators to effectively alter the environment. The purpose of this paper is to identify a type of mental imagery that can be measured and manipulated to assess its effects on an objective performance measure. The objective performance measure for this investigation was intercollegiate forensic competition (academic debate), mental imagery was operationalized as imagined interactions. This paper will: 1) summarize the theory of imagined interactions, 2) identify how imagined

Mental Imagery, Edited by R.G. Kunzendorf
Plenum Press, New York, 1990

interactions can be used to alter actual communication interactions, and 3) propose future research possibilities.

IMAGINED INTERACTIONS

Mental imagery processes have been studied by Honeycutt, et al. (1989) in terms of "imagined interactions". These researchers defined imagined interactions as a "process of social cognition whereby actors imagine themselves in anticipated or recently recalled interaction with others" (p. 168). Imagined interactions may precede or follow actual communicative encounters. Honeycutt and his associates (1989) have noted how imagined interactions may be used as a type of simulation in preparing for expected communicative encounters. Sherman and Corty (1984) discuss simulation as a type of cognitive heuristic that affects individuals' skills in making accurate judgements. Kahneman and Tversky (1982) listed five tasks in which mental simulation can be used to facilitate communication. Communication simulation can be used for problem solving; predicting a future event; assessing the probability of a specific event; assessing conditional probabilities; counterfactual assessments; and assessments of causality. During imagined interactions, individuals actually work through representations of communication events and prepare responses based on those contingencies.

Honeycutt (1990) discusses how imagined interactions are grounded in symbolic interactionism. Mead (1934) showed how individuals develop representations of self through imaginary conversations and cited an individual's ability to monitor social action as an essential mark of human intelligence. This type of mental activity, according to Manis and Meltzer (1978), "is a peculiar type of activity that goes on in the experience of the person. The activity is that of the person responding to himself, of indicating things to himself" (p. 21). What is important about this type of mental activity is that one may consciously take the role of others, imagining how they might respond to one's messages, and thus one can test and imagine the consequences of alternative messages prior to communication.

Imagined interactions are functionally related to actual communication in that they are instantiations or exemplars of cognitive scripts. Imagined interactions provide communicators with verbal and perhaps visual representations of past or anticipated communication behavior and should facilitate script development and enactment. Imagined interactions are theorized to function as rehearsal and review devices; individuals mentally replay earlier conversations (analyzing them for alternative outcomes) and "practice" for important upcoming conversations (Honeycutt et al., 1989-90). The communicative behaviors occurring in the imagined interaction provide the individual with a plan for actual interaction.

Honeycutt and his associates (1989) proposed that, as individuals have imagined interactions, "procedural records are activated (and perhaps reconstituted) which may inform behavior related to specific situational exigencies" (p. 170). The research findings reported by Honeycutt et al. (1989) indicated: 1) that individuals vary in the activity or frequency of how many imagined interactions they may have, 2) that imagined interactions are often with the same person, 3) that imagined interactions perform a rehearsal function, and 4) that the self dominates the interaction. The results in previous research exploring imagined interactions have focused on the imagined interactions of individuals not engaged in a particular task (Edwards, Honeycutt, & Zagacki, 1988). But in order to determine whether individuals utilize imagined interactions to alter/create reality, it was necessary to examine imagined interactions in an environment in which the participants desire a certain outcome. The environment utilized was intercollegiate forensics.

INTERCOLLEGIATE FORENSICS

Intercollegiate athletic competition requires the individual to control his/her body in order to perform certain movements and obtain particular outcomes. The athlete with the best control usually wins the event. In intercollegiate forensics, control is also of great importance but not muscular control, message control. Forensics requires participants to be aware of the communication environment. First, competitors are engaged in an activity that rewards the most appropriate communication behavior. In the area of academic debate, debaters are rewarded with a win (the ballot) when they present good reasons, advance effective arguments, demonstrate superior cross-examination skills, and effectively adapt to the judge.

Second, in the competition environment, message selection is in a continuous process of evaluation and reevaluation. In a tournament setting, debaters may compete against teams from 5 or 6 different colleges and universities. While the debate topic is the same for all the competitors, the interpretation of the topic varies from team to team. For example, the topic of foreign investment being detrimental to the United States was interpreted from a variety of perspectives. Topic interpretation ranged from investment causing racism to investment causing unemployment to investment causing AIDS to investment causing prison overcrowding to investment causing drug abuse, etc. Consequently, debaters must be prepared to comprehend and evaluate different meanings of words, phrases, and interpretations of broad topic areas.

To cope with the changing communication environment, debaters perform a variety of functions. Debaters are required to choose from a repertoire of potential arguments to counter opposing positions. Debaters are required to engage in cross examination, deal with case areas that vary, and answer arguments that reflect the idiosyncrasies of the competition. As a result, debaters are required to engage in mental simulations and select argumentative strategies that they think will defend their position and be well received by the critic.

In addition to message selection, debaters must consider the communicative environment. The communicative environment includes analyzing such things as the acoustics of the room, audience size, position of the critic, and room furnishings. Honeycutt and his associates (1989) discussed how imagined interactions not only use verbal imagery but also visual images. Using both visual and verbal stimulants, imagined interactions can enable forensic participants to mentally rehearse messages and prepare for possible exigencies.

PREVIOUS FINDINGS

In order to explore how intercollegiate debaters utilized imagined interactions in competition, Gotcher and Honeycutt (1989) surveyed 73 debaters competing at 3 different debate tournaments in the south. The researchers were interested in identifying what functions of imagined interactions were useful to the participants.

Briefly the results indicated: 1) debaters used imagined interactions to rehearse for potential communication exigencies, 2) the frequency of imagined interactions decreased the discrepancy between imagined interaction and real interactions, 3) proactive imagined interactions correlated with imagined success in the rounds, and 4) the functions of imagined interactions did not correlate with actual success in debate rounds. The implications of these findings suggest some important insights into the role of mental imagery and actual communication interactions.

First, debaters used imagined interactions as a rehearsal process for testing and evaluating potential messages. Due to the interactive nature of the debate activity, imagined interactions enabled the debaters to practice possible messages in light of the contingencies of the situation.

Second, as the frequency of the imagined interactions increased, the discrepancy between imagined and real interactions decreased. Through imagined interactions, debaters were able to construct a reality that mirrored the one imagined. Mental simulation enabled inexperienced debaters to gain experience by imagining a debate round. The rehearsal function tended to compensate for lack of experience. Imagined interactions acted as a substitute for actual performance.

Third, the proactivity of the imagined interaction significantly correlated with imagined success. When an individual experienced the imagined interaction before the actual encounter, they tended to experience more success in the imagined interaction. This result corroborated Rosenthal and Jacobson's (1968) theory of self-fulfilling prophecy. Before the actual encounter, participants imagined the best possible outcome. Imagined interactions seemed to assist the debaters in psychologically preparing for actual competition.

Finally, the functions of imagined interactions did not correlate with actual success. Self-report categories were used to assess whether imagined interactions correlated with actual success in the debate rounds. The self-report tapped whether the participants thought they were: extremely successful in debate, somewhat successful, or not very successful. The discrete categories proved inadequate because the participants were very hesitant to rate themselves extremely successful or not very successful; despite their actual records.

PRESENT RESEARCH

Due the to failure to link actual performance with mental simulation, it is difficult to pinpoint the legitimate role of imagined interactions in actual communication activity. Even though it is important for imagined interactions to project a perception of improved performance for the participant, it is merely a placebo if mental simulation does not actually affect performance; therefore, the on-going research project explores an unbiased measure of success with the functions of imagined interactions.

Since the debate environment is one in which actual performance is easily measured (a winner and a loser), then it is a prime environment for assessing the role of imagined interactions and actual performance. If mental simulation affects the performance of debaters, then one could posit that imagined interactions could affect other communication interactions.

The preliminary results of the present project indicate that the functions of imagined interactions correlate with actual success. An analysis of the reported imagined interactions of 20 debaters revealed that activity, dominance, and proactivity correlated with actual success. As the debaters reported increased use of imagined interactions, their success in academic debate improved. Of course, additional subjects will be examined and additional data analysis will be necessary to establish a stronger foundation, but the findings do suggest that imagined interactions can affect actual communication behavior.

FUTURE IMPLICATIONS

If mental simulations can enable individuals to construct reality, then imagined interactions could be used by salesmen to meet their goals or educators to better instruct students or ministers to better reach their congregations. Overall, imagined interactions could improve the communication process by enabling individuals to be prepared for contingencies of the situation.

What should be noted about the intercollegiate debate situation is that the locus of control was in the hands of the debaters. The debaters were required to shape the communication encounter. The debaters had the responsibility as well as the power to determine the key issues and to establish how those issues were to be decided. However, when the locus of control was not in the hands of the interactants, imagined interactions proved to be less frequent and more discrepant from reality (Gotcher & Honeycutt, 1989).

Locus of control needs further examination before one actively encourages the use of imagined interactions in real world scenarios. For example, cancer patients could be encouraged to utilize imagined interactions to create a "reality" of healing. Unfortunately, the locus of control for recovery may not be in the hands of the patient. The disease may have already spread and unsuccessful mental simulation could cause the patient to experience a deep state of depression. The state of depression could significantly decrease the patient's ability to cope with disease (Goodkin, Antoni, & Blaney, 1986). Consequently, mental simulation could be more harmful than beneficial.

Second, it is important to note that the debate environment is not "real" world. Debate is a game. Debaters utilize strategies that would not be acceptable in normal communicative encounters. For example, debaters speak at a rate of 200-350 words per minute. They argue the benefits of nuclear war, the advantages of world government, the wonders of totalitarianism and the harmful effects of democracy. Debaters actively seek unique interpretations to gain an advantage over an opponent. Thus, imagined interactions may be necessary to prepare for the presentation of such strategies as well as preparation for arguments against such positions.

In the real world, such preparations are unnecessary. Individuals are not faced with unique or unusual situations requiring quick and creative responses. To most, the world is predictable and stable, thus imagined interactions may not be necessary. To some, imagined interactions may even be dysfunctional. Before recommendations can be made concerning the usefulness of mental simulations, future research should explore the possible dysfunctional aspects of imagined interactions.

SUMMARY

Imagined interactions of intercollegiate debaters were examined in a tournament setting. The results indicate that debaters used imagined interactions to prepare for environmental exigencies and to control the communicative encounter. Imagined interactions were significantly correlated with imagined success and substituted for actual experience. Preliminary findings indicate that imagined interactions also correlate with actual success in the debate environment. Mental imagery enabled college debaters to imagine a communicative exchange and then reproduce the exchange in an actual encounter. The implications of the findings are explored and the limitations of the research concerning mental simulations are identified.

REFERENCES

Bombeck, E. (1989). *I want to grow hair, I want to grow up, I want to go to Boise: Children surviving cancer*. New York: Harper & Row, Publishers.

Cousins, N. (1988). Intangibles in medicine: An attempt at balancing perspective. *Journal of the American Medical Association, 260*, 1610-1612.

Edwards, R., Honeycutt, J.M., & Zagacki, K.S. (1988). Imagined interaction as an element of social cognition. *Western Journal of Speech Communication, 52*, 23-45.

Fishbein, M., & Ajzen, I. (1975). *Belief, attitude, intention, and behavior*. Reading, MA: Addison-Wesley.

Goodkin, K., Antoni, M.H., & Blaney, P.H. (1986). Stress and hopelessness in the promotion of cervical intraepithelial neoplasia to invasive squamous cell carcinomia of the cervix. *Journal of Psychosomatic Research, 30*, 67-76.

Gotcher, J.M., & Edwards, R. (in press). Coping strategies of cancer patients: Actual communication and imagined interactions. *Health Communication.*

Gotcher, J.M., & Honeycutt, J.M. (1989). An analysis of imagined interactions of forensic participants. *National Forensic Journal, 7*, 1-19.

Honeycutt, J. M. (1990). A functional analysis of imagined interaction activity in everyday life. In Joseph E. Shorr, Pennee Robin, Jack A. Connelia, & Milton Wolpin (Eds.), *Imagery: Current Perspectives* (pp.13-25). Baywood/Plenum Press.

Honeycutt, J. M., Zagacki, K. S., & Edwards, R. (1989). Intrapersonal communication and imagined interactions. In Charles Roberts & Kittie Watson (Eds.), *Readings in Intrapersonal Communication* (pp. 167-184). Scottsdale, AZ: Gorsuch Scarisbrick Publishers.

Honeycutt, J. M., Edwards, R., and Zagacki, K. S. (1989-1990). Using imagined interaction features to predict measures of self-awareness: Loneliness, locus of control, self-dominance, and emotional intensity. *Imagination, Cognition, and Personality, 9*, 17-31.

Kahneman, D., & Tversky, A. (1982). The simulation heuristic. In D. Kahneman, P. Slovic & A. Tversky (Eds.), *Judgment under uncertainty: Heuristics and biases*. New York: Cambridge University Press.

Manis, J.G. & Meltzer, B.N. (1978). *Symbolic interaction: A reader in social psychology*. Boston: Allyn and Bacon.

May, J.R., & Asken, M.J. (1987). *Sports psychology*. New York: PMA Publishing Corp.

Mead, G.H. (1934). *Mind, self and society*. Chicago: University of Chicago Press.

Miller, G.R., & Steinberg, M. (1975). *Between people: A new analysis of interpersonal communication*. Chicago: Science Research Associates.

Orlick, T. (1980). *In pursuit of excellence*. Champaign, IL: Human Kinestics Publishers, Inc.

Ornstein, R., & Sobel, D. (1988). *The healing brain* . New York: Simon & Schuster, Inc.

Pettingale, K.W., Burgess, C., & Greer, S. (1988). Psychological response to cancer diagnosis-I. Correlations with prognostic variables. *Journal of Psychosomatic Research, 32*, 255-261.

Schank, R., & Abelson, R. (1977). *Scripts, plans, goals, and understanding: An inquiry into human knowledge structures*. Hillsdale, NJ: Lawrence Erlbaum.

Siegel, B.S. (1988). *Love, medicine, and miracles*. New York: Harper & Row, Publishers.

Sherman, S. J. & Corty, E. (1984). Cognitive heuristics. In R. S. Wyer, Jr. & T. K. Srull (Eds.), *Handbook of social cognition* (Vol. 1). Hillsdale, NJ: Lawrence Erlbaum.

Stavraky, K.W., Buck, C.N., Lott, J.S., & Worklin, J.M. (1968). Psychological factors in the outcome of human cancer. *Journal of Psychosomatic Research, 12*, 251-259.

PSYCHOPHYSIOLOGICAL STUDIES AND APPLICATIONS OF CONSCIOUS IMAGES

THE CAUSAL EFFICACY OF CONSCIOUSNESS IN GENERAL,

IMAGERY IN PARTICULAR: A MATERIALISTIC PERSPECTIVE

Robert G. Kunzendorf, Ph.D.

Department of Psychology
University of Lowell
Lowell, MA 01854

PART I: INTRODUCTION TO SYMPOSIUM ON "IMAGERY AND HEALTH"

It is my pleasure to introduce this keynote symposium on the relationship between physical health and mental imagery. Historically, attempts to relate physical health to anything mental have been resisted by the scientific and medical establishments. The tenacity of this resistance is perhaps best illustrated by Carol McMahon's (1975) historical case study of a soldier who died from fright, as an enemy cannon ball passed right before his eyes--without touching him. Because the medical examiners refused to believe that this soldier's death could have been caused by a mental variable like fright, they concluded that the wind of the cannon ball had sucked the air out of his lungs.

And if the establishment's resistance to mentally induced infirmities has been tenacious, its resistance to mentally induced cures has been even stronger. To this day, many medical researchers assert that mental imaging can have a curative effect only on illnesses that are imaginary or psychosomatic, not on diseases that are physical in origin. And many behavioristic researchers make similar assertions, in their campaign to reduce mental phenonmena to epiphenomena with no causal effects: These behavioral scientists assert that physical diseases can be psychologically cured only through 'objective treatments' like biofeedback and Palovian conditioning, not through subjective regimens of conscious imaging. *Ironically, such epiphenomenalist assertions imply that consciousness is something spiritual rather than something physical--because if conscious images were physical events in the brain, then they could innervate at least some bodily responses.*

In other words, if one believes that specific mental images are identical with particular neural events, as I believe, then one must posit that vivid imagers are better able to innervate those neural events and are better able to control whatever bodily responses are affected by those neural events. And given such a position, it makes more sense to reduce biofeedback and Pavlovian conditioning to special cases of vivid imaging, than the other way around.

Indeed fifteen years ago, Gary Schwartz (1975) reported that biofeedback subjects who could raise their heart rate in one feedback session and could lower it in another session were subjects who spontaneously imaged emotional agitation in the former session and emotional tranquillity in the latter session. Subsequently, Hirschman and Favaro (1977, 1980) reported that biofeedback subjects who could raise their heart rate were subjects who possessed more vivid imagery. And over thirty researchers reported that *mental imagery with no biofeedback* could be used to control heart rate (Ahsen, 1978;Arabian, 1982; Bauer & Craighead, 1979; Bell & Schwartz, 1973, 1975; Blizard, Cowings, & Miller, 1975; Boulougouris, Rabavilas, & Stefanis, 1977; Carroll, Baker, & Preston, 1979; Carroll, Marzillier, & Merian, 1982, Craig, 1968; Favill & White, 1917; Furedy & Klajner, 1978; Gottschalk, 1974; Grossberg & Wilson, 1968; Jones, 1977; Jones & Johnson, 1978, 1980; Jordan & Lenington, 1979; Kunzendorf, 1984; Lang, 1979; Lang, Kozak, Miller, Levin, & McLean, 1980; Leber, 1979; Leigh, 1978; Marks & Huson, 1973; Marks, Marset, Boulougouris, & Huson, 1971; Marzillier, Carroll, &

Newland, 1979; McCanne & Ierrarella, 1980; Roberts & Weerts, 1982; Schwartz, 1971; Schwartz & Higgins, 1971; Schwartz, Weinberger, & Singer,1981; Shea, 1985; Taylor & Cameron, 1922; Waters & McDonald, 1973; Wein, 1979). Douglas Carroll's research, Peter Lang's research, and my own research confirmed that those subjects who successfully used imagery to control heart rate were subjects who possessed more vivid imagery. When one looks back at behaviorism's mixed success with heart-ratebiofeedback in animal subjects, one is sobered by the scientific consequences of shunning human subjects and dismissing their subjective reports of mental imagery.

If biofeedback has become the scientific establishment's 'objective' approach to controlling heart rate, then Pavlovian conditioning has become its 'objective' approach to controlling immunoreaction. In two recent attempts to classically condition an enhanced immunoreaction, both Spector (1987) and Gorczynski, Macrae, and Kennedy (1982) reported statistically significant enhancement in animal subjects. But the latter group of researchers reported that such conditioned enhancement was clearly successful in only half of their subjects. In explaining why Pavlovian conditioning is never successful in all subjects, Hobart Mowrer (1977) theorized that conditioned responses are really unconditioned responses...to vivid anticipatory images of the unconditioned stimulus. By implication, *only dogs with vivid anticipatory images of food* should salivate to a bell with no food, and *only mice with vivid anticipatory images of immunity-enhancing stimuli* should exhibit enhanced immunoreactions to a conditioned stimulus. Although this implication was not tested in animal studies of conditioned salivation or conditioned immunoreaction, it was tested in human studies of heart-rate conditioning and GSR conditioning. In these human studies, Arabian and Furedy (1983) and Mangan (1974) found that Pavlovian conditioning was more effective in human subjects with more-vivid images. Presumably, similar findings would be obtained if conditioned immunoreactions were studied in human subjects (with measurable images). Indeed, in human immunoreaction experiments to be described later in this symposium, John Schneider found that immune responsiveness was increased by certain mental images--without any conditioning--and was increased most in subjects with the most vivid images. Truly, the most 'scientific' psychological research is that which examines not only objective factors, but also subjective factors.

PART II: THE CAUSAL EFFICACY OF CONSCIOUS IMAGES

In my own presentation, I want to focus on the causal efficacy of conscious events in general and conscious images in particular. When one is dealing with newly discovered relationships between mental imagery and physical health, one is really dealing with the historically controversial relationship between mind and body. And historically, there have been some compelling theoretical arguments against the causal efficacy of any conscious event. So, those of us who believe in the efficacy of the conscious image need to respond not only with data which refute these arguments, but also with alternative theories which clarify the causal role of conscious events such as images. Let us consider three historically influential arguments against the causal efficacy of any conscious event.

First, let us consider the argument of the animal behaviorist, John Watson: an argument which focuses on the conscious image--and which relies on empirical data, but which has important theoretical implications. In Watson's 1913 article on "Image and Affection in Behavior", he noted that close to a dozen studies had failed to find a positive correlation between the subjective vividness of visual imagery and the objective accuracy of visual memory. Based on the results of these studies, Watson concluded that conscious events in general and conscious images in particular are *epiphenomena, with no causal effects on behavior.* Moreover, even though a dozen recent studies have found a positive correlation between the subjective vividness of imagery and the objective control of bodily processes like heart rate and immune functioning, another dozen studies from the last 25 years still have not found a positive correlation between vividness of imagery and memory for detail (Berger & Gaunitz 1977; Danaher & Thoresen, 1972; Ernest & Paivio, 1971; Hall, Talukder, & Esposito, 1989; Rehm, 1973; Richardson, 1978, 1980; Rimm & Bottrell, 1969; Sheehan & Neisser, 1969; Stewart, 1966; Wagman & Stewart, 1974; Walczyk & Hall, 1988). Thus, Watson's argument must be taken into account by us today, because it implies that certain theories of the relationship between conscious images and brain events are inadequate theories. Clearly, Watson's argument reveals the inadequacy of theories which liken the brain's subjective experiences to 'impressions in a block of wax'-- theories which predict that people with deeper, stronger impressions should possess both more vivid images and more detailed memories. Of course, modern theories have replaced the 'block of wax' with a visual memory store which is located somewhere in the right hemisphere, and which is more strongly activated by vivid imagers and/or primary-process thinkers. Indeed, a right-hemisphere origin for images seems to explain why pathological images more often affect the left side of the body, as Paul Bakan (in press) has shown us. But, a right-hemisphere memory-store for all conscious images does not stand up to Watson's correlational evidence, and it does not speak to the remaining arguments against the efficacy of consciousness.

The first of these remaining arguments has been put forth not by animal behaviorists like John Watson (1913) and B. F. Skinner (1974), but by computer behaviorists like Zenon Pylyshyn (1973, 1978) and John Kemeny (1955). The latter theorists believe that it is possible to study objective behavior inside a computer's 'black box' or a human's brain, but that it is still not necessary to take into account the brain's conscious sensations or the computer's subjective states. Pylyshyn (1973, p. 22) asserts that the imager's conscious "experience of imaging has no causal role" and is just a subjective by-product of the neural process of imaging. In other words, the physical process of imaging in a person or a computer is what influences all resulting behaviors, and any subjective experience of conscious images is epiphenomenal. Suppose for a moment that we have two robots containing subroutines that simulate the neural processes of visual imaging and emotional imaging, *but only one of our robots contains wires that glow with subjective qualities like greenness and redness, pain and pleasure.* According to Pylyshyn, the behavioral output of the subroutine that glows with conscious images has to be the same as the behavioral output of the unconscious subroutine. To see why Pylyshyn's argument is wrong, we need to take our two robots one step further. Kemeny points out that--if we give a robot a lot of wire, some scrap metal, a warm soldering gun, and some subroutines for building another robot--then it should be able to reproduce itself. So, let's suppose that we do this with both of our robots. Now, I am not a gambling man, but I am willing to bet big bucks that the robot whose wires glow with pleasure every time it produces robotic offspring will engage in more reproductive behavior....And if both of our robots were only pre-programmed to produce partial robots *and were still randomly evolving subroutines to produce full robots,* then I know which robot would be consciously motivated to 'fool around' until it developed subroutines to complete both its objective offspring and its subjective climax.

Through this thought-experiment with robots, we can see that conscious sensations like 'pleasure' *are sometimes necessary* to motivate biologically adaptive behavior. The biological wires or nerves that glow with this subjective quality of pleasure *are also necessary* to induce reproductive behavior. But without the subjective quality, objective neural structures *would not always be sufficient* to induce reproduction. *Only when objective brain structures and their subjective qualities are taken together is there a sufficient cause of every behavioral development.*

Thus, conscious experience does have a causal effect on behavior--or at least, the subjective experience of conscious pleasure does. But what about the subjective experience of redness or greenness? Let's consider a third argument against the efficacy of consciousness: a classic argument against the efficacy of redness and greenness. Jerry Fodor (1981) has transformed this third argument into a thought-experiment with two human observers, one of whom has had his brain rewired so that his private sensation of redness corresponds to the other observer's subjective experience of greenness...and his greenness corresponds to the other observer's redness. As Fodor notes, this subjective difference between the observers will not differentially affect their objective behaviors--because both of them will see Macintosh apples and stop signs as similar in color, and both of them will learn verbally to identify that color as *red.* And perhaps both of them will associate Macintosh apples with images of Little Red Riding Hood, and Granny Smith Apples with feelings of envy. No matter how red or green or blue or purple the rewired observer's experience of an apple is, his subjective experience will not lead to behaviors that are noticeably different from those of the normally wired observer. So according to Fodor, conscious redness and conscious greenness are epiphenomena, even if conscious pleasure and conscious pain are not.

Ironically, a rebuttal to this last epiphenomenalist argument can be found in Oswald Kulpe's historically misunderstood theory of imageless thought. Behaviorist histories of psychology would have us believe that Kulpe' (1893) arguments for imageless thought are arguments against the efficacy of conscious imagery. But listen to what Kulpe actually argued back in 1893:

> Anatomical investigations show that the sensory centres [of the cortex] are very uniform in structure; whereas the peripheral sense organs present obvious differences, which are plainly of importance for the differences in the conscious processes which they mediate. If we continue to speak of specific energies, we must consequently localise them in the peripheral sense organs. Look at the two higher senses, and see

how admirably the structure of the eye is adapted to its spatial duty, and the structure of the ear to its qualitative function! The specific significance of the external organs is also evidenced by the fact, that their removal absolutely prevents the appearance of sensible qualities in consciousness, while extirpation of the corresponding central organs may to a certain extent be compensated by the activity of others. We are, therefore, justified in supposing that the nerve fibres [in sensory centres of the cortex] are... to be regarded *not as* the inevitable substrate of [a conscious] sensation...on the same plane with the peripheral organ, but *only as* a condition of its appearance. [Moreover], one recent discovery...seems to throw light upon many points of difficulty in the theory of sensation,--the discovery of sensory nerve fibres with centrifugal conduction...sensory fibres, originating in the brain and ending in the sense-organ. This fact [suggests] that the 'centrally excited' sensations --memorial images, as they have also been very inappropriately named--are at least in many instances correlated with a co-excitation of the peripheral organs. We thus have a comparatively simple explanation of the fact that in certain cases these sensations may take on the character of peripherally excited mental processes. (pp. 84-85)

Thus Kulpe hypothesizes that, in all people, the central nervous system is the locus of *imageless* memories and *imageless* thoughts. And in vivid imagers, the peripheral nervous system is the locus of sensory images, including those images that are constructed from imageless memories and those that are constructed from imageless fantasies.

Furthermore, this hypothesis counters both Watson's and Fodor's arguments against the efficacy of consciousness. In accounting for Watson's evidence that imagery vividness and memory accuracy are uncorrelated, Kulpe's hypothesis simply explains that *all people can retrieve their imageless memories*, but only vivid imagers can construct sensory images of their imageless memories! And unlike Watson's epiphenomenalist argument, Kulpe's hypothesis correctly predicts that imagery vividness and bodily control are positively correlated. For inasmuch as vivid imagers have better centrifugal control over sensory organs, they should be more likely, also, to have better centrifugal control over peripheral processes like heart rate and immunoreaction.

In addition, Kulpe's hypothesis rebuts Fodor's epiphenomenalist argument against the causal efficacy of sensory qualities like redness and greenness. Fodor is right that, if redness and greenness are qualities of cortical neurons, then 'subjectively red' and 'subjectively green' neurons can be switched without disrupting the causal chain of neural events and behavioral outcomes. But if redness is the subjective quality of *retinal hardware that responds to 650 nanometer light-waves*, and if greenness is the subjective quality of *retinal hardware that evolved for 500 nanometer light-waves*, then red and green qualities cannot be switched. Indeed, to the extent that conscious redness is a subjectively necessary component of the retinal response to 650-nanometer light-waves, the subjective experience of redness is a logically necessary (but not sufficent) cause of the retina's responsiveness.

Finally, Kulpe's hypothesis asserts that conscious sensations have scientifically discernible substrates in the nervous system. According to materialist theories of consciousness, each conscious sensation is the subjective quality of a particular set of nerves in their excited state, and the entire 'stream of consciousness' in the mind *subjectively changes* as the whole pattern of excitation in the nervous system *objectively changes*. Thus, as the philosopher Stephen Pepper (1960) notes, scientists ought to be able to look at an exposed nervous system and to distinguish those neural states with sensory qualities from those with sensationless qualities, those neural states with visual sensations from those with auditory sensations, those neural states with the subjective quality of redness from those with the subjective quality of greenness. Although exposed neural structures with the subjective quality of redness need not reflect 650-nanometer light waves and need not produce a red quality in the nervous system of the scientist observing the exposed nervous system, some structural characteristic unique to neural states with the subjective quality of redness ought to be objectively discernible by the scientist. But as Kulpe noted, only neurons in the peripheral nervous system--in the retina, the cochlea, the olfactory bulb, and the corpuscular system--are structurally distinguishable across sensory modalities and structurally variable within each modality.

So according to Kulpe's hypothesis, *visually perceived* sensations are the subjective qualities of peripherally innervated retinal structures, and *visually imaged* sensations are the subjective qualities of centrifugally innervated retinal structures. Likewise, *auditorily imaged* sensations are the subjective qualities of centrifugally innervated cochlear structures. And the tacit location of an image and other sensationless characteristics of the image are subjective qualities of the central nervous system. The remainder of this presentation will focus on recent evidence supporting Kulpe's hypothesis, as it applies both to the mental image itself and to the control of physical health through mental imaging.

From an anatomical perspective, Kulpe's hypothesis presumes that centrifugal pathways from the brain to the sensory transmitters exist. And such a presumption is supported by evidence for centrifugally conducting neurons in the optic nerve (Van Hasselt, 1973-1973; Reperant, Vesselkin, Rio, Ermakova, Miceli, Peyrichoux, & Weidner, 1981), the auditory nerve (Klinke & Galley, 1974), the olfactory tract (Broadwell & Jacobowitz, 1976), and the somatic sensory tracts (Angel, 1977). Let's begin with with the visual system.

The specific proposition that retinal structures are centrifugally innervated during visually imaged sensations, most notably during vividly imaged sensations, is supported by both the earliest studies of visual imagery and the latest studies of its psychophysiology. At the beginning of the nineteenth century, Erasmus Darwin (1803) and F. P Gruithuisen (1812) observed that a negative after-image follows a vivid visual image, just as it follows a visual percept. Moreover, Gruithuisen observed that the after-images of vivid visual images--like the *retinal* after-images of visual percepts--maintain a *fixed location on the retina* as the eye moves. And 150 years later, Ian Oswald (1957) confirmed that the afterimages of vivid visual images also maintain a *fixed size on the retina* and, thus, appear larger when projected against backgrounds farther away. Recently, in replicating and extending Oswald's retinal effect, I found that images vivid enough to induce lasting after-images of fixed retinal size are experienced by only 5% of the college population, but by 40% of the elementary school population (Kunzendorf, 1989).

Like these studies of image-induced after-images, studies of electroretinograms or ERGs also show that retinal structures are centrifugally innervated during vivid visual imaging. In a study of drug-induced imagery in human subjects with surface electrodes on their eyes, Krill, Wieland, and Ostfeld (1960) observed significant changes in the electroretinograms of subjects who experienced hallucinatory images and no change in the ERGs of control subjects who received either nonhallucinogenic doses or nonhallucinogenic analogues of two drugs. Similarly, in a study of hallucinatory imagery in a suggestible patient with implanted electrodes, Guerrero-Figueroa and Heath (1964) observed larger and then smaller evoked potentials in the optic tract, when the evoking light was hallucinated to be brighter and then dimmer. In research on the Pavlovian conditioning of human electroretinograms, Bogoslovskii and Semenovskaya (1959) and Freedman and Ronchi (1964) obtained increases in both the subjective brightness and the ERG amplitude of a dim light, when the light was accompanied by a conditioned stimulus that had previously been paired with a bright light. And in biofeedback research on visual evoked potentials, Roger and Galand (1981) found that human subjects could augment the peripherally generated components of such potentials, by associating "the [evoking] flash with complex imagined sights such as bomb explosions" (p. 481). Finally, in a study of color imagery in vivid imagers and control subjects with electrodes on one eye (Kunzendorf, 1984), I obtained the results depicted in Figure 1: specifically, unimodal ERGs when the vivid imagers and control subjects viewed green flashes; bimodal ERGs when the vivid imagers and control subjects viewed red flashes; bimodal ERGs when the vivid imagers imagined that green flashes were vivid red flashes; and unimodal ERGs when the vivid imagers imagined that red flashes were vivid green flashes. Such evidence strongly suggests that visual sensations are the subjective qualities of retinal structures.

Going beyond the psychophysiology of visually imaged sensations, recent research by Walter Freeman suggests that olfactively imaged sensations are centrifugally innervated qualities of the olfactory bulb. Employing animal subjects, Freeman found that the olfactory bulb exhibits a particular "spatial pattern of bulbar activity" not only when a particular odor occurs, but also when a search image for the odor occurs.

In addition, two lines of research with humans suggest that auditorily imaged sensations are centrifugally innervated qualities of the cochlea. First, in hypnosis research with auditory evoked potentials, Deehan and Robertson (1980) found that the waveform of such potentials is 'cancelled out' by negative hallucinations, like suggested deafness. Second, in imagery research with brain-stem auditory evoked potentials, my students and I recently found that Wave 5--emanating from the inferior colliculus just 7 milliseconds after stimulus onset--becomes larger not only when the evoking tone is actually perceived to be louder, but also when the evoking tone is vividly imaged to sound louder (Kunzendorf, Jesses, Michaels, Caiazzo-Fluellen, & Butler, in press).

All of the preceding evidence confirms Kulpe's psychophysiological theory of imagery: that vividly imaged sensations are the subjective qualities of centrifugally innervated states in the sensory organs. But the question remains as to the causal role played by sensory images that are

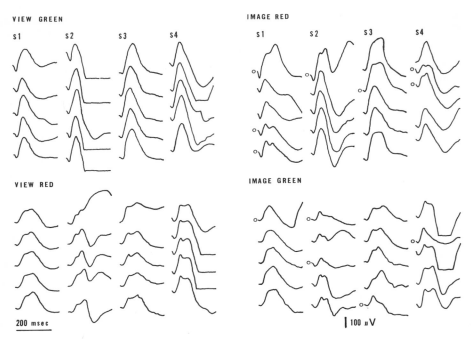

VIEW GREEN   IMAGE RED

s1   s2   s3   s4   s1   s2   s3   s4

VIEW RED   IMAGE GREEN

200 msec | 100 μV

Fig. 1. Electroretinograms (ERGs) from Kunzendorf's (1984) vivid imagers (S1-S4):
         Five successive ERGs from each green-flash condition ('view green' and
         'image red') and from each red-flash condition ('view red' and 'image green').
         (The ERGs that were judged to be complementary to the color of the flash are
         preceded by unfilled circles.)

retinal. Possibly, the act of constructing percept-like images on the retina allows most young
children and some artistic adults to generate, test, and refine their *visual rules for transforming
retinal sensations into percepts* --just as babbling allows young children to generate, test, and
refine their *linguistic rules for transforming auditory sensations into phonemes* (Liberman, 1970;
Liberman, Cooper, Harris, & MacNeilage, 1963). Consistent with this possibilty is my
previously mentioned finding that younger people's images are more vivid and are more likely to
induce after-images of *fixed retinal size* . And another of my own studies plus two of Martin
Lindauer's studies show that artistic adults with more vivid imagery exhibit greater mastery of
visual rules like the rules of linear perspective, which transform visual sensations into three-
dimensional percepts (Kunzendorf, 1982; Lindauer, 1977; Bilotta & Lindauer, 1980). So,
perhaps the imaging of peripheral sensations plays a causal role in the early development and
artistic refinement of such transformational rules.

　　In any event, to the extent that the centrifugal construction of conscious sensations in the
sensory organs correlates with centrifugal control in general, young people--and adults with vivid
imagery--should exhibit better control of their autonomic nerves. Indeed, developmental research
on autonomic processes shows that younger people exhibit better imaginal control of heart rate
(Lang, Troyer, Twentyman, & Gatchel, 1975) and vasodilation (Lynch, Hama, Kohn, & Miller,
1976). And other research shows that adults with more vivid imagery exhibit better centrifugal
control of heart rate (Carroll, Baker, & Preston, 1979; Hirschman & Favaro, 1977, 1980),
vasodilation (Kunzendorf, 1981), immunoreaction (Achterberg, Lawlis, Simonton, & Matthews-
Simonton, 1977; Hall, 1984; Schneider, Smith, Minning, Whitcher, & Hermanson, in press),
and electrodermal activity (Ikeda & Hirai, 1976; Kunzendorf & Bradbury, 1983). Accordingly,
the ability to centrifugally innervate conscious sensations may be a sufficient cause of other
centrifugally mediated abilities.

　　But according to present theorizing, only the ability to generate the *peripheral* sensations of
imagery should be related to the control of these *peripheral* autonomic processes. The ability to
generate the sensationless *cortical* qualities of imagery should not necessarily be related to such
control. For example, whether one can experience tactually imaged sensations 'on one's skin'--
or whether one can only experience tactile images 'in one's mind'--need not be related to the

peripheral control of skin temperature, GSR, or immunoreaction (Kunzendorf, 1990). Research on the ability to locate tactile sensations indicates that the *locative* qualities of such sensations are cortically represented and are phenomenally independent of the tactile sensations themselves, which are peripherally represented. In particular, Cronholm (1951) notes that an amputee's tactile sensations of a phantom limb can be elicited by stimulating the stump, and can be extinguished by anesthetizing the stump. Also, he notes that cortical lesions can eliminate the amputee's tendency to mislocate his tactile sensations in a 'phantom limb'.

Cronholm's evidence that sensory qualities are phenomenally and neurally separate from locative qualities is philosophically quite important, because it negates a common argument against materialist theories of consciousness. Commonly, it is argued that if an imaged sensation is a neural event, then we should experience the sensation and the neural event in the same location: we should experience a tactile sensation, for example, in some nerve--not on the skin. But in fact, neural states with tactile subjective qualities would be experienced as having *no location*, if there were *no separate neural states with locative qualties* . These separate neural states happen to be cortical states with sensationless qualities of bodily location and spatial location, rather than nerve location.

In conclusion, my presentation has focused not only on the physiological relationship between mental imagery and physical health, but also on the philosophical relationship between mind and body. I strongly believe that, if we are to foster a better understanding of the imagery/health relationship both for ourselves and for our critics, then we cannot afford to ignore metaphysical and other philosophical issues. I hearken back to the words with which William James (1892/1961) concluded his abridged version of *The Principles of Psychology* :

> When...we talk of 'psychology as a natural science,'...it means a psychology particularly fragile, and into which the waters of metaphysical criticism leak at every joint, a psychology all of whose elementary assumptions and data must be reconsidered in wider connections and translated into other terms....it is only the hope of a science. The matter of a science is with us. Something definite happens when to a certain brain-state a certain 'sciousness' corresponds. A genuine glimps into what it is would be *the* scientific achievement....But at present psychology is in the condition of physics before Galileo and the laws of motion....We don't even know the terms between which the elementary laws would obtain if we had them....When they do come, however, the necessities of the case will make them 'metaphysical'. (p. 335)

REFERENCES

Achterberg, J., Lawlis, G. F., Simonton, O., & Matthews-Simonton, S. (1977). Psychological factors and blood chemistries as disease outcome predictors for cancer patients. *Multivariate Experimental Clinical Research*, 3, 107-122.

Ahsen, A. (1978). Eidetics: Neural experiential growth potential for the treatment of accident traumas, debilitating stress conditions, and chronic emotional blocking. *Journal of Mental Imagery*, 2, 1-22.

Angel, A. (1977). Processing of sensory information. *Progress in Neurobiology*, 9, 1-122.

Arabian, J. M. (1982). Imagery and Pavlovian heart rate decelerative conditioning. *Psychophysiology*, 19, 286-293.

Arabian, J. M., & Furedy, J. J. (1983). Individual differences in imagery ability and Pavlovian heart rate decelerative conditioning. *Psychophysiology*, 20, 325-331.

Bakan, P. (in press). Imagery and the sinistrality of symptoms. In R. G. Kunzendorf, (Ed.), *Mental imagery*. New York: Plenum.

Bauer, R. M., & Craighead, W. E. (1979). Psychophysiological responses to the imagination of fearful and neutral situations: The effects of imagery instructions. *Behavior Therapy*, 10, 389-403.

Bell, I., & Schwartz, G. E. (1973). Cognitive and somatic mechanisms in the voluntary control of human heart rate. In D. Shapiro, T. X. Barber, L. V. DiCara, J. Kamiya, N. E. Miller, & J. Stoyva (Eds.), *Biofeedback and self-control 1972*. Chicago: Aldine.

Bell, I., & Schwartz, G. (1975). Voluntary control and reactivity of human heart rate. *Psychophysiology*, 12, 339-48.

Berger, G. H., & Gaunitz, S. (1977). Self-rated imagery and vividness of task pictures in relation to visual memory. *British Journal of Psychology*, 68, 283-288.

Bilotta, J., & Lindauer, M. S. (1980). Artistic and nonartistic backgrounds as determinants of the cognitive response to the arts. *Bulletin of the Psychonomic Society*, 15, 354-356.

Blizard, D., Cowings, P., & Miller, N. E. (1975). Visceral responses to opposite types of autogenic-training imagery. *Biological Psychology*, 3, 49-55.

Bogoslovskii, A., & Semenovskaya, E. (1959). Conditioned reflex changes in the human electro-retinogram. *Bulletin of Experimental Biology and Medicine* (translated from Russian), 47, 265-269.

Boulougouris, J. C., Rabavilas, D. D., & Stefanis, C. (1977). Psychophysiological responses in obsessive-compulsive patients. *Behaviour Research and Therapy*, 15, 221-230.

Broadwell, R. D., & Jacobowitz, D. M. (1976). Olfactory relationships of the telencephalon and diencephalon in the rabbit: III. The ipsilateral centrifugal fibers to the olfactory bulbar and retrobulbar formations. *Journal of Comparative Neurology*, 170, 321-346.

Carroll, D., Baker, J., & Preston, M. (1979). Individual differences in visual imaging and the voluntary control of heart rate. *British Journal of Psychology*, 70, 39-49.

Carroll, D., Marzillier, J. S., & Merian, S. (1982). Psychophysiological changes accompanying different ypes of arousing and relaxing imagery. *Psychophysiology*, 19, 75-82.

Craig, K. D. (1968). Physiological arousal as a function of imagined, vicarious, and direct stress experience. *Journal of Abnormal Psychology*, 73, 513-520.

Cronholm, B. (1951). *Phantom limbs in amputees* (R. Cameron, Trans.).Copenhagen: Ejnar Munksgaard.

Danaher, B. G., & Thoresen, C. E. (1972). Imagery assessment by self-report and behavioral measures. *Behaviour Research and Therapy*, 10, 131-138.

Deehan, C., & Robertson, A. W. (1980). Changes in auditory evoked potentials induced by hypnotic suggestion. In M. Pajntar, E. Roskar, & M. Lavric (Eds.), *Hypnosis in psychotherapy and psychosomatic medicine* (pp. 93-95). Ljubljana: University Press.

Ernest, C. H., & Paivio, A. (1971). Imagery and sex differences in incidental recall. *British Journal of Psychology*, 62, 67-72.

Favill, J., & White, P. D. (1917). Voluntary acceleration of the rate of the heart beat. *Heart: A Journal for the Study of the Circulation*, 6, 175-188.

Fodor, J. A. (1981). The mind-body problem. *Scientific American*, 244, 114-123.

Freedan, S. J., & Ronchi, L. (1964). Adaptation and training effects in ERG: IV. Overview of eight years. *Atti della Fondazione Giorgo Ronchi*, 19, 542-565.

Furedy, J., & Klajner, F. (1978). Imaginational Pavlovian conditioning of large-magnitude cardiac decelerations with tilt as US. *Psychophysiology*, 15, 538-548.

Gorczynski, R. M., Macrae, S., & Kennedy, M. (1982). Conditioned immune response associated with allogeneic skin grafts in mice. *Journal of Immunology*, 129, 704-709.

Gottschalk, L. A. (1974). Self-induced visual imagery, affect arousal, and autonomic correlates. *Psychosomatics*, 15, 166-169.

Grossberg, J. M., & Wilson, K. M. (1968). Physiological changes accompanying the visualization of fearful and neutral situations. *Journal of Personality and Social Psychology*, 10, 124-133.

Gruithuisen, F. v. P. (1812). *Beytrage zur Physiognosie und Eautognosie, fur Freunde der Naturforschung auf dem Erfahrungswege*. Munchen: I. J. Lentner.

Guerrero-Figueroa, R., & Heath, R. G. (1964). Evoked responses and changes during attentive factors in man. *Archives of Neurology*, 10, 74-84.

Hall, H. (1984). Imagery and cancer. In A. Sheikh (Ed.), *Imagination and healing*. Farmingdale, NY: Baywood.

Hall, V. C., Talukder, A. B. M. N., & Esposito, M. (1989). Individual differences in the ability to learn and recall with or without imagery mnemonics. *Journal of Mental Imagery*, 13, 43-54.

Hirschman, R., & Favaro, L. (1977). Relationship between imagery and voluntary heart rate control. *Psychophysiology*, 14, 120.

Hirschman, R., & Favaro, L. (1980). Individual differences in imagery vividness and voluntary heart rate control. *Personality and Individual Differences*, 1, 129-133.

Ikeda, Y., & Hirai, H. (1976). Voluntary control of electrodermal activity in relation to imagery and internal perception scores. *Psychophysiology*, 13, 330-333.

James, W. (1961). *Psychology: The briefer course* (G. Allport, Ed.). New York: Harper & Row. (Originalwork published 1892)

Jones, G. E. (1977). The influence of stimulus context and somatic activity on phasic heart rate response during imagery (Doctoral dissertation, Bowling Green State University, 1976). *Dissertation Abstracts International*, 37, 4208B-4209B.

Jones, G. E., & Johnson, H. (1978). Physiological responding during self-generated imagery of contextually complete stimuli. *Psychophysiology, 15,* 439-446.

Jones, G. E., & Johnson, H. Heart rate and somatic concomitants of mental imagery. *Psychophysiology, 17,* 339-347.

Jordan, C. S., & Lenington, K. T. (1979). Physiological correlates of eidetic imagery and induced anxiety. *Journal of Mental Imagery, 3,* 31-42.

Kemeny, J. G. (1955). Man viewed as a machine. *Scientific American, 192,* 18-67.

Klinke, R., & Galley, N. (1974). Efferent innervation of vestibular and auditory receptors. *Physiological Reviews, 54,* 316-357.

Krill, A. E., Wieland, A. M., & Ostfeld, A. M. (1960). The effect of two hallucinogenic agents on human retina function. *Archives of Ophthalmology, 64,* 724-733.

Kulpe, O. (1893). *Outlines of psychology* (E. B. Titchener, Trans.). New York: Macmillan.

Kunzendorf, R. G. (1981). Individual differences in imagery and autonomic control. *Journal of Mental Imagery, 5,* 47-60.

Kunzendorf, R. G. (1982). Mental images, appreciation of grammatical patterns, and creativity. *Journal of Mental Imagery, 6,* 183-202.

Kunzendorf, R. G. (1984). Centrifugal effects of eidetic imaging on flash electroretinograms and autonomic responses. *Journal of Mental Imagery, 5,* 47-60.

Kunzendorf, R. G. (1989). After-images of eidetic images: A developmental study. *Journal of Mental Imagery, 13,* 55-62.

Kunzendorf, R. G. (1990). Mind-brain identity theory: A materialistic foundation for the psychophysiology of mental imagery. In R. Kunzendorf & A. Sheikh (Eds.), *The psychophysiology of mental imagery: Theory, research, and application* (pp. 9-36). Amityville, NY: Baywood.

Kunzendorf, R. G., & Bradbury, J. L. (1983). Better liars have better imaginations. *Psychological Reports, 52,* 634.

Kunzendorf, R., Jesses, M., Michaels, A., Caiazzo-Fluellen, G. & Butler, W. (in press). Imagination and perceptual development: Effects of auditory imaging on the brainstem evoked potentials of children, adult musicians, and other adults. In R. G. Kunzendorf (Ed.), *Mental imagery.* New York: Plenum.

Lang, P. J. (1979). Emotional imagery and visceral control. In R. J. Gatchel & K. Price (Eds.), *Clinical applications of biofeedback: Appraisal and status.* New York: Pergamon.

Lang, P. J., Kozak, M. J., Miller, G. A., Levin, D. N., & McLean, A. (1980). Emotional imagery: Conceptual structure and pattern of somato-visceral response. *Psychophysiology, 17,* 179-192.

Lang, P. J., Troyer, W. G., Twentyman, C. T., & Gatchel, R. J. (1975). Differential effects of heart rate modification training on college students, older males, and patients with ischemic heart disease. *Psychosomatic Medicine, 37,* 429-446.

Leber, W. R. (1979). Stimulus familiarity and muscular involvement as determinants of image-produced arousal (Doctoral dissertation, Bowling Green State University, 1979). *Dissertation Abstracts International, 40,* 1928B-1929B.

Leigh, H. (1978). Self-control, biofeedback, and change in'psychosomatic' approach. *Psychotherapy and Psychosomatics, 30,* 130-136.

Liberman, A. M. (1970). The grammars of speech and language. *Cognitive Psychology, 1,* 301-323.

Liberman, A. M., Cooper, F. S., Harris, K. S., & MacNeilage, P. F. (1963). Motor theory of speech perception. *Journal of the Acoustical Society of America, 35,* 1114.

Lindauer, M. S. (1977). Imagery from the point of view of psychological aesthetics, the arts, and creativity. *Journal of Mental Imagery, 1,* 343-362.

Lynch, W. C., Hama, H., Kohn, S., & Miller, N. E. (1976). Instrumental control of peripheral vasomotor responses in children. *Psychophysiology, 13,* 219-221.

Mangan, G. L. (1974). Personality and conditioning: Some personality, cognitive and psychophysiological parameters of classical appetitive (sexual) GSR conditioning. *Pavlovian Journal of Biological Sciences, 9,* 125-135.

Marks, I., & Huson, J. (1973). Physiological aspects of neutral and phobic imagery: Further observations. *British Journal of Psychiatry, 122,* 567-572.

Marks, I., Marset, P., Boulougouris, J., & Huson, J. (1971). Physiological accompaniments of neutral and phobic imagery. *Psychological Medicine, 1,* 299-307.

Marzillier, J. S., Carroll, D., & Newland, J. R. (1979). Self-report and physiological changes accompanying repeated imaging of a phobic scene. *Behaviour Research and Therapy, 17,* 71-77.

McCanne, T. R., & Iennarella, R. S. (1980). Cognitive and somatic events associated with discriminative changes in heart rate. *Psychophysiology, 17*, 18-28.

McMahon, C. E. (1975). The wind of the cannon ball. *Psychotherapy and Psychosomatics, 26*, 125-131.

Mowrer, O. H. (1977). Mental imagery: An indispensable psychological concept. *Journal of Mental Imagery, 1*, 303-325.

Oswald, I. (1957). After-images from retina and brain. *Quarterly Journal of Experimental Psychology, 9*, 88-100.

Pepper, S. C. (1960). A neural-identity theory of mind. In S. Hook (Ed.), *Dimensions of Mind*. New York: Collier.

Pylyshyn, Z. W. (1973). What the mind's eye tells the mind's brain. *Psychological Bulletin, 80*, 1-24.

Pylyshyn, Z. W. (1978). Imagery and artificial intelligence. In C. Savage (Ed.), *Minnesota studies in the philosophy of science* (Vol. 9, *Perception and cognition: Issues in the foundations of psychology*). Minneapolis: University of Minnesota Press.

Rehm, L. P. (1973). Relationships among measures of visual imagery. *Behaviour Research and Therapy, 11*, 265-270.

Reperant, J., Vesselkin, N. P., Rio, J. P., Ermakova, T., Miceli, D., Peyrichoux, J., & Weidner, C. (1981). La voie visuelle centrifuge n'existe-t-elle que chez les oiseaux? *Revue Canadienne de Biologie, 40*, 29-46.

Richardson, J. T. E. (1978). Mental imagery and memory: Coding ability or coding preference? *Journal of Mental Imagery, 2*, 101-115.

Richardson, J. T. E. (1980). *Mental imagery and human memory* . New York: St. Martins.

Rimm, D. C., & Bottrell, J. (1969). Four measures of visual imagination. *Behaviour Research and Therapy, 7*, 63-69.

Roberts, R. J., & Weerts, T. C. (1982). Cardiovascular responding during anger and fear imagery. *Psychological Reports, 50*, 219-230.

Roger, M., & Galand, G. (1981). Operant conditioning of visual evoked potentials in man. *Psychophysiology, 18*, 477-82.

Schneider, J., Smith, C. W., Minning, C., Whitcher, S., & Hermanson, J. (in press). Guided imagery and immune system function in normal subjects: A summary of research findings. In R. G. Kunzendorf (Ed.), *Mental imagery* . New York: Plenum.

Schwartz, G. E. (1971). Cardiac responses to self-induced thoughts. Psychophysiology, 8, 462-467.

Schwartz, G. E. (1975). Biofeedback, self-regulation and the patterning of physiological processing. *American Scientist, 63*, 314-324.

Schwartz, G. E., & Higgins, J. (1971). Cardiac activity preparatory to overt and covert behavior. *Science, 173*, 1144-46.

Schwartz, G. E., Weinberger, D. A., & Singer, J. A. (1981). Cardiovascular differentiation of happiness, sadness, anger, and fear following imagery and exercise. *Psychosomatic Medicine, 43*, 343-364.

Shea, J. (1985). Effects of absorption and instructions on heart rate control. Journal of *Mental Imagery, 9*, 87-100.

Sheehan, P. W., & Neisser, U. (1969). Some variables affecting the vividness of imagery in recall. *British Journal of Psychology, 60*, 71-80.

Skinner, B. F. (1974). *About behaviorism*. New York: Knopf.

Spector, N. H. (1987). Old and new strategies in the conditioning of immune responses. *Annals of the New York Academy of Sciences, 496*, 522-531.

Stewart, J. C. (1966). An experimental investigation of imagery. *Dissertation Abstracts, 27*, 1285B.

Taylor, N. B., & Cameron, H. G. (1922). Voluntary acceleration of the heart. *American Journal of Physiology, 61*, 385-398.

Van Hasselt, P. (1972-1973). The centrifugal control of retinal function: A review. *Ophthalmic Research, 4*, 298-320.

Wagman, R., & Stewart, C. G. (1974). Visual imagery and hypnotic susceptibility. *Perceptual and Motor Skills, 38*, 815-822.

Walczyk, J. J., & Hall, V. C. (1988). The relationship between imagery vividness ratings and imagery accuracy. *Journal of Mental Imagery, 12*, 163-172.

Waters, W. F., & McDonald, D. G. (1973). Autonomic response tp auditory, visual and imagined stimuli in a systematic desensitization context. *Behaviour Research and Therapy, 11*, 577-585.

Watson, J. B. (1913). Image and affection in behavior. *Journal of Philosophy, Psychology, and Scientific Methods*, 10, 421-428.

Wein, K. S. (1979). The effects of direct and imaginal stimulation on physiological and self-report measures: A test of the continuity assumption (Doctoral dissertation, University of North Carolina at Greensboro, 1978). *Dissertation Abstracts International*, 39, 6149B-6150B.

IMAGINATION AND PERCEPTUAL DEVELOPMENT:
EFFECTS OF AUDITORY IMAGING ON THE BRAINSTEM EVOKED POTENTIALS OF
CHILDREN, ADULT MUSICIANS, AND OTHER ADULTS

Robert G. Kunzendorf, Ph.D., Michael Jesses, B.A., Athena Michaels,
Gina Caiazzo-Fluellen, and William Butler, B.A.

Department of Psychology
University of Lowell
Lowell, MA 01854

In the present research, we examined the effects of auditory imaging on the brainstem
reponses of children, adult musicians, and other adults. Previously, researchers have looked for
efferent effects of attention on the brainstem auditory evoked potentials of adults, but have
neglected to look for efferent effects of auditory imaging.

Auditory evoked potentials are obtained from EEG measurements, by repeatedly stimulating
the ears with an auditory signal, and by computer-averaging the signal-evoked EEGs. With
sufficient computer-averaging, signal-unrelated components of the 30-50 microvolt EEG are
averaged out, and signal-evoked waveforms of lesser amplitude are left. The earliest and
smallest of these signal-evoked waves appear within 10 milliseconds of signal onset, while the
underlying innervation travels through the brainstem. The most prominent waveform of the
brainstem evoked potential is the negatively charged trough of Wave 5--which occurs 6-8
milliseconds after a weak signal, exhibits an amplitude of less than 1 microvolt, and originates in
the inferior colliculus. Like all cochlear and brainstem responses, Wave 5 displays progressively
shorter latencies and progressively greater amplitudes, as the acoustic signal becomes
progressively more intense (Hughes,1985; Picton, Hillyard, Krausz, & Galambos, 1974).

Several recent studies of the brainstem evoked potential have tested for an efferent effect of
attention on Wave 5, in attempts to elucidate the functional role of efferent nerves to the cochlea
(Klinke & Galley, 1974; Ross, 1971). Unfortunately, these studies have simply assumed that
attention is an unconscious 'gating' process, in accordance with the computer metaphor for mind,
and have completely neglected evidence that attention is a process of conscious 'anticipatory
imaging' (Mowrer, 1977; Piaget & Inhelder,1971). Inasmuch as all imaging, 'anticipatory' and
otherwise, is subject to *individual differences*, it should come as no surprise that three brainstem
studies of attention obtained longer Wave 5 latencies during inattention (Brix, 1984; Lukas,
1980, 1981) and the three other studies obtained no significant brainstem changes during
inattention (Collet & Duclaux, 1986; Davis & Beagley, 1985; Picton, Stapells, & Campbell,
1981). Indeed, in a direct study of individual differences in the efferent effects of attention,
Sommer (1985) found that inattention increases Wave 5 latency in electrodermal nonresponders,
but not in responders. Electrodermal nonresponders constitute less than ten percent of the
general population (Venables, 1977), but they constitute half of the schizophrenic population
(Gruzelier & Venables, 1972, 1973)--an abnormal population whose images are subject to
confusion with perceptual representations and, thus, are candidates for efferent representation in
the peripheral nervous system (PNS). In addition, electrodermal nonresponding is found in half
of all three-year-old children (Venables, 1978), a population whose mental images are as vivid as
perceptual representations (Kunzendorf, 1989) and, also, are candidates for efferent
representation. Our current research examines both children's brainstem evoked potentials and
normal adults' brainstem evoked potentials, not only when the evoking click is attended and
unattended, but also when it is imaged louder and imaged softer.

But if it should turn out that children's brainstem responses are enhanced by anticipatory images of sound, and enhanced even more by vivid images of louder sound, then surely it need not follow that the developmental function of these efferent images is to minimize PNS differences between imagination and perception. Apparently, for cases where such differences are minimized, the central nervous system (CNS) has evolved 'source monitoring' mechanisms-- mechanisms through which normal people differentiate the *central source* of imaginal sensations and the *peripheral source* of perceptual sensations (Kunzendorf, 1987-1988; Kunzendorf & Hoyle, 1989). Still, these monitoring mechanisms merely compensate for efferent images, and suggest no reason why such images should occur in the first place. One possible reason why efferent imaging should be useful, especially during childhood, is suggested by Piaget and examined by our present research.

As Piaget and Inhelder (1971) note, the sensory image is not a copy of perception, but is a reconstruction of perceptual sensations:

> According to the hypothesis that the image is a prolongation of perception, the image would tend to reproduce everything that had been perceived in the past, and would then anticipate situations not previously perceived by analogy...We adopt the other hypothesis that the images originate in the internalization of imitation, [and that] the child imitates only what he can understand or is well on the way to understanding. (p. 367).
>
> The fact that the image is able to reproduce the content of perceptions, their shape, color, etc., if not their 'vividness' - proves nothing either for or against the hypothesis in question. For, if the image derived from imitation, it would, in any case, imitate perceptual impressions, and would induce the partial reafference explaining the simili-sensible aspects, in exactly the same way as if it were merely a prolongation. (p. 365)

Extending this Piagetian hypothesis to efferent images and their functions, Kunzendorf (1982, 1990) suggests that the construction of cochlear and retinal images allows evolving minds to develop and test the rules of auditory and visual perception. For example, the retinal imagery which is constructed by children (Kunzendorf, 1989) allows them to develop and test basic rules of linear perspective--rules which everyone needs in order to translate retinal sensations into three-dimensional percepts. Likewise, the retinal imagery which is constructed by imaginative and artistic adults (Kunzendorf, 1984) allows them to develop and test refined rules of linear perspective--rules which artists need in order to perceive new visual relationships and to imagine new visual possibilities. Based on this functional interpretation of efferent visual imagery, the present study of efferent auditory imagery examines children's and musicians' brainstem image-evoked potentials, and compares them to randomly sampled adults' image-evoked potentials.

Presently, four brainstem auditory evoked potentials (BSAEPs) were obtained from 13 children, 13 adult musicians, and 13 other adults. One of the four BSAEPs was obtained while subjects listened attentively to the evoking clicks, and another was obtained while subjects counted backwards and ignored the clicks. Still another BSAEP was sampled while subjects imaged the clicks sounding louder, and the remaining BSAEP was sampled while subjects imaged the clicks sounding softer. It was predicted that children's and musicians' imaging would have the greatest effect on Wave 5 of the BSAEP.

METHOD

Subjects

BSAEPs were sampled from three groups of subjects--adult musicians, other adults, and children--until a discernible Wave 5 was obtained for 13 adult musicians, 13 other adults, and 13 children. The adult musicians were students in the College of Music at the University of Lowell, and were between 18 and 29 years of age. The other adults were students in General Psychology classes at the University of Lowell, and were between 18 and 20 years of age. The children, who had written parental permission to participate, were relatives of the latter adults, and were between 7 and 12 years of age (9.7 years on the average).

Every adult and child was tested individually. Every child was asked to observe his or her adult relative being tested and, thereafter, was tested in the presence of this relative.

Apparatus

Each subject's brain potentials (EEGs) were recorded at the vertex from a miniature disc electrode, referenced to one ear-clip electrode and grounded by another ear-clip electrode. EEG recordings between 0.3 Hz and 3kHz were amplified with a Grass Instruments 7P511 AC Amplifier.

In order to evoke brain potentials for computer averaging, an 8000 Hz click lasting .25 msecs was generated 500 times in succession--once every 200 msecs--by a computer-interfaced Coulbourn Instruments signal generator and audio amplifier. The individual clicks were transmitted through air-conduction earphones and, 11.0 msecs after their generation, were presented to both ears at 55 dBHL.

Upon every presentation of the evoking click, amplified EEGs were sampled 100 times, once every 0.1 msec, and were digitized with a Tecmar PC-Mate Lab Master. If any of the 100 sampled digits for a particular click was below the digital floor (-2047) or above the digital ceiling (-2047), then all 100 sampled digits were rejected by computer.

Following each bout of 500 successive clicks, all unrejected 100-digit EEGs were summed in an IBM Personal Computer. Throughout each subject's testing, 13 such 100-digit EEGs were summed for 13 different 500-click bouts--1 practice bout, plus 3 bouts in each of 4 experimental conditions. After 3 bouts (1500 evoking clicks) per experimental condition, all unrejected 100-digit EEGs from each condition were computer-averaged, and the resulting BSAEP for each condition was plotted on an IBM Graphics Printer.

Procedure

At the outset of the experiment, the individually tested subjects participated in a practice bout, before which they had been instructed "to notice how loud the bout's 500 clicks are". Thereafter, subjects participated in three blocks of experimental bouts. The first block, like the second and third, contained a randomly ordered succession of 4 experimental bouts: 1 'attentive listening' bout, 1 'inattentive counting' bout, 1 'imaging louder' bout, and 1 'imaging softer' bout.

Before each of the three 'attentive listening' bouts, subjects were instructed "to listen attentively to the 500 clicks and to notice how loud they really are". Before each of the three 'inattentive counting' bouts, adults were instructed "to silently count backwards by threes, starting at [1700, e.g.], and to ignore the clicks"; children were instructed "to silently count backwards by ones, starting at [250, e.g.], and to ignore the clicks". Before each of the three 'imaging louder' bouts, subjects were instructed "to image the clicks sounding much louder than they really are". Finally, before each of the three 'imaging softer' bouts, subjects were instructed "to image the clicks sounding much softer, either by imaging background music that drowns out the clicks or by imaging silence, whichever method of imaging works best".

RESULTS

The brainstem effects of attention and imagery are exemplified in Figure 1, where the BSAEPs of an adult musician are depicted. In order to quantify the four BSAEPs from this and other subjects, latencies of the BSAEPs were measured from click onset to the most reliably observed wave--the negatively charged trough at the end of Wave 5. In addition, amplitudes of the BSAEPs were measured from the positively charged peak of Wave 4 or Wave 5, whichever was higher, to the negatively charged trough of Wave 5. Table 1 describes the Wave 5 latencies and Wave 5 amplitudes of the 13 adult musicians, the 13 other adults, and the 13 children; Table 2 summarizes the Wave 5 latencies and Wave 5 amplitudes of all 39 subjects.

For the musician whose BSAEPs are depicted in Figure 1, imaging softer clicks dramatically increased the latency of Wave 5 and dramatically decreased the amplitude of Wave 5; to a lesser extent, counting backwards did the same. Consistent with this depiction, the 13 musicians in Table 1 exhibited a significantly longer Wave 5 latency when imaging softer clicks than when attentively listening. Moreover, a multivariate analysis of variance confirmed that, for the Wave 5 latencies in Table 1, there was a significant interaction between the three subject groupings and the four experimental conditions, $F(6,68)=2.38$, $p=.038$.

Whereas musicians' images of softer clicks were more effective in modifying BSAEPs, children's images of louder clicks were more effective. When the 13 children in Table 1 imaged louder clicks, they exhibited both a significantly shorter Wave 5 latency and a significantly

Table 1. Effects of Imagination and Attention on Brainstem AEPs of 13 Children, 13 Adult Musicians, and 13 Other Adults: Means (and SDs) of Wave 5N Latency and Wave 5P-5N Amplitude

		Attend to the clicks	Count back- wards	Image clicks louder	Image clicks softer
Latency in milliseconds					
	Children	7.87 (.92)	7.80 (.90)	7.45a (.93)	7.78 (.87)
	Musicians	7.04 (.44)	7.09 (.41)	7.05 (.41)	7.23b (.39)
	Others	7.23 (.80)	7.34 (.78)	7.18 (.75)	7.28 (.49)
Amplitude in microvolts					
	Children	0.32 (.19)	0.37 (.32)	0.45c (.25)	0.34 (.18)
	Musicians	0.35 (.27)	0.29 (.27)	0.42 (.34)	0.35 (.34)
	Others	0.36 (.16)	0.30 (.22)	0.38 (.18)	0.30 (.21)

a This 'image louder' lat. is significantly less than children's 'attend' lat., p=.003.
b This 'image softer' lat. is reliably greater than musicians' 'attend' lat., p=.008.
c This 'image louder' amp. is reliably greater than children's 'attend' amp., p<.032.

greater Wave 5 amplitude. Although the interaction between subject groupings and experimental conditions was significant for Wave 5 latencies, as noted above, it was not significant for Wave 5 amplitudes, $F(6,68)=0.69$. Nevertheless, the main effect of experimental conditions was significant both for amplitudes, $F(3,34)=2.88$, p=.050, and for latencies, $F(3,34)=4.96$, p=.006. Thus like the children, all 39 subjects in Table 2 exhibited a significantly shorter Wave 5 latency and a significantly greater Wave 5 amplitude, when imaging louder clicks.

Although the 13 children in Table 1 generally had a longer Wave 5 latency than the 26 adults, the main effect of subject groupings on latency was not quite significant, $F(2,36)=3.10$, p=.057. Also, the main effect of subject groupings on amplitude was not significant,

Table 2. Effects of Imagination and Attention on Brainstem AEPs of All 39 Subjects: Means (and SDs) of Wave 5N Latency and Wave 5P-5N Amplitude

	Attend to the clicks	Count back- wards	Image clicks louder	Image clicks softer
Latency in milliseconds				
	7.38 (.82)	7.41 (.77)	7.22a (.73)	7.43 (.65)
Amplitude in microvolts				
	0.34 (.21)	0.32 (.27)	0.42b (.26)	0.33 (.25)

a This 'image louder' latency is significantly less than the 'attend' latency, p=.010.
b This 'image louder' amplitude is reliably greater than the 'attend' ampl., p=.014.

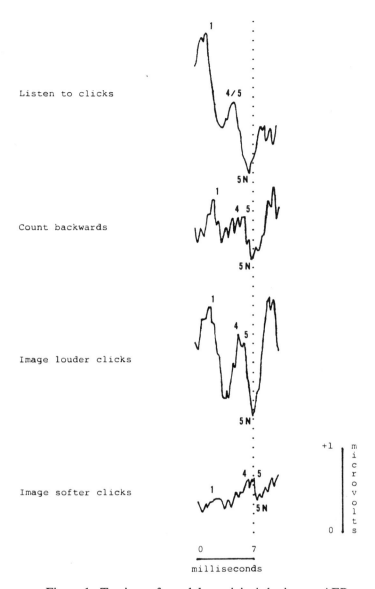

Listen to clicks

Count backwards

Image louder clicks

Image softer clicks

Figure 1. Tracings of an adult musician's brainstem AEPs.

F(2,36)=0.09. In previous research comparing adults and children, the latter have exhibited both a longer Wave 5 latency and a smaller Wave 5 amplitude (Salamy, Mendelson, & Tooley, 1982).

DISCUSSION

In the present study of brainstem auditory evoked potentials (BSAEPs), no Wave 5 differences between the 'attentive listening' condition and the 'inattentive counting' condition were found. Yet, relative to the 'attentive listening' condition, the 'imaging softer' condition increased the Wave 5 latency evoked by 55 dBHL clicks--just as perceiving softer clicks would do. Also, relative to the 'attentive listening' condition, the 'imaging louder' condition decreased the Wave 5 latency and increased the Wave 5 amplitude--just as perceiving louder clicks would

163

do. Furthermore, these percept-like effects of imaging on Wave 5 of the BSAEP were greatest in children and in adult musicians.

In order for our present effects of imaging to be attributed to efferent innervation of the brainstem and cochlea, the possibility that such effects are attributable to other efferent mediators needs to be considered and ruled out. In particular, the possibility that our effects are due to image-induced contractions of middle ear muscle needs to be considered. Our use of 8000 Hz clicks at 55 dBHL appears to rule out this possibility, inasmuch as the contractions in question do not affect brainstem responses to tones as high-pitched as 8000 Hz or as soft as 55 dBHL (Lukas, 1980, 1981). In the absence of other possibilities of image-induced mediation, we attribute our results to the efferent effects of imaging on the brainstem.

Finally, our finding that children's and adult musicians' auditory images produce percept-like effects in the brainstem, whereas other adults' images do not, suggests that efferent images serve a developmental function. In this regard, Kunzendorf (1982, 1990) has suggested specifically that, by constructing efferent images, the developing perceiver can efficiently generate and test the rules that he or she needs in order to decode cochlear sensations into perceptual relationships. Indeed, recent research confirms that highly imaginative artists are better perceivers of aesthetic relationships (Bilotta and Lindauer, 1980; Lindauer, 1977). Still, further research needs to be addressed to this suggested function, and other possible functions, of efferent cochlear innervation. And should "other possible functions" have anything to do with attention, then--given our current findings--the operational definition of attention must shift from computer-based 'gating' operations to image-based 'anticipatory' operations.

ACKNOWLEDGMENT

The authors thank Stuart Smith, Professor of Computer Science at the University of Lowell, for designing the auditory system used in this study.

REFERENCES

Bilotta, J., & Lindauer, M. S. (1980). Artistic and nonartistic backgrounds as determinants of the cognitive responses to the arts. *Bulletin of the Psychonomic Society*, 15, 354-356.

Brix, R. (1984). The influence of attention on the auditory brainstem evoked responses. *Acta Oto-Laryngologica*, 98, 89-92.

Collet, L., & Duclaux, R. (1986). Auditory brainstem evoked responses and attention. *Acta Oto-Laryngologica*, 101, 439-441.

Davis, A. E., & Beagley, H. A. (1985). Acoustic brainstem responses for clinical use: The effect of attention. *Clinical Otolaryngology*, 10, 311-314.

Gruzelier, J., & Venables, P. (1972). Skin conductance orienting activity in a heterogeneous sample of schizophrenics. *Journal of Nervous and Mental Disease*, 155, 277-287.

Gruzelier, J., & Venables, P. (1973). Skin conductance responses to tones with and without attentional sig-nificance in schizophrenic and nonschizophrenic psychiatric patients. *Neuropsychologia*, 11, 221-230.

Hatanaka, T., Shuto, H., Yasuhara, A., & Kobayashi, Y. (1988). Ipsilateral and contralateral recordings of auditory brainstem responses to monaural stimulation. *Pediatric Neurology*, 4, 354-357.

Hughes, J. R. (1985). A review of the auditory system and its evoked potentials. *American Journal of EEG Technology*, 25, 115-158.

Klinke, R., & Galley, N. (1974). Efferent innervation of vestibular and auditory receptors. *Physiological Reviews*, 54, 316-357.

Kunzendorf, R. G. (1982). Mental images, appreciation of grammatical patterns, and creativity. *Journal of Mental Imagery*, 6, 183-201.

Kunzendorf, R. G. (1984). Centrifugal effects of eidetic imaging on flash electroretinograms and autonomic responses. *Journal of Mental Imagery*, 8, 67-76.

Kunzendorf, R. G. (1987-1988). Self-consciousness as the monitoring of cognitive states: A theoretical perspective. *Imagination, Cognition, and Personality*, 7, 3-22.

Kunzendorf, R. G. (1989). Afterimages of eidetic images: A developmental study. *Journal of Mental Imagery*, 13, 55-62.

Kunzendorf, R. G. (1990). Mind-brain identity theory: A materialistic foundation for the psychophysiology of mental imagery. In R. G.Kunzendorf & A. A. Sheikh (Eds.), *The *psychophysiology of mental imagery: Theory, research, and application* (pp. 9-36). Amityville, NY: Baywood.

Kunzendorf, R. G., & Hoyle, D. (1989). Auditory percepts, mental images, and hypnotic hallucinations: Similarities and differences in auditory evoked potentials. In J. E. Shorr, P. Robin, J. A. Connella, & M. Wolpin (Eds.), *Imagery: Current perspectives* (pp. 1-12). New York: Plenum.

Lindauer, M. S. (1977). Imagery from the point of view of psychological aesthetics, the arts, and creativity. *Journal of Mental Imagery*, 1, 343-362.

Lukas, J. H. (1980). Human auditory attention: The olivocochlear bundle may function as a peripheral filter. *Psychophysiology*, 17, 444-452.

Lukas, J. H. (1981). The role of efferent inhibition in human auditory attention: An examination of the auditory brainstem potentials. *International Journal of Neuroscience*, 12, 137-145.

Mowrer, O. H. (1977). Mental imagery: An indispensable psychological concept. *Journal of Mental Imagery*, 2, 303-326.

Piaget, J., & Inhelder, B. (1971). *Mental imagery in the child* (P. A. Chilton, Trans.). New York: Basic Books. (Original work published 1966)

Picton, T. W., Hillyard, S. A., Krausz, H. I., & Galambos, R. (1974). Human auditory evoked potentials. I: Evaluation of components. *Electroencephalography and Clinical Neurophysiology*, 36, 179-190.

Picton, T. W., Stapells, D. R., & Campbell, K. B. (1981). Auditory evoked potentials from the human cochlea and brainstem. *Journal of Otolaryngology*, Supplement 9, 1-41.

Ross, M. D. (1971). Flueorescence and electron microscopic observations of the general visceral, efferent innervation of the inner ear. *Acta Oto-Laryngologica*, Supplement 286, 1-18.

Salamy, A., Mendelson, T., & Tooley, W. H. (1982). Developmental profiles for the brainstem auditory evoked potential. *Early Human Development*, 6 331-339.

Sommer, W. (1985). Selective attention differentially affects brainstem auditory evoked potentials of electrodermal responders and nonresponders. *Psychiatry Research*, 16, 227-232.

Venables, P. H. (1977). The electrodermal psychophysiology of schizophrenics and children at risk for schizophrenia: Controversies and developments. *Schizophrenia Bulletin*, 3, 28-48.

Venables, P. H. (1978). Psychophysiology and psychometrics. *Psychophysiology*, 15, 302-315.

IMAGERY AND THE SINISTRALITY OF SYMPTOMS

Paul Bakan, Ph.D.

Psychology Department
Simon Fraser University
Burnaby, British Columbia, Canada V5A 1S6

INTRODUCTION

I would like to consider a phenomenon which has been observed over many years, namely, the greater likelihood of symptoms, especially psychogenic symptoms, on the left side of the body, i.e. the sinistrality of symptoms. The symptom is at the heart of all medical encounters. This encounter begins with one symptom and then goes on to diagnosis, prognosis and treatment. But at the very core of this encounter, in the very conception of the symptom, there is a semantic confusion which becomes obvious in distinctions between organic and functional, real and imaginary, organic and hysterical and so on. It was the problem of hysterical symptoms which gave rise to psychoanalysis and its many psychotherapeutic offshoots. The possibility of a relationship between imagination and symptom formation was seriously considered well before the nineteenth century. Let us consider Robert Burton's seventeenth century work, *The Anatomy of Melancholy* (Burton, 1948), for some historical perspective on this matter. Burton was a Christian minister, whose book was referred to by the famous physician William Osler as "a medical treatise, the greatest indeed written by a layman..." (Jackson, 1989). Burton saw the root cause of melancholy or depression, as well as other symptoms, in a "damaged imagination", i.e. an imagination which somehow had escaped from the control of reason to become a faculty that "is most powerful and strong, and often hurts...". The faculty of imagination when corrupted, hurt, misaffected, depraved, or damaged, he saw as the cause of melancholy. The damaged imagination, he said, misrepresents matters to the understanding, and makes patients see and hear "that which indeed is neither heard nor seen". Burton seems to be distinguishing here between imagery and perception. In reviewing the work of other physicians Burton singles out the work of Thomas Fienus (1567-1631) for whom he had the highest regard, referring to him as "worth all of them together" (Rather, 1967). Fienus presented a model in which the imagination was seen to stir up the emotions--leading to bodily changes in the humours and spirits, which in turn lead to bodily symptoms. This is essentially a psychosomatic model, wherein a disturbed imagination produces physiological changes leading to psychogenic symptoms. This sixteenth century model prefigures contemporary understanding of the relationship between imagination and symptoms.

SINISTRALITY OF SYMPTOMS

I would like now to address the question: Why do psychogenic symptoms preferentially show up on the left side of the body? I introduce this topic by describing an experiment I have recently completed. Standing before a class of 278 students, I read to them a script designed to suggest and induce a feeling of tingling in the hand. I then asked the subjects to indicate on a 3 x 5 card which hand was the first to feel the tingle..right, left, both simultaneously, or no tingle at all. Results: 63% of the right-handed Ss who reported a unilateral tingle reported that it was the left hand that first felt the tingle. This differed statistically at the .001 level from a 50% chance expectation.

This is hardly a new discovery. There is a long history of similar findings of an excess of left-sided unilateral psychogenic or hysterical symptoms (Harrington, 1987; Stern, 1983). Following a review of this history I would like to consider symptom sinistrality in the light of a late twentieth century understanding of imagery, cerebral hemispheric asymmetry and some related matters.

There is an early description of left-sided imaginal symptomatology in a work written in 1747 by Julien de la Mettrie (Harrington, 1987). He tells how the philospher Blaise Pascal "always required a rampart of chairs or else someone close to him at the left, to prevent his seeing horrible abysses into which he ...feared that he might fall...Great man on one side of his nature, on the other half he was mad." He goes on to say "Madness and wisdom each had its compartment, or its lobe, the two separated by a fissure." Note that as early as 1747 de la Mettrie already anticipates the importance of a relation between hemispheric asymmetry and this lateralized disturbance of the imagination. This case of Blaise Pascal is discussed a century and a half later by Sigmund Freud, who refers to it as a case of "obsession and phobia...allied to the symptoms of hysteria..."

Nineteenth Century

In the early nineteenth century phrenologists reported on cases of unilateral mental disorder. Gall reported the case of a Viennese minister who was tortured by insults coming from his left side, so that he kept looking to the left. Gall also reported a case of a young woman who claimed that everything felt different on her left side than on her right side, and she also claimed that sometimes her power of thinking would stop on her left and an icy torpor would grip her skull (Harrington, 1987).

Probably the first scientific study of this problem is found in Briquet's work, the *Traite Clinique et Therapeutique de l'Hysterie* (Briquet, 1859). It is because of this work that hysteria is sometimes referred to as Briquet's disease. Briquet reported on an extensive series of 430 cases in which hysterical hemianesthesias and hemiplegias were observed three times as often on the left side as on the right. Later he extended this finding to hysterical pain symptoms as well. Despite these observations of laterality Briquet resisted an explanation in terms of hemispheric asymmetry of the brain. Rather he felt that the muscles on the left side were weaker as a result of education and habits, and that this weakness resulted in easier fatigue which is responsible for the hysterical symptoms. In 1864, Trousseau, the neurologist who contributed the word "aphasia" to our language, also reported that unilateral hysteria was more likely on the left side of the body. He could offer no reason for this. This was the year when Broca asserted a hemispheric asymmetry for language in the left hemisphere.

The problem was taken up again by Armand de Fleury in 1871. He accepted the finding of an excess of left-sided hysterical symptoms and he offered possibly the earliest explanation in terms of hemispheric asymmetry. His argument was that there is an asymmetry between the cerebral hemispheres, in that the right hemisphere, which controlled the left side, had a less plentiful blood supply than the left hemisphere. Consequently it was weaker and less powerful in its reactions, and more vulnerable to hysterical afflictions. Three years later in 1874, Charles Edouard Brown-Sequard, an influential neurologist of the time, reported on his collection of 121 cases of unilateral hysterical paralysis; 97 of these were left-sided and only 24 were right-sided. In his explanation of this finding he associated the right hemisphere with emotional reactivity. "The right side of the brain", he said, "serves chiefly the emotional manifestations, hysterical manifestations included". This right brain/emotionality relationship is a recurring theme in the history of hemispheric asymmetry.

In France the name of Charcot was very closely associated with hysteria. It was in Charcot's clinic at Salpetriere that Freud had his early exposure to hysterical conditions. Charcot believed in the asymmetry of hysterical symptomatology. In 1881 Paul Richer, of the Charcot school, actually referred to the notion of hysteria's predilection for the left side of the body as Charcot's Rule. But by this time Charcot had already expressed his doubts about it since he now thought that hysteria could be found almost as frequently on the right side as the left side (Harrington, 1987) .

Further reports of left side vulnerability to hysterical symptoms came from Pitres in 1891 and Gilles de la Tourette in 1891 and Clarke in 1892 (Clarke, 1892). One of the most influential studies of the left side/hysteria connection was that of Pierre Janet in 1899 (Harrington, 1987). Janet systematically studied the case records of 388 hysterical patients with anaesthesias and paralyses. Of these 388 there were 138 with bilateral symptoms, 148 with unilateral left-sided symptoms, and 102 with unilateral right-sided symptoms. Considering the unilateral cases the left/right ratio was about 3 to 2, somewhat less than Briquet's 3 to 1 ratio. Janet took his analysis a step further as he examined other symptoms and their relationship to the side affected by the major hysterical symptom. Thus he found differences between right and left-side hysterics in associated symptoms. Patients with right-sided hysteria were more likely to have language related disorders such as loss of voice and aphasia. Right-sided hysteria was also associated with disturbances of limb movement, and with respiratory disorders such as coughing and hiccups. Patients with left-sided hysteria were more likely to manifest somnambulism, fugue, and epileptiform attacks.

Twentieth Century

During the twentieth century the interest in left-sided symptoms continues, positive findings continue to accumulate, there are some references to hemispheric asymmetry, and a psycho-analytic flavor shows up in explanations for the asymmetry favoring the left side. In 1905 Whiting reported a 4 to 1 left/right ratio in symptoms, but was unable to explain it. In contrast Ernest Jones (the biographer of Freud and psychoanalyst) in 1908 studied 277 cases of hysterical hemiplegia and found no evidence of asymmetry. A year later in 1909 Dubois noted how striking it was to see so many hysterics avow feeling less on the left side (Harrington, 1987).

Purves-Stewart (1924) reported the frequent occurrence of hysterical hyperesthesia in "little islands of the skin", and "when not in the middle line, (they) are generally left-sided". Regarding hysterical anesthesia he said that "its commonest distribution is a hemianesthesia" usually left-sided. In 1926 the psychoanalyst Ferenczi accepted the fact that hysterical symptoms appear more often on the left side and argued that "in right-handed people...the sensational sphere for the left side shows...a certain predisposition for unconscious impulses" and the left side is placed at the service of unconscious libidinal fantasies (Ferenczi, 1926). In this view the unconscious itself is asymmetrically organized to favor left-sided expression, and thus the tendency to left-sided hysterical expression becomes integrated with psychoanalytical thinking.

In 1937 Halliday described a group of 21 cases of what he called "psychosomatic rheumatism". These patients reported pain in muscles, joints, tissues of the neck, shoulder, arms, stiffness, numbness, pricking sensations and sudden attacks of loss of power, but with no apparent evidence of organic disease. In 14 of the 21 cases the symptoms were lateralized, and in 13 of these 14 lateralized cases the symptoms were predominately on the left side. This study was followed by that of Boland and Carr in 1943, but with less dramatic results. In 50 cases of what they call "pure psychogenic rheumatism" they found 16 with lateralized symptoms, 9 on the left and 7 on the right (Stern, 1983).

In 1947 Edmonds reported on 87 "neurotic" patients from his general medical practice with symptoms of pain in the absence of any discernble organic origin (Edmonds, 1947). The pain symptom was unilateral in 51 of the 87 cases, and in 44 of the 51 lateralized cases the pain was mainly on the left side. Taking these three studies of psychogenic pain together we have 81 cases of lateralized pain, lateralized to the left in 66 cases or 81% of the cases. Edmonds provided an interesting theoretical account of his results in terms of functional hemispheric asymmetry. He argued that because of the left hemispheric dominance for language in right-handed persons, the emotional or what he called the "thalamic" impulses directed to the right side were under "cortical restraint". The right hemisphere is unable to provide such restraint and as a result the expression of emotion has more access to the left side of the body. He is presenting a theory of a hemispheric asymmetry of cortical restraint of emotional expression. The absence of such restraint in the right hemisphere, leads to more left-sided expression of symptoms with an emotional origin. This asssociation of the right hemisphere with emotional expression seems to revive the earlier view of Brown-Sequard in 1874 (Harrington, 1987).

By 1950 we find this kind of thinking reflected in the writings of Paul Schilder, a neurologist with a strong psychoanalytic bias (Schilder, 1950). In a discussion of non-perception in one half of the body he says: "One might assume that only centers in the right hemisphere have a sufficiently close relation to central emotional activities." The association of the right hemisphere with the unconscious is echoed by Werner (1952). He says: "If an injury weakens the left brain dominance, the right hemisphere can become active, releasing primitive and symbolic processes characteristic of the unconscious, which thus seems to be centered in the non-dominant hemisphere".

By the middle of the twentieth century there emerged a psychoanalytic account to explain the tendency to left-sided expression of psychogenic symptoms. These symptoms were deemed to be manifestations of unconscious emotional forces which have their home in the right hemisphere, and find expression on the left side of the body, which is intimately related to, and controlled by, the right hemisphere. This psychoanalytic view reaches full fruition in the work of Galin. Galin argues that certain aspects of right hemisphere functioning are congruent with the mode of cognition that psychoanalysts refer to as primary process. This is the form of thought said to characterize the unconscious mind in psychoanalytic theory. Galin considers the possibility that repression is a deconnection of certain psychic material, located in the right hemisphere, from the language centers of the left hemisphere. Since the right hemisphere is the locus for the unconscious mental contents, somatic representations, psychosomatic disorders, and somatic delusions should occur primarily on the left side of the body (Galin, 1974; Galin, 1976; Galin, Diamond, & Braff, 1977).

Before considering some other contemporary theoretical possibilities to account for the left-sided symptom proclivity, I would like to briefly review some of the empirical findings since 1950. Magee (1962) reported on a syndrome of paralysis and loss of sensation on a whole half of the body. He found that this syndrome was present on the right side of the body in only three of more than 50 cases observed. Kenyon found that 58 of 83 (70%) hypochondriac patients with lateralized symptoms experienced them on the left side (Kenyon, 1964). Prick is quoted as saying in 1965 that when a person develops a conversion paralysis it is as a rule manifested on the left and that if a bilateral conversion syndrome exists then one finds the conversion symptoms are more pronounced on the left side (Stern, 1983).

Merskey (Merskey, 1965) studied 100 psychiatric patients with persistent pain and found a trend toward more left-sided pain. Merskey and Spear (1967) studied a sample of 132 English psychiatric patients with pain most being depressed or anxious/hysterical. Of 92 lateralized pains 65 or 71% were on the left side. Stern (1977) studied all cases diagnosed "hysterical reaction, conversion type" at University of Iowa Hospitals in 1966-67. Of 114 patients with unilateral sensory symptoms 78 or 68% had them on the left (p=.001); of 81 with unilateral motor symptoms 52 or 64% had them on the left (p=.02). Galin studied hysterical patients and found that 36 of 55 or 66% had left-sided symptoms (p=.05) (Galin et al., 1977). Ley in an archival study of case histories of early writers on hysteria, such as Freud, Breuer, Janet, Charcot found that 66 of 100 cases had left-sided symptoms in cases of unilateral hysteria (Ley, 1980).

Fleminger (Fleminger, McClure, & Dalton, 1980) studied lateralized psychogenic somatic symptoms in 106 psychiatric outpatients. Eighteen of 24 (75%) with clearly lateralized sensory symptoms had them on the left side, and 9 of 14 or 65% with lateralized motor symptoms had them on the left-side. Merskey and Watson (1979) cited 10 clinical studies that consistently report left lateralization of pain symptoms at all body sites except for the face. These authors say that "the right hemisphere may play a special role in producing pain, conversion symptoms and disordered emotional expression". Axelrod, Noonan and Atanacio (1980) surveyed published reports of unilateral psychogenic symptoms and found a greater frequency of left-sided symptoms.

Blau, Wiles, and Solomon (1983) followed up on the work of Tavel (1964) who reported that 12 of 14 healthy subjects reported left-sided somatic symptoms when they engaged in hyperventilation. They reported on neurological referrals with possible diagnoses of migraine, multiple sclerosis, brachial neuritis, angina etc., where examination showed no organic disease, and where symptoms could be produced by hyperventilation and cured by breathing instruction. They found that 12 of 16 (75%) had left-sided symptoms. Keane (1989) studied gait disorders that were referred for neurological investigation and turned out to be hysterical. Of 60 patients, 13 were hemiparetic and 9 of these 13 had hemiparesis on the left side.

On the phantom experience

In 1551 a physician named Ambrose Pare referred to "..patients who have many months after the cutting away of the leg, grievously complained that they yet felt exceeding great pain of the leg so cut off". The reporting of awareness of a non-existent bodily part in a mentally competent individual is called a phantom; if the body part is a limb, then it is a phantom limb. It is usually associated with amputation of the body part. The phantom experience varies from acute pain, pricking, itching, burning, cramp, uneasiness and numbness to feelings which are hardly perceptible. Whether this is hysteric, psychogenic, or possibly organic in origin is a matter of dispute, but it turns out that the phantom experience is also one which is preferentially associated with the left side of the body (Weinstein, 1969).

In a study of a group of limb amputees it was found that the left-sided amputee was more likely to develop the phantom experience. High levels of phantom pain after amputation were found in 45% of left amputees, in contrast to only 24% of right amputees (Morgenstern, 1970). In a study of phantom experiences after mastectomy in females it was found that left breast phantoms appeared significantly earlier than did right breast phantoms (Weinstein, 1969). There is also evidence that the left breast is more often affected by cancer than is the right breast (Kramer, Albrecht, & Miller, 1985).

TOWARD AN EXPANDED MODEL

I would like to turn now to a consideration of some factors and variables which might be relevant in constructing a model that would account for the left-sided expression of symptoms. Perhaps we can, in the light of recent research, go beyond the simple psychoanalytic model. According to this model the right hemisphere is the repository of the emotional unconscious, which tends to find expression, not in words, but in the psychogenic or hysterical symptoms on the left side of the body. This may be due to the fact that, in the left hemisphere sensory data undergo a complex conceptual elaboration by means of language, while in the right hemisphere where there is less representation of language, they are processed in a more primitive way, so that they retain their immediateness and affective value. Though this model may represent a fair first approximation of an explanation for left-sided symptom expression, I believe that there have been research findings in recent years which can extend the model.

Emotion and the Hemispheres

The two cerebral hemispheres appear to have an asymmetric role in the mediation of emotions. Research on this problem has taken two pathways. The first suggests that the right hemisphere is essential to the regulation of emotion in general. The second is that the hemispheres are differentiated for handling emotion, the right hemisphere mediating negative affect, and the left hemisphere mediating positive affect (Davidson, & Fox, 1982; Sackeim, & Weber, 1982b).

The neuropsychological evidence suggests that the right hemisphere is essential for normal emotional communication (Flor-Henry, 1979; Heilman & et al, 1985; Sackeim et al., 1982b). It is needed for understanding emotion from tone of voice or facial expression. The left side of the face shows greater intensity of emotional expression than the right side of the face (Borod, Koff, & Caron, 1983). The left ear which is well-connected to the right hemisphere seems to have an advantage for interpreting emotion in tone of voice. The right hemisphere has more skill in dealing with non-verbal, analogical representation of information.

Relevant to the second approach, that of asymmetry of the hemispheres with respect to kind of emotion, is an experimental study of differential emotional response from right and left hemispheres (Dimond, Farrington, & Johnson, 1976). It was found that when people viewed unpleasant emotionally provocative films with an apparatus that allowed only the right hemisphere to see them, the films were perceived to be very unpleasant, significantly more unpleasant than when viewed by the left hemisphere. In their discussion of this result the authors say that "the right hemisphere adds its own emotional dimension which represents the thing perceived as more unpleasant and horrible, and thus aligns itself more with the characteristic perception of the depressive patient than with that of the normal individual."

There is good reason to believe that just as the right hemisphere has a depressive bias, the left hemisphere may have a manic bias. It has been shown that the manic state is characterized by greater left side activation. There is a form of epilepsy known as gelastic epilepsy in which the seizure activity takes the form of fits of uncontrollable laughter. EEG examination shows that in these cases the epileptic focus is on the left side of the brain (Sackeim et al., 1982a); left hemisphere hyperactivity seems to be involved in the laughter seizure. This suggests left hemisphere mediation of manic emotion.

Pain Thresholds and the Left Side

If there is a greater number of symptoms on the left side could this be due to a generally greater sensitivity of the left side? There is evidence of right-left asymmetry in sensory threshold for pain, with lower thresholds for pressure and pain on the left side (Weinstein & Sersen, 1961). In one study sensitivity for pressure was measured on the palms, forearms and soles of the feet. A majority of subjects were found to have greater sensitivity on the left side than on the right side. Greater pain sensitivity in the left than the right hand has also been shown for electrical stimulation (Wolff & Jarvick, 1964) and cold pressor pain (Murray & Safferstone, 1970).

The difference in pain thresholds between the right and left side of the body may be related to the hemispheric asymmetry of neurotransmitters (Glick & Shapiro, 1985). It is likely that much of the difference between the hemispheres has molecular correlates at the level of asymmetries in neurochemistry (Tucker & Williamson, 1984). Thus norepinephrine pathways and norepinephrine itself are more prevalent in the right hemisphere, whereas the dopamine pathway system is more closely associated with the left hemisphere. This seems to be related to a sensory vs. motor dichotomy, with norepinephrine pathways having a greater role in sensory functioning and dopamine pathways having a greater role in motor functioning. The norepinephrine system augments responses to sensory stimulation, especially novel stimuli. The greater norepinephrine activity of the right hemisphere may result in a bias leading to amplification of sensory activity and amplification of symptom activity on the left side of the body. The greater norepinephrine activity of the right hemisphere is thus consistent with greater sensitivity to stimuli on the left side. I expect that further understanding of lateralized neurochemistry will greatly enhance our understanding of the asymmetrical functioning of the hemispheres.

The Hypnosis Connection

Hysteria and hypnosis have a history of being lumped together somehow in the thinking of psychologists and psychiatrists. Such an association is found in the writings of Charcot, Breuer and Freud, Janet, and Lombroso. Perhaps the relationship is related to the fact that both hysteria and hypnosis are mediated by right hemisphere functioning. Both hysteria and hypnosis can produce psychogenic symptoms, and hypnosis has been used as a therapy to remove psychogenic symptoms.

Earlier in my talk today I described an experiment in which a script was used to induce by suggestion a feeling of tingling in the hand. The script was modelled after those used in hypnotic suggestion, and the tingle when it occurred unilaterally was found more frequently in the left hand. If this was akin to a hypnotically induced symptom, then why the preference for the left side. Could it be that hypnosis is somehow mediated by the right hemisphere? There is a study which shows that after a real hypnotic induction, it is easier to induce suggested responses on the left side of the body than on the right (Sackeim, 1982). Or putting it another way, the left side of the body is actually more hypnotizable than the right side. There seems to be a parallelism between left-sided preference for hysteric or psychogenic symptoms and left-sided preference for hypnotically induced symptoms.

Furthermore, there is a body of literature which suggests a close association between hypnosis or hypnotizability and the right hemisphere (Bakan, 1969; Crawford, 1981; Frumkin, Ripley, & Cox, 1978; Gruzelier et al., 1984). I first suggested a relationship between hypnosis and the right hemisphere in 1969 when I found that subjects who in response to a question would move their eyes to the left, a movement produced by right hemisphere activity, were more likely to be hypnotizable than those who made the eye movement to the right.

Right hemisphere activity may have an important role in the mediation not only of hypnosis, but of other altered states of consciousness as well. The states of REM sleep, dreaming and daydreaming, so heavily loaded with imagery and fantasy, have been linked to relative increase in right hemisphere activation (Bakan, 1977). There is evidence that drugs such as alcohol and marihuana which produce changes in the state of consciousness have their effects largely by producing changes in the functioning of the right hemisphere (Stillman et al., 1977).

The Depression-Pain Connection

In trying to understand the left-side/symptom connection, it seems that one has to come to grips with the depression/pain connection (Romano & Turner, 1985). Pain figures prominently in the left-sided symptom family. Pain is also a prominent feature of the syndrome of depression. There is a frequent co-occurence of pain and depression, since about 60% of depressed patients present a complaint of pain without apparent organic etiology. It has been found in recent years that anti-depressant drugs and ECT are effective not only in relieving depression, but also for the relief of pain (Ward, Bloom, & Friedel, 1979). It is well known that the right hemisphere is significantly involved in depression, and the proclivity for psychogenic symptoms to occur on the left side suggests that these symptoms also have a right hemisphere involvement. There is a psychiatric category called masked depression where pain, appearing without obvious depression, is interpreted as a manifestation of a depressive state. There is an implication of an equivalence between pain and depression. This line of thinking suggests that psychogenic symptoms other than pain may also be part of a masked depression syndrome.

A recent paper on depression, pain, and hemispheric activation (Otto, Dougher, & Yeo, 1989) proposes the following hypothesis: "The right hemisphere is specialized to become activated by and to process negative emotional stimuli. If the right hemisphere is involved in the processing of negative affective material, then greater pain sensitivity might be expected on the side of the body contralateral to this hemisphere." A vicious cycle is suggested, wherein pain or other negative affective stimuli activate the right hemisphere, and once right hemisphere activation occurs, there is a negative bias in the processing of subsequent stimuli. If the right hemisphere plays a unique role in processing aversive emotional stimuli, greater pain sensitivity to pain might be expected on the left side because of greater activation of the right hemisphere.

Merskey and Watson (1979) have said that "the right hemisphere may play a special role in producing pain, conversion symptoms, and disordered emotional expression." There is some experimental support for this line of thought. DeBenedittis and De Gonda (1985) compared patients with psychogenic and organic pain on EEG measures of hemisphere activation. They defined psychogenic pain patients in terms of the following criteria: absence of demonstrable organic cause of pain, discrepancy between physical findings and pain behavior, evidence of abnormal psychopathological patterns such as conversion reaction, somatization reaction and masked depression. They found that the psychogenic pain patients showed greater right hemisphere activation when doing a *verbal* task than did somatogenic pain patients or controls. The psychogenic pain patients exhibited a trend toward reduced left hemisphere dominance or relative right hemisphere activation during both verbal/mathematical and visuospatial tasks. Thus the tendency to pain lateralization and possibly lateralization of other psychogenic symptoms to the left side may be due to generally greater right hemisphere activation in these patients.

Cubelli and his associates (Cubelli, Caselli, & Neri, 1984) distinguish between *pain threshold*, the minimal stimulus intensity perceived as painful in an ascending series of stimuli, and *pain tolerance*, the point at which a subject withdraws from or terminates a noxious stimulus. They use the extent of the interval between pain threshold and pain tolerance as a measure, and compare patients with left and right brain damage on this measure. What they found was that this measure, the interval between pain threshold and pain tolerance, was significantly greater in patients with right brain damage, "as if they were slack at setting up an emotional reaction". It appears that the normal role of the right hemisphere to perceive and react to the emotional feature of pain is impaired after right hemisphere damage.

The Life of the Right Hemisphere

I think it is now possible to go beyond the simple psychoanalytical model relating the right hemisphere to left-sided expression of unconscious matters. In light of the massive outpouring of research on hemispheric asymmetry we can begin to address the problem of the life of the right hemisphere, and then ask whether there are individual differences in people's relative dependence on one or the other of their hemispheres in overall psychological functioning. This individual difference approach is represented by the concept of *hemisphericity*, in contrast to the more traditional notion of functional hemispheric asymmetry (Bakan, 1969). To put it in simple language I would like to suggest the possibility that some people "live" more in their right hemispheres than in their left hemispheres or "live" more in their left hemispheres than in their right hemispheres. This is the notion of hemisphericity. I suggest that the occurrence of left-sided psychogenic symtoms is more likely to be found in those people who manifest right hemisphericity, i.e. those who "live" in the right hemisphere.

I have presented some ideas about what life is like in the right hemisphere. It is the place which seems to be relatively more important than the left hemisphere in the mediation of hysteria, hypnosis and other altered states of consciousness, depression, dreaming, left-sided psychogenic symptoms, and perhaps psychogenic symptoms in general, lower sensory thresholds, and a neurochemical system more dependent on norepinephrine pathways. Future research in neuropsychology, neuroanatomy, neuroimmunology (Renoux, Biziere, Renoux, & Gulliaumin, 1983; Shavit, Lewis, Terman, Gale, & Liebeskind, 1984), and neurochemistry are sure to turn up differences between the hemispheres that will enable us to characterize the life of both the left and the right hemispheres with greater precision (Ottoson, 1987).

Treatment Approaches

The analysis in terms of a relationship between psychogenic symptoms and life in the right hemisphere suggests a possible treatment approach for the amelioration of these symptoms. I suggest that treatments which will be successful are those that can somehow turn off or turn down right hemispheric activity. Psychopharmacology which differentially affects the hemispheres is one possibility (Myslobodsky & Weiner, 1988). In fact there is some suggestive evidence that anti-depressants have their effect by doing just this. But there may be non-pharmacological ways of doing this. I suggest several of these as possibilities. At this time, of course, these are hunches and I make no therapeutic claims. In theory these techniques should reduce right hemisphere activity and possibly engage left hemisphere activity.

There is evidence that turning of the head or eyes to the right leads to relatively increased activation of the left hemisphere as compared to the right hemisphere (Bakan, 1969; Drake, 1986; Drake, 1987). Since this may facilitate left hemisphere psychological activity, it may counteract the depression, pain, and left-sided symptomatology resulting from an overactive right hemisphere. It might be worth exploring a program of right turning "exercises" for the treatment of conditions based on right hemisphere overactivity. This might be combined with breathing exercises which feature unilateral right nostril breathing. There is some evidence to suggest that right nostril breathing tends to activate the left hemisphere and thus favors left hemisphere psychological functioning (Backon, 1989). The use of lateralized breathing exercises to produce psychological changes was long ago advocated as part of the Yoga system (Johari, 1989).

There are other techniques which may be useful in changing hemispheric dynamics so as to favor the left hemisphere. Among the possibilities that come to mind are unilateral listening through the right ear which preferentially accesses the left hemisphere; biofeedback techniques which reinforce left hemisphere activity; use of special lenses to preferentially engage the left hemisphere by viewing the right visual field (Dimond et al., 1976; Sivak, Sivak, and MacKenzie, 1985); arranging the position of the patient in psychotherapy so as to require the patient to turn right during the therapeutic interaction; and use of positive and reinforcing imagery (Davidson et al., 1982).

The proposed techniques constitute suggestions for research rather than prescriptions for application. If there is potential value in these techniques, it will be necessary to develop optimal content and "dosage" schedules for their application. It would also have to be demonstrated that they produce no negative effects.

Some Remaining Problems

There are a number of variables which require systematic study in connection with symptom sinistrality. One potentially important variable is sidedness. This includes things like handedness, footedness, eye dominance etc. There is a body of evidence showing that the cerebral hemispheric organization of left-handers, for example, is different from that of right-handers (Bakan, 1990). Left and right handers may have different susceptibility to physical or psychogenic diseases. The interaction between symptom laterality and other aspects of laterality needs to be examined.

There appear to be important gender differences in lateral brain organization (Durden-Smith & deSimone, 1983; McGlone, 1980). In symptom laterality research it is important to look separately at results for males and females. Finally, it is necessary to consider developmental factors in studies of symptom laterality. What is true for adults may not be true for children. There is at least one study of psychogenic symptoms in children where an excess of right-sided symptoms was found (Regan & LaBarbera, 1984). This is in contrast to the frequent finding of an excess of left-sided symptoms in adults.

SUMMARY

The problem of an excess of symptoms on the left side of the body is reviewed from historical, empirical, and theoretical perspectives. A psychoanalytic account of sinistral symptoms has associated the right hemisphere with an emotional, non-verbal, unconscious aspect of the mind, that finds expression in physical, psychogenic or hysterical symptoms on the left side of the body. This paper examines recent work in the neuropsychology of hemispheric asymmetry and related areas in an attempt to formulate a model that goes beyond the traditional psychoanalytic approach. The results point to a complex of interrelated factors which include sinistral symptoms, pain, depression, and right hemisphericity. It is suggested that a common element underlying these factors is relatively increased right hemisphere activity. Potentially applicable treatment approaches designed to increase the relative activity of the left hemisphere are proposed. Research aimed at the development of these approaches is suggested.

REFERENCES

Axelrod, S., Noonan, B. S., & Atanacio, B. (1980). On the laterality of psychogenic somatic symptoms. *Journal of Nervous and Mental Disease, 168,* 517-525.
Backon, J. (1989). An animal analogue of forced unilateral nostril breathing: relevance for physiology and pharmacology. *Medical Hypotheses, 28,* 173-175.
Bakan, P. (1969). Hypnotizability, laterality of eye movements, and functional brain asymmetry. *Perceptual and Motor Skills, 28,* 927-932.
Bakan, P. (1977). Dreaming, REM sleep and the right hemisphere: a theoretical integration. *Journal of Altered States of Consciousness, 3,* 285-307.
Bakan, P. (1990). Non-right-handedness (NRH) and the continuum of reproductive casualty. In S. Coren (Ed.), *Left-Handedness: Behavioral Implications and Anomalies* (pp. 33-74). Amsterdam: Elsevier.
Blau, J. N., Wiles, C. M., & Solomon, F. S. (1983). Unilateral somatic symptoms due to hyperventilation. *British Medical Journal, 286,* 1108.
Borod, J. C., Koff, E., & Caron, H. S. (1983). Right hemispheric specialization for the expression and appreciation of emotion: a focus on the face. In E. Perecman (Ed.), *Cognitive Processing in the Right Hemisphere.* New York: Academic Press.
Briquet, P. (1859). *Traite Clinique et Therapeutique de l'Hysterie* . Paris: Bailliere et Fils.
Burton, R. (1948). *The Anatomy of Melancholy* . New York: Tudor.
Clarke, J. M. (1892). On hysteria. *Brain, 15,* 522-612.
Crawford, H. J. (1981). Hypnotic susceptibility and Gestalt closure. *Journal of Personality and Social Psychology, 40,* 376-383.
Cubelli, R., Caselli, M., & Neri, M. (1984). Pain endurance in unilateral cerebral lesions.*Cortex, 20,* 369-375.
Davidson, R. J., & Fox, N. A. (1982). Asymmetrical brain activity discriminates between positive and negative affective stimuli in infants. *Science, 218,* 1235-7
DeBenedittis, G., & DeGonda, F. (1985). Hemispheric specialization and the perception of pain: a task-related EEG power spectrum analysis in chronic pain patients. *Pain, 22,* 375-384.
Dimond, S. J., Farrington, L., & Johnson, P. (1976). Differing emotional response from right and left hemispheres. *Nature, 261,* 690-692.
Drake, R. A. (1986). Left cerebral hemisphere contributions to tachycardia: evidence and recommendations. *Medical Hypotheses, 19,* 261-266.
Drake, R. A. (1987). Effects of gaze manipulation on aesthetic judgments: hemisphere priming of affect. *Acta Psychologica, 65,* 91-99.
Durden-Smith, J., & deSimone, D. (1983). *Sex and the Brain* . New York: Arbor House.
Edmonds, E. P. (1947). Psychosomatic non-articular rheumatism. *Annals of Rheumatic Disease, 6,* 36-49.
Ferenczi, S. (1926). An attempted explanation of some hysterical stigmata. In S. Ferenczi (Ed.), *Further Contributions to the Theory and Technique of Psychoanalysis* (pp. 110-117). London: Hogarth Press.
Fleminger, J. J., McClure, G. M., & Dalton, R. (1980). Lateral response to suggestion in relation to handedness and the side of psychogenic symptoms. *British Journal of Psychiatry, 136,* 562-566.
Flor-Henry, P. (1979). On certain aspects of the localization of the cerebral systems regulating and determining emotion. *Biological Psychiatry, 14,* 677-698.
Frumkin, L. R., Ripley, H. S., & Cox, G. B. (1978). Changes in cerebral hemispheric lateralization with hypnosis. *Australian Journal of Hypnosis,13,* 741-750.
Galin, D. (1974). Implications for psychiatry of left and right cerebral specialization. *Archives of General Psychiatry, 31,* 572-583.
Galin, D. (1976). Hemispheric specialization: implications for psychiatry. In R. G. Grenell, & S. Gabay (Ed.), *Biological Foundations of Psychiatry* (pp. 145-176). New York: Raven Press.
Galin, D., Diamond, R., & Braff, D. A. (1977). Lateralization of conversion symptoms: more frequent on the left. *American Journal of Psychiatry, 134,* 578-581.

Glick, S. D., & Shapiro, R. (1985). Functional and neurochemical mechanisms of cerebral lateralization in rats. In S. D. Glick (Ed.), *Cerebral Lateralization in Nonhuman Species* (pp. 157-183). New York: Academic Press.

Gruzelier, J., Brow, T., Perry, A., Rhonder, J., & Thomas, M. (1984). Hypnotic susceptibility: a lateral predisposition and altered cerebral asymmetry under hypnosis. *International Journal of Psychophysiology, 2,* 131-139.

Harrington, A. (1987). *Medicine, Mind and the Double Brain: A Study in Nineteenth Century Thought* . Princeton, N.J.: Princeton Univ. Press.

Heilman, K. M., Bowers, D., Valenstein, E., & Watson, R.T. (1985). The right hemisphere: neuropsychological functions. *Journal of Neurosurgery, 64,* 693-704.

Irwin, P. (1985). Greater brain response of left-handers to drugs. *Neuropsychologia, 23,* 61-67.

Jackson, S. W. (1989). Robert Burton and psychological healing. *Journal of the History of Medicine and Allied Sciences, 44,* 160-178.

Johari, H. (1989). *Breath, Mind, and Consciousness* . Rochester, Vermont: Destiny.

Keane, J. R. (1989). Hysterical gait disorders: 60 cases. *Neurology, 39,* 586-589.

Kenyon, F. E. (1964). Hypochondriasis: a clinical study. *British Journal of Psychiatry, 110,* 478-488.

Kramer, M. A., Albrecht, S., & Miller, R. A. (1985). Handedness and the laterality of breast cancer in women. *Nursing Research, 34,* 333-337.

Ley, R. G. (1980). An archival exploration of an asymmetry of hysterical conversion symptoms. *Journal of Clinical Neuropsychology, 2,* 1-9.

Magee, K. (1962). Hysterical hemiplegia and hemianaesthesia. *Postgraduate Medicine, 31,* 339-345.

McGlone, J. (1980). Sex differences in human brain asymmetry: a critical review. *Behavioral and Brain Sciences, 3,* 215-263.

Merskey, H. (1965). The characteristics of persistent pain in psychological illness. *Journal of Psychosomatic Research, 9,* 291-298.

Merskey, H., & Spear, F. G. (1967). *Pain, Psychological and Psychiatric Aspects* . London: Bailliere, Tindall and Cassell.

Merskey, H., & Watson, G. D. (1979). The lateralization of pain. *Pain, 7,* 271-280.

Morgenstern, F. S. (1970). Chronic pain: a study of some general features which play a role in maintaining a state of chronic pain after amputation. In O. W. Hill (Ed.), *Modern Trends in Psychosomatic Medicine* (pp. 225-245). New York: Appleton-Century Crofts.

Murray, F. S., & Safferstone, J. F. (1970). Pain threshold and tolerance of right and left hands. *Journal of Comparative and Physiological Psychology, 71,* 83-86.

Myslobodsky, M. S., & Weiner, M. (1988). Directed drug distribution: adding controlled brain activity to a drug. *International Journal of Neuroscience, 42,* 7-19.

Otto, M. W., Dougher, M. J., & Yeo, R. A. (1989). Depression, pain and hemispheric activation. *Journal of Nervous and Mental Disease, 177,* 210-218.

Ottoson, D. (Ed.) (1987). *Duality and Unity of the Brain: Unified Functioning and Specialisation of the Hemispheres.* New York: Plenum Press,

Purves-Stewart, J. (1924). *The Diagnosis of Nervous Diseases* . London: Arnold.

Rather, L. J. (1967). Thomas Fienus' (1567-1631) "Dialectical Investigations of the Imagination as a Cause and Cure of Bodily Disease". *Bulletin of the History of Medicine, 41,* 349-367.

Regan, J., & LaBarbera, J. D. (1984). Lateralization of conversion symptoms in children and adolescents. *American Journal of Psychiatry, 141,* 1279-.

Renoux, G., Biziere, K., Renoux, M., & Gulliaumin, J. M. (1983). The production of T-cell inducing factors in mice is controlled by the brain neocortex. *Scandinavian Journal of Immunology, 17,* 45-50.

Romano, J. M., & Turner, J. A. (1985). Chronic pain and depression: does the evidence support a relationship. *Psychological Bulletin, 97,* 18-34.

Sackeim, H. A. (1982). Lateral asymmetry in bodily response to hypnotic suggestions. *Biological Psychiatry, 17,* 437-447.

Sackeim, H. A., Gur, R. C., Weiman, A. L., Gur, R. C., Hungerbuhler, J. P., & Geschwind, N. (1982a). Hemispheric asymmetry in the expression of positive and negative emotions: neurological evidence. *Archives of Neurology, 39,* 210-218.

Sackeim, H. A., & Weber, S. L. (1982b). Functional brain asymmetry in the regulation of emotion: implications for bodily manifestations of stress. In L. Goldberger, & S. Breznitz (Ed.), *Handbook of Stress: Theoretical and Clinical Aspects* (pp. 183-199). New York: Free Press.

Schilder, P. (1950). *The Image and Appearance of the Human Body* . New York: John Wiley.

Shavit, Y., Lewis, J. W., Terman, G. W., Gale, R. P., & Liebeskind, J. D. (1984). Opioid peptides mediate the suppressive effects of stress on natural killer cell cytotoxicity. *Science, 223*, 188-190.

Sivak, B., Sivak, J. G., & MacKenzie, C. L. (1985). Contact lens for lateralizing visual input. *Neuropsychologia, 23*, 801-803.

Stern, D. B. (1977). Handedness and the lateral distribution of conversion symptoms. *Journal of Nervous and Mental Disease, 164*, 122-128.

Stern, D. B. (1983). Psychogenic somatic symptoms on the left side: review and interpretation. In M. S. Myslobodsky (Ed.), *Hemisyndromes* (pp. 415-445). New York: Academic Press.

Stillman, R. C., Wolkowitz, O., Weingarten, H., Waldman, I., DeRenzo, E. V. & Wyatt, R. J. (1977). Marijuana: differential effects on right and left hemisphere functions in man. *Life Sciences, 21*, 1793-1799.

Tavel, M. E. (1964). Hyperventilation syndrome with unilateral somatic symptoms. *Journal of the American Medical Association, 187*, 301-303.

Tucker, D. M., & Williamson, P. A. (1984). Asymmetric neural control systems in human self-regulation. *Psychological Review, 91*, 185-215.

Ward, N. G., Bloom, V. L., & Friedel, R. O. (1979). The effectiveness of tricyclic antidepressants in the treatment of coexisting pain and depression. *Pain, 7*, 331-341.

Weinstein, S. (1969). Neuropsychological studies of the phantom. In A. L. Benton (Ed.), *Contributions to Clinical Neuropsychology* (pp. 73-106). Chicago: Aldine Publishing Co.

Weinstein, S., & Sersen, E. A. (1961). Tactual sensitivity as a function of handedness and laterality. *Journal of Comparative and Physiological Psychology, 54*, 665-669.

Wolff, B. B., & Jarvick, M. E. (1964). Relationship between superficial and deep somatic thresholds of pain with a note on handedness. *American Journal of Psychology, 77*, 589-599.

Wolff, W. (1952). *The Threshold of the Abnormal: a basic survey of psychopathology*. London: Medical Publications.

GUIDED IMAGERY AND IMMUNE SYSTEM FUNCTION IN NORMAL SUBJECTS:

A SUMMARY OF RESEARCH FINDINGS

John Schneider, Ph.D., C. Wayne Smith, M.D., Chris Minning, Ph.D.,
Sara Whitcher, Ph.D., and Jerry Hermanson, Ph.D.

Colleges Of Medicine
Michigan State University
East Lansing, MI 48824

INTRODUCTION

Since ancient times, guided imagery has been reported to have effects on bodily processes (Achterberg, 1985; McMahon, 1976), especially on the person's capacity to overcome disease and infection. In modern times, there have been clinical confirmations that this relationship applies to all bodily systems, including the immune system (Achterberg, Lawlis, Simonton, & Simonton, 1977; Achterberg & Lawlis, 1981; Siegal, 1986; 1988; Borysenko, 1987). Thus, Achterberg (1984, p. 2) has noted that:

> virtually all the diseases that remain mysterious with regard to cause or cure involve the immune system. . . cancer, persistent viral, bacterial and yeast infections, genital herpes, mononucleosis and even acquired immune deficiency syndrome (AIDS) are one category, ...along with the autoimmune disorders...which represent conditions when the immune system fails to recognize self from non-self and attacks specific tissue, such as in lupus, multiple sclerosis, rheumatoid arthritis and juvenile onset diabetes...a final group of disorders is the allergic reactions or cases when the immune system acts with excessive vengeance toward substances which are normally not harmful (such as is seen in environmental or chemical sensitivity reactions).

However, traditional immunologic theory has held that the immune system operates in a reflex-like manner, with the central nervous system playing little, if any, role in modulation of immune functions (Ader, 1981). Numerous summaries of clinical and experimental observations (Locke & Hornig-Rohan1983; Rogers, Dubey & Reich, 1979; Riley, 1981) challenge this view, and suggest that psychological and emotional factors may profoundly alter resistance to disease in general (Holden, 1978) and white blood cell function (Palmbad, 1981; Sklar & Anisman, 1979) in particular.

This type of research is variously called "psychoneuro-immunology" (Ader,1981; Solomon, 1985). It owes its emergence to current investigations of the relationship between the central nervous system (CNS) and immunity. As the immune system is influenced by CNS factors, it is a potential mediator of psychosomatic phenomena (Ader, 1981).

Most psychoneuroimmunological research has focused on psychological stress as an immunosuppressive agent (Solomon, 1985). Experiments with animals indicate stress causes increased susceptibility to bacterial infections (Amkraut, Solomon & Kaster, 1974). Stressors such as bereavement may reduce host resistance, and possibly lead to increased susceptibility to cancer (Bartrop, Lazarus, Luckhurst, et al., 1977).

Despite the existence of a vast literature supporting the role of psychological factors in both the onset and exacerbation of all these immune disorders, many of the findings are unclear, and still others are based on weak methodology. Many results are correlational, with little evidence of cause-effect relationships between mental events and changes in the immune system.

The series of studies reported here represent one attempt to provide such systematic data. One part of this series is the investigation of a relationship between a mental process (i.e. imagery) and changes in the function of a particular type of white blood cell (neutrophils).

DISEASE IMAGERY AND THE IMMUNE SYSTEM

This series of studies was stimulated by the research of Jeanne Achterberg and Frank Lawlis on the relationship between disease imagery and cancer progression and remission. Achterberg and Lawlis (1984) proposed that belief and attitudes, as well as stress, affect the immune system. They conducted a series of studies (Achterberg & Lawlis, 1979; Achterberg , Lawlis, Simonton & Simonton, 1977) with patients diagnosed with Stage IV (i.e. prognosis of six months or less to live) cancer. They point out that there are many allegorical accounts in the medical literature about patients who have attained remission from cancer seemingly because of their beliefs.

Other studies have shown that the image can also represent basic threats to the person's ability to survive. Smith (1987), for example, found a significant correlation between the number of reported dreams of death and separation and the severity of heart disease and later mortality. Most physicians realize that their treatments are far more effective if their patients "believe in them", and they respect the "will to live" as a powerful determinant of survival.

In preliminary research, Achterberg and Lawlis (1978) attempted to quantify beliefs and attitudes about cancer by obtaining objective ratings of patients "disease imagery" to statistically investigate the potential of imagery as a predictor of survival time in critically ill cancer patients. In developing their objective measure of disease imagery (Achterberg & Lawlis, 1979), they administered a battery of psychological tests, and obtained informal disease imagery ratings for 126 cancer patients with a five percent chance of five year survival, (patients with Stage IV cancer). They compared the efficacy of these instruments for predicting disease status two months later. The results showed that disease imagery was a far better predictor than any of the standard psychological instruments, and also better than blood chemistry.

On the basis of this research, they developed a psychological instrument, the IMAGE-CA (Achterberg & Lawlis, 1984), to standardize the measurement of disease imagery. The procedure for administering the IMAGE-CA is to have patients listen to a tape recording of suggestions to relax and image their cancer, their immune system, and their treatment. Afterwards, they draw pictures of these aspects of the imagery, and respond to a structured interview designed to elicit a verbal description. The imagery is then rated on 14 dimensions thought to reflect the patients' attitudes about the virulence of their cancer and the efficacy of their immune system and medical treatment against cancer. This procedure yields a final score that reflects what Achterberg and Lawlis call "quality of disease-related imagery".

In a validation study of the IMAGE-CA with 58 Stage IV cancer patients, Achterberg and Lawlis (1979) found that the instrument predicted a favorable prognosis with 93% accuracy, and an unfavorable prognosis with 100% accuracy. The overall correlation between Image CA score and disease response was .78, a highly significant finding. A second normalization study with a low-socioeconomic population indicated that the instrument's predictive potential was generalizable to individuals other than those who opted to use imagery and visualization.

As is true in any pioneering efforts, certain basic questions remained unanswered in their study. Was there a demonstrable effect on the actual cells that were being imaged? Were there specific, directly measurable effects in the body immediately after the visualization? Was the effect due to the nature of the imagery or some other factors (e.g. changes in lifestyle, or depth of relaxation which might be reflected in the imagery)? Could similar effects take place in normal subjects on normal immune system functions, where the motivation for change was not centered on a life-threatening process (i.e. cancer)?

To address these questions, the first two investigators (JMS & CWS), who were the primary investigators for the entire series of studies, decided to examine how imagery and related states, such as biofeedback, exercise, naturally occurring stress and relaxation might affect one type of white blood cells i.e., neutrophils. Normal, rather than diseased subjects were chosen to determine if these changes could take place in circumstances other than life-threatening ones. A pre-post treatment design was used both to test for the immediacy of the effect and to limit other possible explanations of change (raised by the time interval in the Achterberg and Lawlis study).

180

Role of Neutrophils

Neutrophils, a particular type of white blood cells, were chosen for the first nine studies for several reasons. First, it has been shown to be a significant part of the immune system's response to bacterial infections and to inflammation. Second, procedures have been developed to reliably determine the behavior of these cells while in the blood stream in ways which can be related to the immune system. Finally, observations in the second investigator's laboratory and elsewhere have indicated that neutrophils, like other white blood cells, appear to be sensitive to stress factors.

Background

Studies of neutrophils have ongoing in the laboratory of the second investigator of this proposal (CWS) for several years. Since these studies have focused on "in vitro" manipulations, only healthy adult subjects had been donors. On separate occasions (see study 2), three routine donors had marked changes in the adhesiveness of their neutrophils following reported episodes of emotional stress. Murphy et al. (1979) observed a significant increase in the chemotactic responsiveness of human neutrophils following exercise (specifically, a five mile run). Though these were incidental observations without experimental control, they opened interest in the relationship of neutrophils to psychological factors.

DEPENDENT VARIABLES: MEASURES OF NEUTROPHIL FUNCTION

The dependent variables used in this study are based on published techniques (Smith, Hollers, et al., 1972, 1979) for evaluating certain aspects of cell behavior. Specifically, changes in white blood count (WBC) and, more precisely in Study 6, neutrophil count (NC) available by means of venipuncture were obtained at twenty-five minute intervals before and after the experimental condition. A second measure used was the percentage of neutrophils sampled which adhered to a protein coated surface (Ad). This adherence capability is hypothesized to correspond to the neutrophil's capacity to migrate from the blood stream to a particular sight of infection. Its absence is associated with the inability to migrate.

PURPOSE OF STUDIES

1. To determine what factors influence "immunocompetent" responses of neutrophils and t-lymphocytes. Examined were the following:
    a. Ability of first author to influence function under differing conditions.
    b. Effects of naturally occurring stress:
        1) trauma.
        2) exercise.
    c. Preliminary sample of subjects trained by first author.
2. To develop a training procedure for enhancing the subject's capacity to influence immune system function.
3. To determine the imagery factors which most strongly relate to changes in immune system function.
4. To attempt to generalize imagery procedures to others aspects of the immune system.

METHOD

Design

In every study, obtain a control/base line blood sample prior to any treatment or training. Then in addition, obtain pre to post treatment blood samples for the following treatments:
Study 1. Experimenter (JMS) as Subject
    Running
    Imagery/relaxation
    Imagery/stress
Study 2. Naturalistic observations: Emotional Stress

Study 3. Jogging (conditioned and unconditioned subjects)
Study 4. Relaxation (guided imagery)
Study 5. Biofeedback/relaxation/specific imagery
Study 6. Imagery with training: *Decrease* white blood count/*Increase* neutrophil adherence
Study 7. Imagery with training: *No change* white blood count/*Increase* neutrophil adherence
Study 8. Reversal of Studies 6 &7: Imagery with training: *Increase* white blood count/*Decrease* neutrophil adherence
Study 9. Affect imagery
Study 10. Imagery with training: *Increase* t-helper activity/*Decrease* t-suppressor activity; reverse.

Subjects

Ss were screened for health and substance use. Ss who reported feeling "ill", who were under stress (e.g. impending exams), or who had used alcohol, marijuana, or even aspirin were excused or their participation delayed.

Ss in studies 1-3 were selected from colleagues and usual donors in the anatomy laboratory. Ss in studies 4 & 5 consisted of friends and church members of one investigator (CM) who were untrained in any meditative technique. Ss in studies 6-8 were vollunteers from classes in the medical schools at Michigan State, volunteers who believed they could influence their immune function. Ss in study 9 were volunteers from acting classes at MSU. In the final study (10), Ss were selected from a pool of Psychology graduate students and oncology nurses who had previous experience with imagery.

Study 1 N= 3 (Routine blood donors)
Study 2 N= 1 Male (Principle investigator)
Study 3 N= 5 (conditioned); N=3 (out of condition) (faculty/staff)
Study 4 N= 3 (untrained community volunteers)
Study 5 N= 18 (9 Male; 9 Female) (untrained community volunteers)
Study 6 N= 16 (8 Male; 8 Female) (medical & graduate students)
Study 7 N= 27 (12 Males; 15 Females) (medical & graduate students)
Study 8a N= 9 (medical students from Study 7)
Study 8b N= 16 (8 males; 8 females) (medical students)
Study 9 N= 18 (9 males; 9 females) (students from acting classes)
Study 10   N= 6 (3 males; 3 females) (grad students -psyc.; Oncology nurses -Denmark)

Dependent Variables

White Blood Count (WBC): (Studies 1-9)
Neutrophil count: (Study 6)
Adherence (Ad): Percentage of neutrophils (Studies 1-9)
Imagery ratings: Adapted from Achterberg & Lawlis IMAGE-CA: (Studies 6-8)
Saliva secretory IgA (Study 9)
t-lymphocyte suppressor & helper cell activity (Study 10)

Independent variables

Study 1. Emotional stress (natural observation)
Study 2. Single subject- experimenter
Study 3. Jogging (with and without conditioning)
Study 4. Guided imagery without prior training
Study 5. Biofeedback/relaxation/guided imagery without training
Study 6. Imagery with training: *Decrease* WBC; *increase* AD
Study 7. Imagery with training: *Don't change* WBC; *increase* AD
Study 8a.Imagery with training: *Increase* WBC; *decrease* AD (aborted)
Study 8b.Imagery with training: *Increase* WBC; *decrease* Ad
Study 9. Affect induction: Happy-neutral-sad affect simulation
Study 10. Imagery with tr: *Increase* t-helper cell activity/*decrease* t-suppressor cell activity.

NORMATIVE DATA

Means and Ranges

1. Average white blood count (variable/seasonal) Range = 4000-12000
2. Average neutrophil adherence = 45% ; S.D. +/- 3%. Pre-study range = 8% to 75%.

Reliability

1. Neutrophil count & adherence percentage (test-retest 20 minute interval): r=.99; N>100.
2. Imagery ratings:
   a. Study 6. Inter-rater reliability (r's = .65 to. 93: N=16)
   b. Studies 7 & 8. Inter-rater reliability (r's = .90 to .95; N=27)

RESULTS: CONTROLS VERSUS TREATMENTS

Control Data

In every study, Ss had a blood sample taken prior to any participation in the study. Table 1 shows the results of this control blood sample in the studies involving neutrophil function. Two samples were taken, with a twenty minute time interval. These control sample showed that no significant changes occurred pre- to post- in the non-experimental condition.

Studies 1-4

The first study resulted from the second investigator (CWS) observing changes in the blood samples of routine donors and following up these observations with questions about current life events. Each S had clearly defined emotional stress within the previous 24 hours.

As a follow-up to this first study, one of the principal investigators (JS), who was experienced at imagery, was given instruction on the function of neutrophils. He attempted to visualize changes in the functions of these cells, with blood samples taken before and after the imaging session (*pre* and *post*).

The third study involved several conditioned and unconditioned joggers running for twenty minutes in order to obtain a measure of the effects of physical stress on neutrophil function.

As a final preliminary study (4), subjects unfamiliar with any form of imagery or hypnosis were given instructions in the function of neutrophils and brief training in imagery and relaxation.

The results of these first four studies suggested that changes in neutrophil function were related to both physical and psychological factors which affected the level of stress or relaxation the person was experiencing. Subsequent studies were designed to test these preliminary findings more systematically.

Study 5. Multiple Experimental Conditions (N = 18)

No significant differences were found in white blood count or adherence of neutrophils pre to post for any of the three conditions (biofeedback; relaxation; guided imagery without training). Very little advanced training was provided for Ss. They were not given specific information about the ways neutrophils functioned, except by suggestion during the experimental session.

Table 1. Control Study (N=32):
Neutrophil Function Tests with 20 Minutes between Samples 1 and 2

	Sample 1 (M ± SD)	Sample 2 (M ± SD)	F-values
Total count (WBC)	74000 ± 2000	72000 ± 1900	NS
Adherence (Ad)	41± 3%	38 ± 4%	NS

Table 2. Studies 1-4:
Factors Effecting Change in Neutrophil Count (WBC) & Adherence (Ad)

Study/Factor	N	Change
1/Emotional Stress	3	Ad decreased from a mean of 45% to 15%. WBC increased from mean of 7200 to 27000.
2/Principal investigator	1	1. Ad increased from 47% to 87%; WBC decreased from 5500 to 3700. 2. Ad decreased from 43% to 12%; WBC increased from 5700 to 12000.
3/Jogging (experienced joggers)	5	Ad (stimulated & unstimulated) remained unchanged: pre=42%; post=43%. WBC increased from 5500 to 12000.
3/Jogging (unconditioned)	3	Ad decreased from 45% to 13%. WBC increased from 4700 to 23,000.
4/Relaxation (guided imagery)	5	Ad increased from 55% to 81%. WBC remained unchanged. Ad still elevated 24 hours later.

Finally, the sessions were held in a psychologist's office in a department of psychiatry. Many of the participants had never been to such a place before the time of the actual experiment. The investigators realized that several factors needed to become standard parts of the experiment:

1. Any control blood samples need to be taken prior to any training or informing of the potential subjects of the exact purpose of the study.
2. Subjects need to know in advance of the experimental session the nature of the immune system function they would later be asked to image.
3. Subjects need some training in imagery and what constitutes effective imagery in advance of the experiment.
4. Familiarity with the site of the experiment in advance is helpful.

Study 6. Guided Imagery with training: Decrease WBC; Increase Ad

Ss were recruited from medical school classes. All Ss were given a lecture/slide presentation on neutrophils and their function in the immune system. Two two-hour imagery training sessions were given, with opportunities for discussion of effective imagery as it related to decreasing white blood count and increasing the adherence of the cells.

Ss were asked to imagine their neutrophils responding as if there were a "crisis". Under such conditions, the desired response would be for the neutrophils to leave the blood stream, stick to the blood vessel walls at the appropriate site, change shape and leave the blood stream. The expected result was that there would be fewer neutrophils available when the blood sample was taken after the imagery than were available in the blood sample immediately prior to the imagery. Table 3 shows the results of the pre to post blood samples in this study.

The drop in total white blood was highly significant. Even more remarkable was the finding that, when the sample was restricted only to neutrophils, the drop was even more dramatic and significant (60% of all the neutrophils were missing in the post sample). When the white blood cells other than neutrophils were evaluated, there was a nonsignificant increase in their numbers. Obviously, the changes were highly specific to the neutrophils.

Table 3. Study 6 (N=16):
Neutrophil Tests before & after Imagery to *Decrease* WBC & *Increase* Ad

	Pre		Post		Multivariate	
	M	SD	M	SD	f-value	p
Total white blood count (WBC)	8200 ± 1500		6400 ± 1300		29.53	<.0001
Neutrophil count	4000 ± 600		1800 ± 400		67.47	<.0001
White blood count (other than neutrophils)	4200 ± 1000		4600 ± 800		1.17	NS
Adherence (ad)	45% ± 12%		32% ± 14%		3.10	<.05

The changes in adherence, however, reached statistical significance in the unpredicted direction. Instead of an increase in adherence, the pre to post sample showed a significant decrease. This finding was totally unexpected.

In order to better understand this combination of results (i.e. how could there be a decrease in the number of neutrophils and a decrease in their adherence when the imagery was to decrease number and increase adherence), the ratings made following the imagery session were correlated with the blood changes. Table 4 shows the results of this analysis.

The rated imagery correlated positively with a decrease in the white blood count. Again unexpectedly, there was a strong negative correlation with the change in adherence (Ad).

The findings from this study were mixed and troubling. Clearly there had been a drop in white blood count specific to neutrophils which corresponded to the images created in the session. The specificity of this shift to neutrophils only suggests that this was not a function of something quite general but a specific effect on a particular cell which the subjects had learned about previously.

On the other hand, the drop in the adherence of the neutrophils was in the opposite, unexpected direction: The more the subject's imagery indicated that the cells were increasing in adherence, the less adherent they were. Such a finding suggests that what we image can actually create the opposite effect, a potentially dangerous outcome of doing imagery for health.

An alternative explanation of these findings was considered. Since there had been a sixty percent drop in the available neutrophils from pre to post treatment, it was suggested that the neutrophils which remained were not the ones which had increased in their adherence. It was the ones that had marginated in the blood vessel which actually were more adherent.

Table 4: Study 6 (N=16; Imagery to *Decrease* WBC & *Increase* Ad)
Correlations between Imagery Measures and Neutrophil Changes

Imagery measures	Blood function changes	
	WBC	Adherence
Vividness	NS	-.38
Adherence	NR	-.57**
Leaving blood stream	.55**	-.49*
Strength	NS	-.49*
Feeling effective	NS	-.46*
Symbolism	.66**	NS
Clinical judgment	NS	-.71**

NS = did not reach statistical significance
NR = not rated
* p < .05
** p <.01

185

Table 5. Study 7 (N=27; Imagery to *Stabilize* WBC and *Increase* Ad)
Neutrophil function tests: Pre-post measures

	Pre	Post	Multivariate f - value	p
WBC	5805 $\pm$ 1331	5747 $\pm$ 1738	0.65	NS
Ad	42% $\pm$ 10%	54% $\pm$ 16%	4.43	<.001

To-test this hypothesis, the same Ss were asked to repeat the experiment, with one alteration in their imagery. They were asked to keep the neutrophils in the blood stream while increasing their stickiness. Ss initially resisted doing this type of imagery, since they felt it might not be "healthy". When they were persuaded that it was only for the time of the study, and subsequently they could "let" the neutrophils do whatever was necessary, they all agreed.

In this study (Study seven), there was no expected change in the number of white blood cells, since they were supposed to all stay in the blood stream. There was an expected increase in adherence.

Study 7. Guided Imagery with Training: Keep WBC Constant; Increase Ad (N=27)

Table 5 shows the results of the pre to post blood sampling. As expected, there were no change in white blood count, while there was a significant increase in adherence (Ad). Table 6 shows the results of the imagery ratings which followed the session. The only imagery variable which was rated for white blood change was strength (i.e., how strong were the cells in being able to resist leaving the blood stream). As expected, imagery ratings correlated positively with neutrophil adherence this time. These results tended to support the hypothesis from the previous study that the reason for the negative correlation between imagery and adherence was due to the unavailability of the cells which had actually responded to venipuncture.

If imagery was actually the key factor in such findings, the investigators hypothesized that the direction of change could actually be reversed. Once again, the same Ss were asked to image changes in their neutrophils. This time, however, they were to increase the number of neutrophils in the blood stream by decreasing the stickiness of the cells. This would be accomplished by those cells already on the blood vessel walls releasing into the blood stream. Study 8a was the result.

Study 8a. Guided Imagery with Training. Increase WBC & Decrease Ad (N = 9; study aborted)

Only nine of the 27 Ss from the previous study completed this study. The study was stopped as a result of the feedback given in the imagery follow-up session. No significant

Table 6. Study 7 (N=27; Imagery to *Stabilize* WBC and *Increase* Ad)
Correlations between Imagery Measures and Neutrophil Changes

Imagery measure	Blood function change	
	WBC	Adherence
Vividness	NR	.46**
Adherence	NR	NS
Strength	.52**	.52**
Feeling effective	NR	.49**
Symbolism	NR	.51**
Clinical Judgment	NR	.41*

NR = not rated in this study
NS = not significant
* p<.05
** p<.01

Table 7. Study 8b (N=18; Imagery to *Increase* WBC & *Decrease* Ad)
Neutrophil Tests before & after 25 min Relaxation/Imagery Session

	Pre		Post			
	M	SD	M	SD	t-value	p-value
WBC	4857 ± 941		4700 ± 1108		-1.16	NS
Ad	38.8 ± 13.0%		24.2 ± 4.8%		-3.17	<.0

differences were found. Variance was quite high. Subjects, who were the same ones from Studies 6 & 7, complained that this type of imagery was "not healthy". Apparently they had been so persuaded that what was healthy was the opposite, they found themselves anxious and conflicted about doing this type of imagery. While a subsequent debriefing allowed them to be reassured that they hadn't done anything unhealthy (in fact, such mobility of the neutrophils is an important function as well), it was decided to start with a new subject pool in Study 8b.

Study 8b. Guided Imagery with Training. Increase WBC & Decrease Ad (N=18)

The same orientation procedure was given to these new subjects as had been done in Study six. Ss were told that imagining the neutrophils increasing in count and becoming less adherent was a healthy response ("going on maneuvers"). Table 7 shows the results of the pre to post blood testing.

The expected increase in WBC did not occur. There was the expected significant drop in adherence. These findings offered only partial support of the hypothesis that either directional change could take place. One reason for the lack of increase in count could be that such increases usually occur only under conditions of emotional or physical stress. In the latter condition (i.e. physical stress), people ordinarily increased their rate of breathing, while in this condition, the imagery induction required relaxation and an actual decrease in the rate of breathing.

Table 8 shows the results of the imagery ratings correlating with the blood changes. Imagery correlated significantly with adherence, but not with WBC. This suggests that what was imaged by the subjects did correspond with the changes in blood cell function. Since there was no change in white blood count, the lack of correlation is difficult to interpret.

Study 9. Affect Induction: Happy-Neutral-Sad Affect Simulation (N=18)

Subsequent to this series of investigations, other studies were planned by different parts of the investigative team. One member (JH) was interested in the relationship of imaged affective states and corresponding changes in neutrophil function. Like the previous studies, Ss were

Table 8. Study 8b (N=18; Imagery to *Increase* WBC & *Decrease* Ad)
Correlations between Imagery Measures and Neutrophil Changes

Imagery measure	Blood function change	
	WBC	Adherence
Vividness	NS	.43*
Adherence	-.39	NS
Leaving blood stream	-.48*	.46*
Strength	NS	NS
Feeling effective	NS	NS
Symbolism	NS	NS
Clinical Judgment	-.33	.50*
Felt Sense	NS	.47*
Playfulness	NS	.47*

NS = not significant
* p<.05

oriented to the functions of neutrophils. Unlike the previous series of studies, Ss were not given a sense of what direction might result from a particular feeling. Neither were they placed in an induced imagery condition.

Only shifts in WBC show any relationship to affect simulation. In light of the number of non-significant correlations, this relationship could have occurred by chance. The author was unable to conclude from this study if affect did related to changes in neutrophil functions.

Study 10

If neutrophils were indeed affected by specific imagery, it was hypothesized that other cells in the immune system might also be affected. The same procedure used in Studies 6-8 was adapted by one of the investigators (JS) for measuring functional changes in t-helper and suppressor cells in a preliminary study conducted in Denmark with a group of psychology graduate students and oncology nurses from a community hospital. In this study, three blood samples were taken at twenty minute intervals, with the second twenty minute period involving a reversal of the first twenty minute activity. All six Ss show expected increase in helper cell activity and decrease in suppressor cell activity in the first twenty minutes. The reverse was true for all six in the second twenty minutes. No statistical tests were run on this sample. The results of this preliminary study were promising, but obviously need a larger sample.

At the present time, investigations are underway to apply the adapted Achterberg-Lawlis procedure to the relationship between imagery and changes in the tuberculin skin (Mantoux) response.

SUMMARY OF IMAGERY RATINGS

The changes in blood samples, for the most part, correspond to the expected direction and outcome of the imagery being used. These findings will be discused more comprehensively in a subsequent section.

Understanding the rated imagery and the blood sample changes is somewhat more complex. A summary of these correlations is show in Table 9.

Table 9. Summary of Significant Correlations Between Imagery Ratings and Pre-to-Post Changes in Blood Function

Imagery measure	Study 6 (N=16)		Study 7 (N=27)		Study 8b (N=16)	
	WBC	Ad	WBC	Ad	WBC	Ad
Vividness	--	-.38	NR	.46**	--	+.43*
Adherence	--	-.57**	NR	--	-.39	--
Leaving the blood stream	.55**	-.49*	NR	NR	-.48*	+.46*
Strength	--	-.49*	.61**	.52**	--	--
Feeling effective	--	.46*	NR	.49**	--	--
Symbolism	.66**	--	NR	.51**	--	--
Clinical judgment	--	-.71**	NR	.41*	-.33	+.50*
Felt sense	NR	NR	NR	NR	--	+.47*
Playfulness	NR	NR	NR	NR	--	+.47*

NR = not relevant in this study
*p < .05
**p < .01

Significant Correlations with White Blood Count:
Total Possible Correlations = 17; Correlations Reaching Significance (p<.05) = 4

Shifts in the activity and availability of white blood cells, corresponding with subjects' imagery, are not much greater than what could be expected by chance. This could in part be explained by the measures of white blood count, which were less specific and less sensitive than measures of neutrophil count.

Also in one study (Study 7), where the subjects were asked to keep the neutrophils available, no measure could adequately be made of the subject's imagery (except for strength, which did correlate with a lack of change).

It could also be that relaxation conditions may have a natural tendency to decrease the activity level of white blood cells. As a result, the studies which did not have an expectation of a decrease in white blood cells (Studies 7 & 8), may have an uncontrolled covariate of relaxation depth affecting the findings. Future studies may wish to develop imagery ratings which more directly reflect the desired changes in activity level of the white blood cells.

Significant Correlations with Adherence:
Total Possible Correlations = 22; Correlations Reaching Significance (p <.05) = 15

With fifteen of a possible twenty-two correlations between imagery and adherence, a relationship does seem to exist. This relationship cannot be explained simply by increased or decreased activation of the neutrophils, since adherence percentage is not dependent on the number of cells available.

Correlations were found in all three studies, and the direction of the correlations correspond to the hypothesized actions of the neutrophils. It is possible that specific functions of cells, in this case neutrophils, can be influenced by imagery. This finding needs extensive testing across other types of cells, both within and outside the immune system.

DISCUSSION OF GENERAL FINDINGS

Replication by another laboratory measuring neutrophil function is necessary. Since the particular way of measuring neutrophil function (i.e. adherence) was unique to the second investigator's (CWS) laboratory at the time of these studies, such replication may be difficult. Application to other types of immune system function which are more standardized (such as the activity level of t-lymphocytes) may be a necessary alternative way to replicate. As measurement of cell functions grows increasingly sophisticated (e.g. the ability not only to measure cellular activity, but cell function, endorphin receptivity and even genetic markers on cells), the relationship of imagery to the subcellular level may also be measurable.

General Conclusion and Implications for Further Research

At the present time, research on the relationship between mental imagery and changes in cellular function has begun. Future studies can profit by taking into account the following:

1. Subjects who believe that they can have an influence on their immune system function under certain circumstances may demonstrate such influences. Research is needed on what distinguishes those who believe they are capable of such influence and those who do not.
2. Knowledge of the specific functions of the cell or bodily process is necessary for effective imagery. Within health limits, some studies might test the effect of systematic misinformation on subsequent changes.
3. Subjects need to be trained in relaxation/guided imagery. The extent and types of this training needs further study.
4. The procedure to be imaged needs to be perceived as potentially stress free and healthy. The subject's perception of the outcome of imaging needs to be systematically studied.
5. Subjects need to believe they are capable of influencing immune system function. Issues of suggestibility, personality, and education need to be investigated to determine how changeable this belief might be.
6. Within the group of subjects who believe that there is a relationship between mind and body, the least effective appear to be those who believe the mind *controls* the body. The

extent to which the imagery process is experienced as work or playfulness is a variable in need of further study.

7. Significant aspects of imagery and specific cellular function appear to include the following:

a. Vividness of the image (which may or may not be visual);
b. Awareness of the functions being altered;
c. Strength/energy of the cells involved;
d. Playfulness. of the imagery;
e. Felt sense (Gendlin, 1977)--was something actually *experienced* during imagery?;
f. General feelings about how the imagery went;
g. Clinical judgment of the experimenter present during the imagery, based on observations of such factors as depth of relaxation, rapid eye movement, and the effects of distractions.

SUMMARY

A sequential series of studies with healthy adult subjects were designed to investigate the relationship of various psychological and physical changes on the functions of neutrophils, a type of cell within the immune system. With increasing sophistication in the procedures, the investigators found that guided imagery, following training in the functions of neutrophils, was significantly correlated ($p<.05$) with the adherence function of neutrophils in three separate studies. It is suggested that specific functions of cells may be influenced by imagery if the subject is aware of those cellular functions. Extensive research is needed on neutrophils and other cells, both within and outside of the immune system in order to test this hypothesis.

REFERENCES

Achterberg, J. (1985). *Imagery and Healing: Shamanism and Modern Medicine*. Boulder, CO: New Science Library/Random House (Imprint of Shambhala Publishing Company).

Achterberg, J. (1984). Imagery and medicine: Psychophysiological Speculations. *Journal Of Mental Imagery, 8(4)*, 1-14.

Achterberg, J. & Lawlis, G.F. (1979). A canonical analysis of blood chemistry variables related to psychological measures of cancer patients. *Multivariate Experimental Clinical Research, 4*, 1-10.

Achterberg, J. & Lawlis, G.F. (1981). *Bridges of the Body/Mind*. Champaign, IL: Institute for Personality and Ability Testing.

Achterberg, J. & Lawlis, G.F. (1984). *Imagery of disease: A diagnostic tool for behavioral medicine*. Champaign, IL: Institute for Personality and Ability Testing.

Achterberg, J. Lawlis, F. Simonton, O.C. & Simonton, S. (1977). Psychological factors and blood chemistries as disease outcome predictors for cancer patients. *Multivariate Experimental Clinical Research, 3*, 107-122.

Ader, R. (1981). *Psychoneuroimmunology*. New York: Academic Press.

Bartrop, R.W., Luckhurst, E., Lazarus, L., Kiloh, L. G., & Penny, R. (1977). Depressed lymphocyte function after bereavement. *Lancet*, 834-836.

Gruber, B.L., Hall, N.R., Hersch, S.P. & Dubois, P. (1988). Immune System and Psychological Changes in Metastatic Cancer Patients Using Relaxation and Guided Imagery: A Pilot Study. *Scandinavian Journal of Behavior Therapy, 17*, 25-46.

Hall, H.R. (1982-1983). Hypnosis and the Immune System: A Review of implications for cancer and the psychology of healing. *American Journal of Clinical Hypnosis*, 25, 92-103.

Holden, C. (1978). Cancer and the Mind: How are they connected? *Science*, 200, 1363-1369.

Locke, S. & Hornig-Rohan, M (eds.) (1983). *Mind and Immunity: Behavioral Immunology: An Annotated Bibliography*. New York: Institute for the Advancement of Health.

MacMahon, C.E. (1976). The role of imagination in the disease process: Pre-Cartesian history. *Psychological Medicine, 6*, 179-184.

Minning, C. (1981). Unpublished doctoral dissertation, Michigan State University, East Lansing, MI.

Murphy, S.A., Shade, D.S. & Vanepps, E.E. (1979). Catacholamine stimulation of neutrophil and monocyte chemotoxins. *Clinical Research*.

Palmbad, J. (1981). Stress and immunologic competence in man. In R. Ader (Ed.), *Psychoneuroimmunology*. New York: Academic Press.

Riley, V. (1981). Psychoneuroendocrine influences on immunocompetence and neoplasia. *Science, 212*, 1100-1109.

Rogers, M.P., Dubey, D. & Reich, P. (1979). The influence of the psyche and the brain on immunity and disease susceptibility: A critical review. *Psychosomatic Medicine, 41*, 243-364.

Rossi, E.L. (1986). *The psychobiology of mind-body healing: New concepts in therapeutic hypnosis*. New York: W.W. Norton.

Rossi, E. L. & Cheek, D.B. (1988). *Mind-body therapy: Methods of ideodynamic healing in hypnosis*. New York: W.W.Norton.

Sklar, L.,& Anisman, H. (1979).Stress and coping factors influence tumor growth.*Science, 205*, 513-515.

Smith, C.W. et al. (1972). Decrease in motility, chemotaxis and glass adherence of PMN's in a child with recurrent infection. *Clinical Research, 20,* 102.

Smith, C.W., Hollers, J.C., Bing, R. & Patrick, R.A. (1979). Effects of human CL inhibitor on complement mediated human Leukocyte chemotaxis. *Journal of Clinical Investigations, 63,* 221-229.

Smith, C.W., Hollers, J.C. (1980). Motility and adhesiveness in human neutrophils: Redistribution of chemotactic factor-induced adhesion sites. *Journal of Clinical Investigations, 65,* 804-812.

Smith, C.W., Hollers, J.C., Dupree, E., Goldman, A.S. & Lord, R.A. (1972). A serum inhibitor of leukotzxis in a child with recurrent infections. *Journal of the Laboratory of Clinical Medicine, 79,* 878-885

Smith R. C. (1987). Do dreams reflect a biological state? *Journal Of Nervous and mental Disease, 175(4),* 201-207.

Solomon, G. (1985). The emerging field of psychneuroimmunolgy with a special note on AIDS. *Advances, 2 (Winter),* 6-19.

Solomon, G. & Amkraut, A. (1981). Psychoneuroendocrinological effects on the immune response. *Annual Review of Microbiology, 35,* 155-184.

THE USE OF IMAGERY IN A MULTIMODAL PSYCHONEUROIMMUNOLOGY PROGRAM FOR CANCER AND OTHER CHRONIC DISEASES

Deirdre Davis Brigham, M.S., M.P.H., and Philip O. Toal, M.S.

GETTING WELL Program
Orlando General Hospital
Orlando, FL 32822

During the past three decades anecdotal reports and research studies suggestive of a connection between imagery/emotions and improved physical functioning have been visible (Klopfer, 1957; Simonton et al. 1978; Cousins, 1976, LeShan, 1958; etc.). In the past decade studies have been tightening, and a scientifically viable body of literature on the mind/body connection is building (e.g., Kiecolt-Glaser et al., 1987; Ader, 1981; Rossi & Cheek, 1988; Green & Green, 1986; Hall, 1983; McClelland, 1988; Achterberg & Lawlis, 1984; Schneider et al., 1984; Norris, 1988; Speigel et al., 1989) The literature in sports psychology, psychology of self esteem, stress management , and psychotherapy (Sheikh, 1983) indicates that imagery can be an effective strategy in a wide range of aspects of a person's life. Norris (1988), among others, suggests that imagery is the blueprint for all voluntary behaviors and exerts a preeminent influence on involuntary physical, emotional and mental behavior.

"However interesting, plausible and appealing a theory may be, it is techniques, not theories, that are actually used on people" (London, 1964). The GETTING WELL program at Orlando General Hospital has translated the literature in the area of psychoneuroimmunology (PNI) into viable life techniques for people with cancer and other chronic diseases such as MS, lupus, HIV, IBS, rheumatoid arthritis, and neurological dysfunctions. This intensive adjunctive inpatient program draws from all areas of cognitive/behavioral medicine to immerse the participant in new ways of living and perception of the world. Although GETTING WELL is comprehensive in its offerings, imagery provides the backbone for the program and is the focus of this paper.

We take a broad view of imagery—seeing it as the salient element of hope, the placebo effect, goal setting, cognitive restructuring, hypnosis, optimism, humor, attitude, and emotional empowerment—involving *all* sensory channels. As Norris (1988) has stated, "We must learn imagery is everything. We create our world or it is created for us. We will be effects if we are not effectors, victims instead of masters of our destiny."

In designing and implementing a responsible program one must consider legitimate potential hazards. A frequent, often justified, criticism of mind-body or even "responsibility for one's health" interventions is that the individual might blame himself for causing his disease and experience guilt if he does not get well. A sense of power and control of one's life appears essential to the healing process, yet guilt is sometimes a side-effect. A credible program needs to take both aspects into consideration. Indeed, the promulgation of simplistic ideas of "cause," "cure," "blame," and "guilt" *can* cause damage to the individual. The complex web of causality for cancer, cardiovascular and other chronic diseases implies there is a myriad of factors ranging from genetics and nutrition to behavioral and emotional components. Some of these factors are essentially unchangeable, yet others are eminently negotiable. However, there is a big difference between "blaming" oneself for past situations and present uncontrollable ones and "accepting responsibility" for a future controllable outcome. Teasing out those factors which can be changed and taking responsibility for them, yet accepting those components beyond one's present control, returns power to the patient and may indeed affect the outcome of the disease or

Mental Imagery, Edited by R.G. Kunzendorf
Plenum Press, New York, 1990

treatment. Frequently, powerful medical treatments have side effects, yet effective treatment is not abandoned because of side effects. We have found that those who truly understand the concept of PNI do not experience guilt; however, if that side effect appears, we as psychotherapists are eminently qualified to deal with it.

Yet another criticism of the argument for a mind/body connection is the issue of false hope. We argue that hope is the image of or desire for a positive outcome and as such there is no "false" hope. We cannot prove without a doubt that a hopeful/powerful image of the future will extend life. Yet, on the other hand, we know that with the diagnosis of "hopeless" conditions such as cancer or HIV positive, immune status plummets precipitously—putatively from loss of hope and of control over one's life (Hall, 1990). "To argue for the *absence* of a mind-body connection could be viewed as offering the patient *false despair* in contrast to the much feared problems of offering false hope " (O'Regan, 1989, p.13).

The philosophy of the authors' program focuses not on outcomes, but on the journey. The emphasis of GETTING WELL is not on physical healing, but on living the most joyous, high quality life one can imagine. Physical healing *may* be a side effect, but it is not a necessary outcome. The focus is on living life to the fullest, and any physiological change is seen as a "lagniappe" or a delightful extra. The person who is focused only on the medical change is less likely to achieve it than the person who focuses on living well and making each day of his life a masterpiece. Seeing one's disease as a *gift* which allows one to image and live one's life in new, more powerful ways, frequently leaves the person able to get one's needs met without having to depend on the disease. Thus the program is designed to provide benefits at several different levels at the same time. Techniques to orchestrate change in one's physiology are not implemented in the GETTING WELL program unless they also have a salubrious effect on quality of life, empowerment, and peace of mind in and of themselves.

This intensive adjunctive psychoneuroimmunology program is residential for a minimum of 10 days to an optimal 28 days. Imagery training *per se* is a daily activity; however the concept of imagery as a blueprint for all voluntary behaviors, for many autonomic functions, and for cognitive /emotional restructuring is inherent in all the six to eight therapy/learning sessions daily. Although we use a variety of cognitive/behavioral techniques, for this paper we are focusing on the aspects of each component which relate directly to imagery. A typical day at GETTING WELL includes "formal" sessions in stress management, group therapy, guided imagery, exercise/nutrition, laughter and play, high-level wellness, expressive therapies, yoga/Therapeutic Touch, and individual/family therapy. In addition video and audio tapes on imagery or other aspects of PNI are scheduled in the evenings, and a well stocked library and a game/art/music room are available to participants at all times.

Initial psychological testing includes not only standard tools such as the MMPI and Rotter Incomplete Sentences, but also imagery-based instruments such as the Image CA (Achterberg & Lawlis, 1984) and a modified House, Tree, Person (HTP). The Image CA involves a brief guided imagery seeing the disease, imaging the immune system mount an attack, and seeing treatment effectively dealing with the disease. The participant is then asked to draw his images which can be scored as to perceived strength of the body's response, effectiveness of treatment, and invasiveness of the disease process. Studies have indicated that the Image CA has better predictive value than blood studies—that a perceived positive outcome will eventuate 93% of the time while a perceived negative outcome is 100% likely to occur (Schneider, 1989). The Image CA generates guidelines for more powerful imagery training throughout the rest of the program. Our revision of the HTP employs a formal evocation of images of a house, a tree, and a person before they are drawn. The drawings generate a good metaphorical view of the person's feelings about himself, his family, his strengths, and his relationship with the world in addition to the traditional pathologic markers such as depression and anxiety. The HTP is an imagery window on some of the emotional conflicts which may be impacting quality of life as well as the healing process *and* frequently reveals unrecognized strengths which can be built upon.

Stress management focuses on reducing the secretion of cortisol and the catacholamines which destroy the balance of the immune system. This daily session makes heavy use of imagery in changing the participants' perceptions of stress through cognitive/imagery restructuring—with the disturbing event being imaged in a manner less stimulating to the sympathetic nervous system. The concepts of stress inoculation (Meichenbaum, 1977) and systematic desensitization (Wolpe, 1969) are combined in strategies where imagery is used to elicit a parasympathetic effect. Graded images of a present or future stressor are conjured, and the participant sees himself feeling powerful, in charge, and successful in handling the situation. Techniques from neurolinguistic programming (NLP) may be employed to distance the individual from a stressful situation; for example, seeing oneself *watching* oneself perform in a panic-frought situation. It could involve imaging one's *bete noire* in diapers, in a hamster ball, or in some other powerless situation. Similarly assertive rights are reinforced by the participant imaging himself accepting the right, being aware of how he feels and looks physically, how he feels emotionally, how people are responding to him, etc. In other aspects of assertiveness training and communication skills imagery rehearsal is used to precede behavioral rehearsal in sessions. Goal setting, an important dimension of stress management, relies heavily on imagery both in breaking down long-term goals into manageable short-term goals and in producing an "inner video" seeing oneself successfully accomplishing the short-term goals and reveling as long-term goals are achieved.

The daily process group focuses mainly on support, expressing feelings, and deepening self esteem and relationship skills. However, it is frequently an arena in which dream work is done—using that wonderful window into the unconscious to more fully understand oneself. Group is another place in which the images of hope and optimism are reinforced and extended.

Imagery training is a daily staple of the GETTING WELL program. First we explore the status of conscious and unconscious imagery (through dialogue and the Image CA) in relation to the participant's disease status and his treatment. Participants are then encouraged to develop creative, idiosyncratic imagery which is consistent with their values and both conscious and unconscious core beliefs. Basic relaxation and breathing are taught, a "special place" is incorporated, and "anchors" are developed. A wide variety of visualization experiences (from a generalized "healing light" to specific immune system "wars" against cancer cells) is offered to expand and develop the patient's individual imagery. An important aspect of the formalized imagery sessions is reframing treatment such as chemotherapy and radiation from uncomfortable, noxious images into seeing it as the "elixir of life" or as "healing beams of light energy from a radiant star." The important connection between PNI and standard medical treatment is empowered during this session particularly, and undesirable side effects of medical treatment may simply disappear. This session is also used to introduce and reinforce images and techniques for pain/discomfort management. Again, a variety of images is presented and individual work may be done to hone the techniques. Participants are encouraged, empowered by input from the group, to craft their own creative imagery tapes.

In recent years the literature increasingly is endorsing nutritional and exercise lifestyles as significant factors not only in prevention, but also in the "treatment" of cancer and chronic diseases (e.g., Sporn & Roberts, 1983). Imagery plays an important role in adherence and compliance as well as enhancing the effects of good nutrition and aerobic exercise. Didactic material is presented as to the role of beta carotene, protective indoles, complementary complex carbohydrates, fresh fruits and vegetables, etc., and the importance of exercise in reducing lean muscle mass loss, stimulating lymphatic circulation, increasing core body temperature, increasing endorphin production, etc. The person is encouraged to image these salubrious changes taking place (such as their carrot juice being directed to a tumor and reducing its size, the tumor area being bombarded by oxygen from aerobic activity, or the weak cancer cells being destroyed by increased core body temperature). Imagining the overall feeling of health and well being during eating or exercising seems to actualize the body's becoming whole, healthy, beautiful, and powerful. Joy (1979, p.127) states, "I believe that if you put fine food into a body with a crummy mind, you get a crummy body; but if you put crummy food into a body with expanded awareness, you get a fine body." Exercise is a particularly difficult behavior to implement, yet it is one of the most important for the cancer or chronic disease patient for the management of pain, depression, and anxiety, and in building feelings of inner power and self control—in addition to the purely physical aspects. Participants are encouraged to use this time of enhanced right brain receptiveness to guide imagery and positive affirmations, or to creatively problem solve. Seeing oneself as a magnificent jaguar exercising effortlessly, frequently taps in to ancient, atavistic memories of being the animal we were designed to be before we were fettered by the configurations of modern, chronic-disease-producing "civilization."

Laughter and non-competitive play are so important physiologically and emotionally that they comprise a formal daily session at GETTING WELL. Physiologically, laughter promotes muscular relaxation as profoundly as relaxation training (Cogan et al.,1987) and produces beta-endorphins which increase pain threshholds and enhance lymphocyte proliferation (Gilman et al., 1982), reduce depression and anxiety, and increase feelings of well being. Berk (1989) indicates that "mirthful laughter" enhances immune function. In a study looking at the effect of laughter on the immune system, those who watched a video of the comedian Gallagher had increased natural killer cell activity. Even anticipation of seeing the video positively affected immune function. At GETTING WELL patients tell funny stories, learn to juggle, watch *Candid Camera*, Gallagher, etc., and play childhood games non-competitively. Laughter and play therapy is frequently the most difficult part of the program for people with cancer and chronic diseases since they have long since "put away childish things" and have entered into the "consensus trance" image of the perfect, competitive adult in our society. Unfortunately, our cultural expectations of the "adult" are not in the best interest of our bodies. Frolicking with a parachute, blowing soap bubbles, or playing "Simon Says" seems to trigger muscle memory and images of the happy child within who is curious, playful, powerful, creative, and able to heal quickly and naturally. Seeing the humorous, ridiculous side of a situation allows a person more options and perspective in handling it. When people have an alternative way of viewing things, they are not helpless. Participants may be encouraged to stage an impossible situation as a farce with themselves in the audience watching themselves as an actor in the play—and enjoying the outrageous and funny aspects of their own human comedy. When we can laugh, we can move from a morbid, unhealthy image stance to an imagery stance of creativity, hope, fun, and fulfillment.

High-level wellness is the philosophical, spiritual, and "metaphysical" component of GETTING WELL which focuses on thriving as opposed to merely surviving. Frequently work may be done on identifying and extirpating psychological weeds (such as guilt, depression, resentment, lack of forgiveness, destructive images/beliefs, helplessness, blame, attachments, co-dependency, poor self esteem, etc.) from the garden of a full, joyous, healthy life. Although many of these "weeds" are identified in a rather analytical, left-brained process, the uprooting is effected more usually with right-brained, guided imagery processes. For example, the group may be asked to identify the part of the body in which they feel "guilt" or "anger." (This is all too frequently the site of the illness.) The participants are then asked to give it a name, shape, texture, color, sound, movement, smell, and even taste. They are then encouraged to uproot and remove the emotional blockage from their beings by whatever method they choose, releasing it "to the light" or "to the universe." Then it is suggested that they fill the remaining space with power, love, healing, light—or whatever feels right. Along with removing the weeds, powerful new seeds are sown—forgiveness, unconditional love for self and others, connecting with the flow of life or the waves of the universe, empowerment, nurturing the child within, a positive world view, joyfulness, mindfulness, love for what the universe presents rather than demanding the universe present what one loves. We prefer to see destructive behavior, attitudes, images, and even disease as having a positive intention (though perhaps unconscious) as far as protecting the individual in the past, and seeing the participant "reframing" (Bandler,1975) or imaging himself using more viable, healthier and creative options to enable the positive intent to be realized in a physically and spiritually healthy way.

Expressive therapies, which daily follow high-level wellness, carry the work to yet another level and tap into unconscious imagery perhaps as effectively as dream work. Through music/sound, movement, drama, poetry, mask-making, journaling, and drawing/painting/sculpture, various imagery channels are opened to the participants for their exploitation. A typical exercise—recreating one's healing imagery in an idiosyncratic medium—consistently yields incredibly meaningful and creative results: from paintings, to collages, to poetry, to a tape created by a jazz pianist of her own jazz creation effectively dissolving her lung tumors. Although many of the exercises are designed to elicit and reinforce the image of perfect, joyful functioning, many are designed to reveal metaphorical blockages to emotional and physical healing. For example, the exercise of "drawing one's family as anything but humans" is a particularly revealing activity with excellent therapeutic potential.

Yoga and Therapeutic Touch (TT) (Kreiger, 1979) are two peace/healing offerings in the program which are in some senses mechanical, yet are deeply eidetic. TT involves the use of intention (intensive directed imagery) for the healing of others as well as oneself. The weekly workshop in TT crackles with the excitement of sharing with each other the individual and collective power of imagery and intention. (It is similar in feeling to sessions spent with Qigong masters in China.) Each session produces a few "miracles" from pain disappearance to increasing light perception in the blind; however, frequently the big "miracle" is the bonding of the patients to each other in a spirit of love and universality. Believing as some physicists that consciousness is the most powerful force in the universe, we see in TT the actualization of the *physical* power of imagery—whether it be seeing oneself as being healthy, touching another with the intention of healing, praying for an enemy, projecting a healing white light around a loved one, or imaging world peace.

Individual therapy frequently focuses on exorcising the demons of earlier trauma/loss which interferes with the healing process in the broadest sense. A variety of imagery techniques including hypnosis, NLP, Transformational Fantasy (Shaffer, 1986), psychosynthesis (Assagioli, 1976), eidetic psychotherapy (Sheikh, 1978), and Gestalt therapy, are used consistently. In family therapy (chronic illness is a family disease) family sculpture, genograms, Gestalt, and other bodymind techniques complement traditional interactional therapies. We have found that the GETTING WELL program provides deep, intensive psychotherapy for its participants— most of whom would *never* have considered "therapy" for the emotional pain they have internalized. They are usually considered the "well adjusted" individuals and families in our society, not needing psychological assistance. The emotional *Zeitgeist* of our culture is a prodigious producer of "the diseases of civilization," and psychological "adjustment" frequently portends physical problems.

Follow-up is important in maintaining gains made in the program. Weekly sessions for problem solving and extending the imagery experience are available for those who live close by. However, since most participants come from other parts of the country, we have developed a two-hour video, *Let the Living Begin,* designed (by one of our participants) to recreate the GETTING WELL experience when a person's engrams begin to fade. Attempts are made to get "graduates" in touch with counselors or support groups in tune with responsible PNI philosophy in their part of the country. Telephone support by participants and staff is always available.

Although we have established a promising research relationship with the University of South Florida, at this point most of our successes are anecdotal. However, with virtually no exceptions participants report exceptional increases in quality of life and living each moment to its fullest. Much more frequently than would be expected dramatic positive physical improvement and "remissions" take place. A couple of examples illustrate scenarios that we commonly see in the program.

R.E., an 11-year old boy came to GETTING WELL 2 1/2 years ago with a brain tumor which had defied radiation, and multiple surgeries had only increased its growth and his neurological dysfunction. He had been taken off all treatment for several months, and his parents were informed that he had little time to live at the time he entered the program. There he reactivated some imagery that his mother had used with him during years with childhood leukemia when he was five, and he added his image of "Ghostbusters zapping the tumor with God's light." During the four weeks spent at the program his imagery became a constant companion, and we saw organicity and paralysis begin to disappear. Several months later an MRI indicated only a small amount of calcification at the site instead of the tumor, and a few months later he celebrated his first *full* year in school in his life. He is now a healthy teenager, playing the sax in the school band, entering into sports, and interested in girls.

T.G., a 27-year-old single mother, entered the program after her oncologist told her there was nothing more he could do for the 50-60 tumors in her abdomen. She was severely depressed and hoped only that she could die where her young daughter would not see her. She found it "impossible" to image at first; however, after exploring her "neatnik" tendencies, she developed an intricate visualization seeing her body as a large hotel and her immune system as the cleaning staff. Maids would go in and clean the rooms, locking the door if they were unable to finish the job so that the debris would not get into the rest of the hotel. Over the past two years her MRIs have given evidence to the effectiveness of her "staff" with tumors receding and disappearing. She was quite pleased when her oncologist finally conceded "spontaneous remission" several months ago; however she questions how "spontaneous" it was. She recently directed and produced our video and is living an inspired life.

The many physical successes are exciting; however, the most important successes are those we see in people living well, seeing themselves as powerful, whole human beings in tune with themselves and the universe. Occasionally participants die; however, we see them really living until they do. Even when a patient dies, the family consistently reports that GETTING WELL was the most important time he spent in his life, and that death was not seen as a failure, but as a transition.

Although a number of centers in the country use one or two of the techniques described herein, GETTING WELL is one of the few which brings virtually all PNI techniques on all levels together in one place. The authors have observed that the interaction of the various components of the program creates a synergy that far exceeds the sum of the parts and is undoubtedly responsible for the powerful results the program yields. Perhaps the weaving of the imagery of hope, creativeness, optimism, and health in the deepest sense into all facets of a person's life effects a world view that creates the most powerful effects (Chopra, 1989).

Research at this point necessarily has had to be reductive and has measured only one aspect or strategy at a time. However, it may be the synergy of aspects or their interrelation which is a (if not *the*) major force in change. Creative means for measuring this interrelation is indeed a paramount research challenge in creating a firm, accepted scientific basis on which imagery and PNI can evolve.

REFERENCES

Ader, R. (Ed.)(1981). *Psychoneuroimmunogy*. New York: Academic Press.

Achterberg, J. & Lawlis, G.F. (1984). *Imagery and disease*. Champaign: IPAT.

Assagioli, R. (1976). *Psychosynthesis*. New York: Penguin.

Bandler, R. & Grinder, J. (1975). *The structure of magic I*. Science and Behavior Books.

Berk, L. (1989). Reported in *Advances*. 6, 2 & 5.

Chopra, D. (1989). *Quantum healing*. New York: Bantam.

Cogan, R., Cogan, D., Waltz, W., & McCue, M. (1987). Effects of laughter and relaxation on discomfort thresholds. *Journal of Behavioral Medicine,* 10, 139-144.

Cousins, N. (1979). *Anatomy of an illness*. New York: W.W.Norton.

Gilman, S.C., Schwartz, J.M., Milner, R.J., Bloom, F.E., & Feldman, J.D. (1982). B-Endorphin enhances lymphocyte proliferative responses. *Proceedings of the National Academy of Science USA,* 79, 4226-4230.

Green, E.E. & Green, A.M. (1986). Biofeedback and states of consciousness. In Wolman & Ullman (Eds.) *Handbook of states of consciousness*. New York: Van Nostrand Reinhold.

Hall, H.R. (1983). Hypnosis and the immune system. *American Journal of Clinical Hypnosis,* 25, 92-103.

Hall, N.R.S. (1990). The immune system: Minding the body and embodying the mind. Symposium presented in Gainesville, Florida.

Joy, W.B. (1979). *Joy's way*. Boston: Houghton Mifflin.

Kiecolt-Glaser, J.K, & Glaser, R. (1987). Psychosocial Moderators of immune function. *Annals of Behavioral Medicine,* 9(2), 16-20.

Klopfer, B. (1957). Psychological variables in human cancer.*Journal of Projective Techniques,* 31, 331-340.

Kreiger, D. (1979). *Therapeutic touch*. Englewood Cliffs: Prentice Hall.

LeShan, L. (1959). Psychological states as factors in the development of malignant disease: A critical review. *Journal of the National Cancer Institute,* 22(1), 1-18.

London, P. (1964). *The modes and morals of psychotherapy*. New York: Holt, p.33.

McClelland, D.C. (1988). The effect of motivational arousal through films on salivary immunoglobulin A. *Psychology and Health, 2,* 31-52.

Meichenbaum, D. (1977). *Cognitive behavior modification*. New York: Plenum

Norris, P.A. (1988). Clinical psychoneuroimmunology. In Basmajian, J.V. (Ed.) *Biofeedback: Principles and practice for clinicians*. Baltimore: Williams & Wilkins.

O'Regan, B. (1989). Barriers to novelty II. *Noetic Sciences Review. 13.*

Rossi, E.L. & Cheek, D.B. (1988). *Mind-body therapy*. New York: Norton.

Schneider, J., Smith, C.W., & Whitcher, S. (1984). The relationship of mental imagery to white blood cell function. Paper presented at 36th annual convention of the Society for Clinical and Experimental Hypnosis, San Antonio, Texas.

Schneider, J. (1989). Imagery and immune function. Paper presented at the 11th annual conference of the American Association for the Study of Mental Imagery, Washington, D.C.

Shaffer, J. T. (1986). Transformational fantasy. In A.A. Sheikh (Ed.) *Anthology of imagery techniques,* Milwalkee: American Imagery Institute.

Sheikh, A.A. (1978). Eidetic psychotherapy. In J.L. Singer & K.S. Pope (Eds.) *The power of human imagination,* New York: Plenum.

Simonton, O.C., Matthews-Simonton, S., & Creighton, J. (1978). *Getting well again*. Los Angeles: Tarcher.

Spiegel, D., Bloom, J., Kraemer, H., & Gottheil, E. (1989). Effect of psychosocial treatment on survival of patients with metastatic breast cancer, *The Lancet,* 10/15.

Sporn, M.B. & Roberts, A.B. (1983). Role of retinoids in differentiation and carcinogenesis.*Cancer Research,* 43:3034-3040.

Wolpe, J. (1969). *The practice of behavior therapy*. New York: Penguin.

DEALING WITH PAIN:

THE PSYCHOLOGICAL MECHANISMS THAT INTENSIFY PAIN

Nicholas E. Brink, Ph.D.

Clinical psychologist, private practice
202 S. Second St.
Lewisburg, PA 17837

A number of hypnotic imagery techniques have been demonstrated to be effective in dealing with pain. Even surgery has been performed using hypnosis as the sole anesthesia. The effectiveness of hypnosis in pain control is due to the high level of motivation to overcome pain (Hilgard & Hilgard, 1975). Yet, many individuals are unable to cope with pain even when using hypnosis. The purpose of this paper is to explore why some people are unable to benefit from hypnotic techniques in dealing with pain.

Melzack and Wall (1965) have presented a widely accepted "gate theory" of pain control. Electro-chemical messages are sent through the network of nerves to the brain from the site of the injury, notifying the brain of the injury. These messages are received by the brain as the sensation of pain. The gate theory describes neural mechanisms that work as a gate to limit or facilitate the message of pain getting to the brain. Various factors work to close this gate. Medication and chemical anesthesia can close the gate. Of concern to this paper are the various psychological mechanisms that have an influence on the position of the gate. Hilgard and Hilgard (1975) presents three hypnotic mechanisms for closing the gate: imagining numbness, altering the experience of pain by redefining it, and directing attention away from the pain. But, first, the patient needs to learn to relax and overcome the fear of pain for these techniques to be effective. The fear of pain intensifies both muscle tension and the inability to direct attention away from the pain. Hypnosis can be effective in teaching relaxation.

Relaxation and hypnotic anesthesia can be very effective in the highly motivated individual, but some individuals do not benefit from these pain relief techniques. This paper presents three psychological mechanisms that work to prevent such pain relief by keeping the gate open: internalization of emotional expression, psychological states that prevent the diversion of attention, and secondary gains.

INTERNALIZATION

Many individuals fear or have difficulty expressing emotions in a direct and open manner. These individuals "internalize" or hold-in their feelings. These internalized feelings are exhibited indirectly in some physical or psychosomatic manner. These psychosomatic problems may be purely the manifestation of some emotional issue or they may be confounded with some real physical problem. Such physical problems as ulcers, headaches, upper back pain, and the various symptoms of generalized anxiety are frequently considered purely psychosomatic. In extreme cases, such severe physical problems as paralysis have been attributed to purely emotional problems in which case the problem is diagnosed as an hysteric conversion reaction.

The manner in which emotions are exhibited somatically may be due to the nature of the emotion, to some inherent weakness in the individual or due to a physical injury. Some individuals typically "carry the weight of the world on their shoulder," they feel great responsibility in many life situations and feel they have no one's shoulder on which to cry.

Mental Imagery, Edited by R.G. Kunzendorf
Plenum Press, New York, 1990

These individuals typically internalize these feelings literally and experience intense shoulder pain. Bruxism is frequently equated to internalized feelings of anger. Frequently, when a person receives an injury, emotional stress finds its outlet at that site of weakness; e.g. lower back pain may initially be experienced as a result of injury but intensified by muscle tension resulting from some emotional issue.

Identifying the reasons why some people internalize feelings and others feel free to express such feelings openly provides suggestions for therapy. A primary reason is fear. Many of these fears may be directly taught by parents, e.g. "boys don't cry." Other fears may develop in a more subtle manner. One young woman did not want to put a burden of emotional expression upon her mother because "her life was difficult enough." For some individuals being emotional is being weak. Such fears as the fear of being weak and the fear that others will be disappointed in one's weakness, are common causes of internalized emotions.

Suggestions for Therapy

One technique to demonstrate the connection between the emotion and the body is biofeedback-- electromylographic (EMG) or Galvanic Skin Response (GSR) biofeedback. When either biofeedback modality is used while discussing pleasant issues, the individual frequently can see and/or hear the body become more relaxed than when painful emotional issues are being discussed. One woman with a real back injury but also involved in a child custody dispute, who had not seen her children for a number of months, denied that this situation had anything to do with her shoulder pain. She was amazed to see how her shoulder tension increased when talking about the situation.

Such emotional tension escalating the pain of an injury can be deconditioned through using biofeedback training. In the case of the woman in the child custody dispute, the EMG sensors were attached to the trapezius muscles, and she was able to observe the tension in those specific muscles. She learned through this feedback to think and talk about her children while maintaining relaxation in that muscle. Mental imagery was effective in teaching her to relax that muscle. Such images as "lying on the sand, between the sun and the sand, and letting the warmth of the sun and the warmth of the sand soak into the muscles of your shoulders" can facilitate such relaxation. The various images of warmth can be very useful for relaxation.

Overcoming the fear of direct emotional expression is generally necessary to break the habit of internalizing feelings. Understanding why the individual internalizes feelings may be necessary to overcome this fear. To gain that understanding, again, mental imagery can be used. Brink (1987) presents a three stage technique to uncover the internal or subconscious language used by the individual preventing direct emotional expression. The client is led to visualize the pain in a metaphoric manner. For example, one individual saw two clawed hands reaching into his lower back, grabbing and twisting. Another individual saw a black form with a cattle prod thrusting it at his back. As these images develop, the client returns to them repeatedly over several therapy sessions. The images are refined in as much detail as possible. Often there is initial resistance in forming these images.

The second stage uses one of several imagery techniques to facilitate a journey while carrying the image of the pain experience. This technique is a variation of Watkins' (1971) affect bridge, using the image of the pain experience as a bridge between the present and what happens on the imagery journey, connecting the image with the subconscious experience. This journey may be one of time regression, or of exploring a hallway or of going down in an elevator and looking behind the doors. The images that develop are, in some manner, related to pain. Generally three such images are developed, that is, going back to three points in time or looking behind three doors. The commonality of these three images reveals a pattern that the client can often understand.

For one young woman with shoulder and neck pain that developed after an automobile accident, hypnotic time regression was used, carrying back in time the hot poker that was used to jab her shoulder. She went to three incidents in her childhood. Two incidents were of her parents fighting and she was trying to rescue her mother. The third was after her mother had been divorced and the family was struggling financially. One day, her mother announced that they were unable to pay bills and that she needed to sell the piano, one of her favorite possessions. The girl was agreeable, though she went to her room and cried. She did not want her mother to see her crying because that would be a burden to her mother and would leave her feeling bad. She was taking the responsibility of protecting her mother on her shoulders. It became very clear that this young woman was an individual who carried the responsibility for everyone on her shoulders, and that she had no one on whose shoulders she could cry.

Once this pattern is identified, the individual then has the opportunity to explore ways of changing. Fears of emotional expression can be understood, yet, letting go of those fears may be more easily said than done. This woman began to experiment with emotional expression with her mother and, with less fear, with her college roommates. Such expression was feared and difficult, and initially she experienced greater emotional tension and greater pain. With time, her confidence grew. She realized she was not going to lose her friends by emotional expression but through this intimacy they grew closer.

When an individual becomes more directly emotionally expressive, it is natural to expect greater anxiety or fear of not knowing how others will respond. As a beginning, the client has the opportunity to try out such expression on the therapist. It is useful to bring a spouse into the therapy session at this point in order to mediate such emotional expression between them. As emotional expression increases, feelings of intimacy and closeness develop, and the health of the marriage improves. As the fear of such expression lessens, tension and pain diminish.

The use of ego state therapy (Watkins, 1981) can be helpful in overcoming fear of emotional expression. When the fear is realized by the client, an image can be developed for each ego state. One state is the strong, emotionally unexpressive individual and the other state is the one seldom seen, the one that can cry and be intimate. It is useful for the client to imagine these two selves sitting in each of two chairs and to describe these selves as completely as possible. For example, the strong ego state may be sitting erect, dressed neatly with every hair in place. The feared ego state may appear sitting with head in hands, with elbows on knees, dressed in a sweatshirt and sweatpants. As these images are developed, such feelings as intimidation are felt towards the stronger ego state and intimacy or warmth towards the weaker ego state. Frequently, the client is led to select an animal for each ego state. Typically a lion, tiger or bear is chosen for the stronger side and a mouse, rabbit or kitten for the weaker side. It is important to work with these images and let them change, until the client realizes that neither are all good or all bad and both are real. Acceptance of both ego states aids in resolving the fear of or battle between them.

The prognosis for overcoming the problem of internalizing feelings is guarded to fair for men and good for women. This distinction between men and women is cultural, because men are expected to be strong and deny feelings. The length of therapy is quite variable. For some, change is rapid and exciting, and for others, change is laborious and slow.

ATTENTION

As discussed in the introduction, Hilgard and Hilgard (1975) presented three hypnotic techniques for pain control. One technique was directing one's attention away from experiencing pain. There are a number of potential reasons why an individual may be unable to divert attention away from the pain. When a football player is injured while playing, attention to the game is so intense that the player may not attend to the pain and continue playing. On the other hand a depressed individual, who is involved in no activities other than lying around the house all day, has more than enough time to dwell on the pain, thus intensifying it. This escalation of pain adds to the depression which, in turn, continues to intensify the pain. The pain and depression become a vicious circle. A second example of when an individual is unable to benefit from using distraction or disassociation is when the individual is in a power struggle. Power struggles will be discussed later in this paper.

Depression

Depression is a normal psychological state in certain life situations, and has the best prognosis in therapy. One factor that inhibits progress in treating back pain is the client's lack of acceptance that strength and a painfree life may never be regained. Even when there appears to be a "cure", the chances are greater that the injury will reoccur, if for no other reason than that the person returns to the same activities and maintains the same attitudes as before. Generally, the injury creates a physical weakness that can be reinjured easily. The greatest hope for an individual with a back injury, or other injury, is to realize that a change in attitude or modification of how an activity is performed can prevent future injuries. Such a change in one's life style takes acceptance that a change is necessary. People seek to be the way they used to be and there is great resistance against change, especially when the injury is not severe. Depression is one sign that the individual is grieving the loss of the old self and is on the verge of making a change in acceptance of the need for a new life. As Elizabeth Kubler-Ross (1969) points out in the process of grieving, reaching acceptance involves five stages: first denial, then anger and bargaining, followed by *depression,* then *acceptance* and finally hope.

The medical model works contrary to this goal of acceptance. The patient goes to the physician to find a cure and the physician provides hope for such a cure. Even when the physician knows that the injury is chronic, the physician generally feels that the best approach is to continue to provide the patient with hope. Many motion pictures have been made of people with severe handicaps that have overcome the hopelessness of the handicap to find ways of living effective lives. By the severity of their disability they are forced to accept their condition. Those people with lesser injuries are more able to deny the hopelessness of the injury. Even physical therapy can support this hope and lead the patient to continue to deny the chronicity of the problem.

One impressive example is that of Joe Montana. After back surgery, he returned to playing football. What impressed me the most is that he had accepted his limitations and had become a different football player than he was before the injury. In watching the 1989 Superbowl, whenever he went to pass, what came first was to avoid being tackled. To avoid being tackled, he would throw the ball away. The sportscaster noted that he was never "sacked."

Suggestions for Therapy

When the client is depressed it is always tempting to provide suggestions of hope. But, the client hears those suggestions for hope as "you do not understand how bad I really feel." Suggestions of hope only add to the alienation between client and therapist and thus to the depression. To fight against such temptation, this therapist finds using his own personal imagery most effective. The client is seen as in a pit. The therapist needs to also be in the pit but even deeper than the client, experiencing the pit as being dreary, damp, dark and frightening. Talking about the misery, pain, despair and fear of the client, using the client's own words but adding to them, provides the client with the feeling of being understood, cared for and supported. The client senses the therapist is not afraid of despair and this lack of fear provides the client with greater strength. The therapist needs to continue to stay deeper in the pit than the client, even as the client begins to climb out. This imagery gives the therapist strength to deal with the despair even with cases of suicidal ideation.

In living through such depression, the client begins to pull together assets and possibilities. The client begins to find ways to continue life but in new ways. Searching for new ways can be exciting but it takes depression and acceptance of the disability first. Even with physical therapy, the greatest hope for the client is to see that physical therapy is providing a new way of life and not a way to return to the old ways. The client needs to realize that exercise and the strengthening and use of new muscles is mandatory to be able to function adequately, that such behaviors as warm-up exercises are necessary before attempting certain activities, etc. Employers and fellow employees in heavy industry may laugh at the employee that does warm-up exercises before attempting tasks, but the employee needs to be ready to accept this laughter and recognize his own limitation. Such a change in one's life style cannot be superficial but needs to be a real commitment to living differently and the old attitudes and life styles necessarily need to die. Grieving and depression are necessary.

Imagery is frequently used to promote this new life style, e.g. the image of going through warm-up exercises and being laughed at when returning to work, or moving and working in a different manner, possibly in a totally different job. Frequently the classified advertisements in the newspaper can be used to provide a stimulus for imagery. An advertisement is read and the client visualizes the job and what it would take to perform such a job. Such visualizations can lead the client into being creative as to how tasks can be performed within the limits of the disability.

For men in particular, their self-image and whole life has been centered around being physically strong and active. Changing that image to one of being sedentary initially seems impossible, frightening and hopeless. Such men feel that they cannot be loved, that they will no longer be men, if a less active job is necessary. Sometimes, marital therapy is necessary to overcome this fear. Facing the fear in the presence of his wife can really strengthen the marriage because, possibly for the first time, the husband is being intimate by expressing his fears. Again grief and depression are necessary before new hope is found. Some men have learned to respect and even thank their disability for forcing them into facing the meaning of real intimacy, the intimacy of being able to talk of their fears and weaknesses, of being real human beings rather than just "human doings," machines that don't feel.

Power Struggles

A second psychological factor that prevents distraction is a power struggle. Power struggles may be internal or external. An internal power struggle can be described as a war within the individual between two ego states.

One common internal power struggle is found within the "perfectionist." The perfectionist is afraid of the imperfect ego state, the ego state that could be lazy or could get in trouble, the ego state that fears not being loved by a parent because love can only be earned. The perfectionist ego state is the one that needs to be in power, that has a very high level of integrity, that is driven to accomplish something in life but can be very abrasive and demanding of family and others. The perfectionist believes that, if defenses are let down, all would collapse. The perfectionist is the "type A" personality who is afraid of being "type B." Such an individual is very vulnerable to any failure, no matter how small it might be. Such a failure can greatly intensify guilt and pain.

Pain can become the excuse for not succeeding and an excuse to "let go." This last statement shows how all three psychological mechanisms can work together to prevent pain relief. Such a power struggle may lead to internalization of feelings, especially feelings of frustration, guilt and fear of failure. Second, the individual is so focused on the struggle that it becomes impossible to distract attention away from the pain. Third, the pain can become a secondary gain (as discussed in the next section) to let go and avoid the struggle.

The external power struggle, e.g., the workers' compensation struggle between the client and the insurance company or employer, can be intense (Brink, 1989) but also has its internal component. The insurance carrier or employer tells the injured employee that the pain is not real and that the employee can work. The employee knows it is real and such confrontation prevents the employee from disassociating from the pain. The pain constantly reminds the employee of the insurance agent or employer which, in turn, brings the employee's mind back to the pain. The pain and the thought of the insurance agent or employer again become a vicious circle.

Confrontation from an employer or insurance agent can also increase fear and anxiety. If the individual is an individual who tends to internalize emotions, then there is a synergistic whammy to intensify the pain. Attention, as well as increased tension from internalizing feelings, increases the pain.

This external form of a power struggle can occur between the person in pain and a frustrated spouse or other close relative. The frustration of the spouse intensifies the anxiety within the patient, thus, intensifying the pain itself. This increase in pain limits the patient's ability to function. This inability to function increases the demands upon the spouse, which in turn increases the frustration of the spouse, again a vicious circle. This same pattern can easily develop with the physician or physical therapist. In each case, the power struggle increases the focus of attention on the pain and not away from it.

Suggestions for Therapy

In each of these cases ways need to be found to break the power struggle and provide the patient/client with an avenue for distraction. Sometimes an attorney can become a buffer between the insurance agent or employer and the employee, giving the employee the feeling of power and the opportunity to find something else in life on which to dwell. Personal empowerment is a concept that may be an important factor in overcoming such a power struggle. If the client is able to find some way to feel personal power, power over his or her own life, then the client has the option to let go of the power struggle. It is extremely difficult for the client to experience this feeling of power. It may be easier for the therapist to become the advocate for the client and attempt to convince the insurance carrier and/or the employer that they are doing more harm than good by continuing the struggle.

The psychologist can help the client see beyond the present depressing situation. Again, imagery can be used. The client can be led to explore the various positive alternatives of the future through imagination. First, though, the individual needs to accept the disability and to assume that the limitations and pain could last for the rest of his/her life. With such acceptance, images or dreams of the future can be developed, new ways of employment within the limitations of the disability. Such dreams depend upon opening the individual's mind to the many possibilities. Biofeedback can be a useful beginning. An individual in a power struggle feels out of control or useless. When the individual discovers that control can be gained over such body functions as temperature or skin moisture, this control provides a beginning of discovering other ways of being in control of one's life.

Behind these power struggles with an external adversary, there are also internal power struggles. The person who is at war with the insurance company is also at war with that self-part or ego state that feels inadequate or fears vulnerability. Such individuals fear others will take advantage of them and they feel a need to stand up and fight. The strategy of the fight is to prove to the other that the pain is real. Working with the individual to overcome the inner power struggle, to not fear vulnerability is another goal of therapy. It takes ego strength to face one's vulnerability.

Again, ego-state therapy techniques are useful. The two ego states to be developed are the one of strength and power, the perfectionist ego state, and the other of vulnerability and weakness. Again, neither ego state is wholly good or bad. By developing both images, again using two chairs and seeking animal representations, the fear of each ego state is diminished through developing greater familiarity with both states. In working towards acceptance of these two ego states, frequently the client is asked to find two objects that can be carried and frequently encountered as a reminder of the battle. One man is carrying in his change pouch a piece of yarn and a chain saw tooth to represent his soft side and his hard-nosed side. Such frequent reminders again aid in lessening the fear and lead the client to have greater respect and compassion for both ego states. When animals are selected to represent each ego state, imagery can be used to explore and manipulate how these animals relate. Such stories are developed not unlike the story of the lion with a thorn in its paw that was removed by a gentle mouse.

Frequently, family therapy is a benefit at this time. The client, demonstrating vulnerability and fear in the presence of a spouse, can work to increase intimacy and health of the marriage. When vulnerability is expressed and met with nurturance from the spouse, trust is greatly increased and fear diminished.

SECONDARY GAIN

For many individuals, pain is intensified because of some secondary gain. Several common secondary gains will be covered in this section: the need for dependency, fear of failure and success, and financial gain for not working.

Dependency

One common secondary gain is one's need for dependency. Such dependency can take several forms. When there is a problem within the family and the family system is in jeopardy, a crisis, such as a back injury, can work to hold the family together. The family pulls together to aid the injured family member and the problems that were tearing them apart are pushed into the background. A second pattern is the pattern of co-dependency. This pattern is seen in alcoholic families but an injury works just as well as alcoholic behavior. The wife may have a need to nurture or to be needed and an injured husband may fill that need, adding to her feelings of satisfaction with life. Some times, an individual who feels unloved finds being injured effective in bringing others closer. Such behavior may have been learned in childhood by the child who was frequently sick and kept home from school. The child learns that it is easy to get mother's love by being sick. Each of these patterns are variations on the dependency pattern.

Suggestions for Therapy

The prognosis for overcoming this pattern is guarded because the injury can turn out to satisfy most everyone in the family system by filling the injured person's need to be dependent and the spouse's or parent's need to be needed. Only when something changes in the family system can this pattern be broken, thus, family therapy is the most appropriate form of therapy. Family members will initially deny a need for dependency, especially the person who seeks dependency, but in confronting the pain experienced within the family, this need becomes clear. When this problem becomes evident to the family, generally, one or more of the family members make the personal decision to seek greater independence and the family begins to change. With the greater independence of some family members, the pain of the one member will generally intensify in an unconscious attempt to pull those others closer. The family will need support in their independence to make a real and healthy change.

Providing the family with metaphoric images through story telling can provide a long range stimulus for change. People find stories less threatening than direct confrontation. Stories are easily remembered, and stay with the listener so that, when the listener is ready, the deeper meanings of the story will be heard. Brink (1983) presents a procedure for creating these stories paralleling the family situation but with new and healthier endings, endings of leading a healthy independent life.

Fear of Failure and Success

A second pattern of secondary gain may be a person's fear of success or fear of failure. Being injured provides the individual with an excuse to avoid either success or failure. Both fears are related or opposite sides of the same coin. Such fears develop out of feelings of inadequacy or possibly a need for dependency as discussed above. One example is of a man who had been a skilled laborer all his life but then succeeded in starting his own business. Yet, he feared the responsibility of success and, thus, needed to fail. He did fail so that more would not be expected of him. He found a laboring job which fit his life style, but after his success in business, such a job was humiliating. He injury on the job provided him with a face saving way to overcome his feelings of humiliation. His injury and pain have become chronic.

Suggestions for Therapy

Clients with such fears are generally more ready to explore these feelings than those clients with a need for dependency. These fears of success and fears of failure may be uncovered and explored through the use of imagery again using Watkins' (1971) affect bridge and time regression and/or looking behind doors. When the source of the client's pattern of fear development is uncovered, change in the pattern takes continued work and support. Frequently, with time regression, while the client is reexperiencing some painful or fear-producing life event, a suggestion is made that the client's adult self go back and be with that younger self and, with all the wisdom and understanding of the adult self, help that younger self to understand (Barnett, 1981). This suggestion can be expanded with such phrases as "your adult self is the only person who can really know how much pain your younger self is experiencing, only you can help that younger self, only you know what that younger self needs. Go back, nurture and love that younger self." Such suggestions frequently provide an emotional release and are useful in dealing with the fear of emotional expression and the fear of being independent.

To help the client deal with this fear, again working with the two ego states, the fearful ego state and the successful ego state, can be of use.

Financial Gain without Needing to Work

There is considerable evidence that people on workers' compensation show greater resistance to overcoming their disability than others who have been injured. The employer and/or the insurance agents are quick to describe such individuals as malingerers. These agents use a learning theory model that the employee is being rewarded with pay for not working, thus, the employee has no need to return to work. I believe that this explanation, though true in some cases, is an oversimplification. A more complete explanation of such chronicity involves the power struggle concept as described above. Yet, the pay for not working is a secondary gain of the injury, and is sufficient to maintain the pain for some individuals. Frequently this secondary gain is confounded by the secondary gain of being dependent. Again the prognosis is poor for overcoming such pain and becoming an independent functioning individual. Frequently improvement is found only after some agreement for commutation is reached between the employee and insurance company and employer.

Suggestions for Therapy

Such individuals on workers' compensation state loudly and clearly that they really do want to return to work and do not like the life of pain and dependency. Learning to express emotions openly, overcoming a need for dependency and gaining power over one's life can lead these individuals into seeking a more effective and productive life. An independent individual who feels some personal power will not be satisfied with doing nothing other than complain about pain. When these deeper changes occur, the secondary gain problem will begin to diminish.

Malingering was mentioned in the above paragraph. Though this word is frequently used in the workers' compensation situation, malingering, as a *conscious* act to avoid returning to work and to collect compensation benefits, has been seen rarely by this therapist. I believe that such secondary gains as mentioned above may occur at a subconscious level and the conscious intent to defraud is rarely present. Understanding why the individual needs to malinger, whether due to the above discussed fears of emotional expression, independence, inadequacy, or success, can help the individual overcome the fears and move towards leading a more productive life.

CONCLUSION

It is impossible to separate an individual into parts, to deal with the emotional or psychological aspects separate from the physical aspects of an injury. One insurance company requested my notes on a client with the intent of paying me for only those sessions where the injury was discussed and not those sessions where other issues were discussed. An individual develops the tendency to internalize pain well before the injury occurred, but such internalization has a significant effect on intensifying the pain. A person's need for dependency developed before the injury occurred, but, again, that need for dependency has a significant effect on the pain. The insurance company's refusal to pay for psychotherapy could be considered discrimination against certain personality types. Only in dealing with those psychological issues in the individual's life, does the individual have the opportunity to find more effective ways of dealing with the pain. Separating psychological issues from the injury is impossible.

REFERENCES

Barnett, E. A. (1981). *Analytic Hypnotherapy, Principles and Practice*. Kingston, Ontario, Canada: Junica.
Brink, N. E. (1983). Imagery and family therapy. In J. E. Shorr, G. Sobel-Whittington, P. Robin & J. A. Connella (Eds.), *Imagery, Vol. 3, Theories and Clinical Applications* (pp.271-283). NewYork: Plenum.
Brink, N. E. (1987). Three stages of hypno-family therapy for psychosomatic problems. *Imagination, Cognition and Personality*, 6(3), 263-270.
Brink, N. E. (1989). The power struggle of workers' compensation - strategies for intervention. *Journal of Applied Rehabilitation Counseling*, 20(1), 25-28.
Hilgard, E. R. & Hilgard, J. R. (1975).*Hypnosis in the relief of pain*. Los Altos, CA: William Kaufmann,.
Kubler-Ross, E. (1969). *On death and dying*. New York: MacMillan.
Melzack, R & Wall, P. D. (1965). Pain mechanisms: a new theory. *Science*, 150, 971-982.
Watkins, J. G. (1971). The affect bridge. *International Journal of Clinical and Experimental Hypnosis*, 19(1), 28.
Watkins, J. G. & Watkins, H. H. (1981). Ego-state therapy. In R. J. Corsini (Ed.), *Handbook of innovative psychotherapies* (pp. 252-270). New York: Wiley.

CLINICAL IMAGERY: HOLISTIC NURSING PERSPECTIVES

Bonney Gulino Schaub, M.S., R.N., C.S., Jeanne Anselmo, B.S.N., R.N., and Susan Luck, R.N., B.S., M.A.

Holistic Nursing Associates
5 Milligan Place
New York, NY 10011

Imagery techniques have the ability to tap the inner healing resources of the body-mind. The richness and variety of imagery approaches allows the practitioner to facilitate changes at a variety of levels of consciousness and, because of this, they are ideally suited to the practioner seeking holistic tools. Many practitioners in the profession of nursing, working from a holistic, bio-psycho-social-spiritual framework, have integrated imagery approaches and concepts into their practice. Major principles within this holistic model of care include the following principles, adapted from Beck, Rawlins, and Williams (1984):

(1) valuing the uniqueness of each individual client's experience;
(2) recognizing the importance of beliefs and cultural values as they relate to health and illness;
(3) viewing illness as an opportunity for self-knowledge and learning;
(4) viewing the therapeutic relationship as an active partnership;
(5) promoting self-care and empowering the client;
(6) focusing on health and health promotion--recognizing what is healthy in the client and supporting this.

With this model as a backdrop, three clinical models of practice will be presented with illustrative case material included. The first example will be that of a nurse-anthropologist working in an urban community health center. The second will be that of a nurse-psychotherapist working in private practice and the third will be that of a nurse therapist specializing in biofeedback and stress management.

IMAGERY AND SYMBOLS WITH A CROSS-CULTURAL CONTEXT

An important element in a holistic model of health is the cultural context within which the symptoms are being experienced. Therefore health care workers should be curious and knowledgeable about culturally held attitudes and beliefs regarding the nature and origin of symptoms and disease processes. Insight into what people believe to be the cause of their illness will offer explanations of client behaviors in response to their symptoms.

Health beliefs and behaviors are deeply held, having been imparted to individuals as part of their earliest experiences. Whether the child's earliest experience was of mother offering the proverbial chicken soup as an antidote to distress or of mother offering a charm to ward off the evil eye, the messages are taken in unquestioningly by the young child. It is also characteristic that people in time of medical crisis tend to feel regressed and more childlike, whether it be because of the stressful effect of their illness or because of the need to give up personal autonomy in the patient role of being cared for. Therefore people who may have thought they had grown

Mental Imagery, Edited by R.G. Kunzendorf
Plenum Press, New York, 1990

away from their early experiences may find themselves seeking out and being comforted by symbols, images and rituals from their past.

Many health practioners work in ethnically and culturally diverse communities where they may not be fully aware of the health beliefs and attitudes of their patients. For example, the western model conceives of illness as "something" entering the body from outside and that "something"--be it viral, bacterial, parasitic, etc.--needs to be destroyed, fixed or protected against. In most other cultural systems of healing, the primary problem is not seen as external, but as a loss of personal power that allows the body's intrusion by other elements, whether these intruders be spiritual or viral. The problem must therefore be addressed at this level of loss of power and it is at this level the use of healing symbols and imagery play a key role.

HEALING IMAGERY WITHIN A LATIN AMERICAN CULTURAL FRAMEWORK

The application of a culturally sensitive approach to working with clients is illustrated in the treatment of Maria, a 30 year old Spanish speaking woman from Guatamala. Maria, who spoke little English, was accompanied by her mother, who spoke no English. Her presenting symptoms included a rapid pulse rate, an elevated blood pressure, stomach pains, nausea, anorexia, insomnia, flu like symptoms, depression and extreme anxiety. Physical exam showed no remarkable findings and laboratory tests were all negative.

Through an interpreter, the following information was obtained. Maria had experienced a terrible fright a few days earlier when her five year old son had just missed being hit by a speeding car. She did not have any other information to offer regarding the onset of her symptoms, but she did share her grave fear that if she was not cured of them, she would die.

Maria expressed a desire to find a local person who might be able to help her. The medical assistant was able to explore with her what might be of help. Reluctantly she asked if her mother could bring a man from her community to help her. After much administrative debate, the staff agreed to allow a healer from her community to come to the unit. Her mother then went to purchase candles, incense, herbs, an egg and fresh flowers. At the bedside, candles were lit and incense was burned. Prayers and chanting, which continued throughout the night, were offered up to evoke the ancestral spirits. The egg was passed over Maria's body as a diagnostic tool, and then the egg was broken into a dish. The healer then studied the pulse as a way of listening to the heart and soul speak to determine the nature of the illness and its cure. Family remained with Maria throughout the ritual. Her body was massaged and blessed water was consumed. She then fell into a deep sleep.

Folk healers, sometimes known as shamans, medicine men or medicine women, are people who provide spiritual and/or psychological counseling, advise, services and rituals directed toward the relief of symptoms and the generalized improvement of functioning and rebalancing. These problems from a western model might be classified as the province of the medical system, the mental health system or social services. The shaman, working from a more inclusive framework, addresses the problem through culturally meaningful images and symbols that allow the individual to move through their crisis and restore homostasis. From the viewpoint of imagery work, it is interesting to note the sensory richness of the shaman's interventions with Maria. He provided olfactory, visual, auditory, gustatory and tactile suggestions in working to evoke an image of healing. Since belief systems have curative power as is evidenced by many studies on the placebo effect, Maria's willingness to be cured was governed by her faith and understanding as to what she needed to promote self-healing.

Maria's culturally designated diagnosis was *susto*. In Latin American Spanish, *susto* comes from the verb *asustar*, meaning "to frighten." From a western model she may have been diagnosed as having severe anxiety or a panic attack, but from the perspective of her culture, Maria's condition included "soul loss." This was perceived as a spiritual crisis that was impacting on an emotional and physical level. It was essential that her soul be returned, and this could only occur through the assistance of one who shared her beliefs and was able to evoke the images necessary to achieve this. When the local healer was with her, engendering faith, confidence and trust in the system, the methods and the practitioner, there was an immediate relaxation response observable in Maria, resulting in a lowered blood pressure and heart rate. Through culturally relevant symbols and images, Maria was empowered and filled with hope and therefore supported in her process of regaining health and well being.

IMAGERY APPLIED WITHIN A HOLISTIC NURSING PSYCHOTHERAPY MODEL

Psychosynthesis is a psychological model that recognizes the bio-psycho-social-spiritual aspects of the person and as such is uniquely applicable to a holistic nursing practice. First developed in 1910 by Roberto Assagioli, M.D., it is a model that while acknowledging the lower unconscious drives elaborated in Freud's model of the psyche, also, acknowledges and works to evoke the client's innate drive towards wholeness (Assagioli, 1965). It is an approach that works to strengthen the healthy evolving aspect of the person's being. Assagioli posited that just as we suffer from repression of our sexuality, human beings suffer from denial and repression of the part of themselves that seeks connection with the ground of being. From this perspective, not all desire for deep connection is about infantile regression and desire for merging with mother. The healthy ego seeks union with a sense of something greater than itself, whether that be the forces of nature, a sense of higher meaning and purpose or a creative power within the universe.

USE OF IMAGERY IN PSYCHOTHERAPY

The application of the holistic model will be illustrated within a case study. Franni was a 35 year old single, white, Jewish woman from an upper middle-class New England background. She had been in psychotherapy with a nurse-psychotherapist for over two years. She was a graduate student and writer with an extensive history of substance abuse, including addiction to narcotics and IV amphetamines. In addition, she had a history of bulimia with purging starting at 12 years old. At the start of working with the nurse-psychotherapist, Franni had been free of narcotic use and other drug use for about six months. About a year into the treatment, the bulimic behavior, which had been present on a daily basis for years was greatly reduced, occurring about once every couple of months. Franni had come to a session in a state of extreme agitation and anger following a disturbing conversation with her mother, who had in the past consistently disappointed her by refusing to acknowledge any role in Franni's pain. She had tried telling her mother that she was willing to take responsibility for her own self-destructive behavior, hoping that her mother, who had always been very defensive, might acknowledge some of her own mistakes. Instead, the mother used this as a vindication for herself, saying Franni had always been depressed, even as a child.

Franni's rage and despair was intense. She kept saying all she could think of doing was using heroin. The nurse-psychotherapist was concerned about the possibility of self-destructive acting out. The desire to use heroin was seen as a reflection of Franni's strong need for self-soothing in response to this disappointment and emotional pain. The powerful calming physical experience of intravenous heroin use had been discussed in therapy numerous times in the past. Franni had been taught to work with breathing techniques, progressive relaxation and autogenic training as stress management techniques, and the therapist thought it would be important to have her reconnect with an experience of physical soothing before going further with the session. The nurse-psychotherapist led Franni through a long grounding and centering exercise with the intention of settling her physically and creating a deep state of relaxation that would be an enhancement to imagery work (Sheikh, 1986).

The client was asked first to focus on diaphragmatic breathing with the instruction to

...Bring all your awareness to a point about four finger widths below your navel... and now be aware of your breathing... the rise and fall of your lower abdomen... if you find yourself distracted by any thoughts, sounds, or sensations, just acknowledge them and then bring your attention back to the rhythm of your breath.

These instructions continued for about ten minutes. Then Franni was instructed to bring all her awareness to physical sensations, and she was systematically led through each body part starting at the top of her head.

Bring all your awareness to the sensations at the top of your head... be aware of all the subtle sensations ... if you find your attention wandering to thoughts or to other experiences, just acknowledge it and then bring your attention back to awareness of the top of your head.

In this way, attention was slowly brought to each part of the body down to the toes. Franni was then instructed to identify all the areas of tightness by breathing into the area and releasing the tightness with each exhaled breath.

The therapist at this point recognized that Franni had achieved a state of deep relaxation. Her breathing had slowed and deepened and body posture has relaxed and was very still. Working from a holistic, health focused model, the nurse-therapist now wanted to mobilize the strengths of the client and connect her consciously with the part of herself that had been motivated to make dramatic and difficult positive changes over the past several years. From a psychosynthesis perspective, Assagioli referred to this as the "personal self," described by him as "a point of consciousness and self awareness, coupled with its realization and the use of its directing will" (Assagioli, 1965).

In other words, from the patient's perspective, there is an ability to observe the the various aspects of oneself from the center of consciousness and then take action that is directed from this point of deep self awareness. As noted earlier, one of the major elements in a holistic nursing model is the promotion of self-care. This concept of helping the client to access resources of inner awareness and inner will is compatible with a model of self-care because the nurse-psychotherapist is giving the client the responsibility of identifying and acknowledging his/her own capabilities. In the case being presented, it was very important to emphasize and reinforce the part of this young woman that had, for the most part, given up the use of drugs, had drastically curtailed her bulimic behaviors and was working fulltime in a responsible position, attending graduate school in creative writing, and in a healthy relationship. Clearly there was a source of strength with which she could connect. An imagery technique of inner dialogue was chosen at this point.

Franni was asked to experience herself in a meadow. She was encouraged to experience this with all her senses, noting the smells, the colors, the sensation of the earth under her feet, the sensation of the air on her skin, the sounds of the birds, insects and breezes. This evocation of nature imagery was a way of fostering an identification with something more powerful than her lone human experience, a connection with something beyond her individual ego. This process of identifying with something greater, begins to strengthen the ability to disidentify from, or objectively observe, the present situation. She was then asked to follow a path through the woods to a clearing with a campfire in the center. She was then asked to sit before the fire and gaze into it, again, emphasizing the fullness of the sensory experience of the fire's heat, sounds, smells and colors. Then her instructions were to become aware of a wise being sitting on the other side of the fire, a wise being that had a great deal of insight and understanding of the present situation. She was then to enter into a dialogue with this wise being, asking for advice. She was told to take as much time as she needed to do this, and when she felt she had gotten all the information she needed she was to open her eyes and discuss the experience. The therapist made very vague suggestions about the nature of the wise being and the questions to be asked because it was important to allow the client to explore the imagery in any way that felt right and to help her to trust her own experience. The therapist, in general, prefers to wait until the imagery experience is completed before asking a client to describe it because the imagery is taking place in an altered state of consciousness and interrupting and asking the client to answer questions would disrupt the depth of the experience.

The client in this case received positive specific information on what to do next. The "wise being" Franni encountered was Doris Lessing, and the advise she received was, "You can always shoot up or commit suicide, that's always an option, but right now you can use this pain to help your writing. Why prove your parents right, that you're a screw-up? Use this energy instead to express your creativity."

When Franni reported this experience, she was truly surprised at the directness and strength of the guidance and felt very relieved and encouraged by it. The therapist's initial internal reaction to the comments that heroin and suicide are always an option, was that this was a negative message, one that would have to be examined more fully in terms of what part of the client's consciousness it was coming from, but in the course of listening to the client discuss it, it became apparent that the overall effect was positive. It was also congruent with this client's process that she would deeply mistrust any answer that seemed too pat or simplistic. The beauty of imagery as a technique is that it allows for an infinite range of possibilities, and is truly respectful of the client's process, allowing information to become available in a way that the client can actually hear it. The therapist's initial internal response came from a preconceived idea of a wise being as a more conventionally benign figure. The image of Doris Lessing however, was perfect for this client. It represented a figure that she deeply respected, a strong woman and a writer and one who did not trivialize the client's experience, but acknowledged it and offered an alternative that was completely compatible with who the client was. From the therapist's perspective, if one is working from a firmly held belief that this client is moving on a path toward healing and actualization, then the therapist can let go of his/her own agenda and trust and support the client.

IMAGERY-ENHANCED BIOFEEDBACK FOR MIND-BODY-SPIRIT INTEGRATION

Imagery for mind-body-spirit healing can be evoked through self-regulation methods such as biofeedback. Clients who typically might not be drawn to psychological approaches are often open to working with a biofeedback therapist because there is usually a physical problem that provides the entry into the work. They are generally feeling out of control of their bodies and their lives.

Using self-regulation as an empowerment technique, clients learn how they can "re-connect" and "re-integrate" their mind, body and spirit. Clients receive information about their body functions via sounds, lights and visual displays from the biofeedback machines. Information that would normally be imperceptible, such as changes in minute levels of muscle activity or one-hundreth of a degree change in extremity temperature or minute changes in sweat gland response (an indication of nervous system activity), are amplified and fed back to the client as the client can learn to:

(1)   become aware of these body signals;
(2)   connect their inner awareness with body functions;
(3)   learn to control dysfunctional psychophysiologic patterns in everyday activity;
(4)   develop the ability to generate deep states of relaxation for healing.

Clients quickly learn that they can control what happens in their body as they watch how their thoughts, feelings, and images create psychophysiological changes on the biofeedback machines. Biofeedback is a paradoxical use of technology, since rather than focusing outward on the machine, the feedback signals from the clients' own bodies help clients to know that "It's safe to go inside." This is especially important when clients feel their own body is a "dangerous place," is "out of control" or has "betrayed them" through illness.

The nurse-client bond of trust is a vital aspect of healing this split within the body. As the client develops a sense of personal inner safety, by learning how to relax and self-regulate the body-mind and experience the safety and security of a healing relationship, the client begins to feel safe embarking into deeper realms of healing imagery.

One such case is Jane, a single teacher of 52 years, afflicted by migraine headaches and hypertension. Jane had a familial history of migraines. Her mother and grandmother both suffered from them without relief. Jane had been treated by her physician for hypertension and was taking a prescribed diuretic for lowering her blood pressure. For the migraines, her physician had prescribed medication which Jane had been very sensitive to and therefore was re-luctant to take unless absolutely necessary. Her main approach to coping with her pain prior to biofeedback therapy, was to sit or lie in a darkened room and to try to "sleep away the pain."

The nurse therapist started Jane on a program which included biofeedback assisted relaxation training, mental imaging and stress management techniques. After her initial evaluation, Jane learned how to warm her hands. A temperature sensor was attached to her fingertip, and visual and audio feedback was given. Jane was asked to "play with inner experiences and physical awareness and see what happens on the machine." After ten minutes, she noticed that her hand temperature would usually hover around 75° F and would occasionally fluctuate to 81° F, but would drop whenever she "tried too hard to warm them." Extremity temperature can drop into the high 60's under stress and can rise as high as 99° F during deep relaxation.

Jane was then taught a basic rooting exercise for relaxation while her hand temperature was monitored. The imagery exercise began with having the client sit comfortably upright on a chair with her feet flat on the floor, shoes removed. She was then asked to imagine a root growing down from each foot into the earth in the same way a tree sends roots into the earth. The client did this exercise and experienced the sensations in her own body, while the nurse-therapist visually monitoring the client's expression, breathing pattern and muscle and facial relaxation. The exercise continues as follows:

After sending a root down through any floors, basements, down through the rocky soil into the deep, rich soil of the earth... draw up the nutrients and energy from the earth, just as a tree would do... and like a tree, bring this energy up your roots and into your trunk, starting at your feet, ankles... going up your calves... to your knees, breathing the energy up to your upper legs... your hips... breathing the energy up your trunk to your abdomen... your back... your chest... your shoulders... drawing the energy down into your branches and leaves... down your arms and into your hands... breathing the energy up through your neck, face, and the rest of your head and hair. Feel the energy and the connection with the earth, just as a tree feels and draws up the nutrients from the earth through its roots. Feel the strength of the tree as you are rooted... breath in relaxation, breath out any tension or discomfort... send any discomfort down into the earth while drawing the air and the warmth of the sun on your leaves, branches, and trunk... drawing in the energy from the sun and feeling the freshness and warmth through your entire body, through your whole trunk. Notice how you are feeling as you feel your strength and connection to the earth through your roots, notice the feelings of warmth from the sun. Be aware of how you are feeling right now, just noticing, paying attention, very gently, very accepting, just noticing how you feel, what you are aware of, there is no right or wrong way of experiencing this exercise, so just be aware and notice what and how you feel right now... (pause). Now gently bring your awareness back to this room, back to the sound of my voice and the other sounds around you.

Following this exercise, client and therapist discussed the experience, paying particular attention to the awareness of physical sensations or images, comfort level during the exercise, and any spontaneous thoughts or feelings. Often the therapist will then have the client draw the images that were evoked.

Most clients demonstrate some shift in extremity (hand) temperature even after their first experience with this rooting exercise. The goal with hand warming is to facilitate the client's ability to (1) recognize signs of vascular changes such as warmth, coolness, tingling, puffiness, throbbing, heaviness, lightness; (2) learn how to use these signals in conjunction with concomitent experiences of relaxation and relaxing imagery to vasodilate and warm the hands to 93-96° F at will.

Jane used the rooting exercise as a way to "stay in her body," slow down from what she called her "hurry sickness" and to help her recognize her connection with the earth, in other words to help keep her feet on the ground. She began to monitor hand temperature by making note of it during everyday activities. She would check the temperature first by touching her hands to her checks. If her hands were warmer or as warm as her face, she noted them as warm, if they were cooler than her face she noted them as cool. She also noted if both hands were the same temperature. She learned to assess her hand temperature by recognizing changes in the color of the hands, the size of the blood vessels on the back of her hands and physical sensations of warming or cooling. This was in addition to awareness training regarding her overall sense of relaxation or hurrying. Jane would subjectively note these changes and she would also, at times, use a small liquid crystal bio-square which would record changes in her hand temperature by changing its color. She would use this to confirm and support her own observations and to help at those times when she felt out of touch with herself.

Jane said she was always working and never allowed herself time off, commenting that she even worked on her school papers in her bedroom. In discussing this issue it became apparent that it was necessary for Jane to look at specific aspects of her belief system and life style in order to restructure her priorities. The ideas of her need for sanctuary came up in an imagery exploration of Jane's work life. The possibility of converting her bedroom into such a place was discussed. With a little bit of guidance, Jane began to generate internal images of her place of sanctuary which she was then able to draw as well. This process, which touched on issues related to life style, beliefs, experiences, and values, resulted in Jane developing a wellness plan for herself. Dietary and nutritional changes, walks in nature, and time to do "nothing" all began to evolve out of the inner awareness of her ongoing imagery and the encouragement and support of the nurse-therapist.

If Jane had difficulty with a personal issue or a self-regulation practice such as a breathing technique, she was taught to ask for guidance in her imagery and then to write or draw about the experiences. She was taught that there was no right or wrong way to do this, rather this was a process of learning to trust herself and the richness of her inner experience. Jane had been having difficulty learning the deep breathing techniques and she became concerned that she was not doing it "right." She was advised to use this process of asking for inner guidance and to observe what happened. The following session Jane said she discovered that she had been having trouble with the breathing because she did not have a personal image for breath that she felt she could connect with. At home, while using imagery to explore this idea, Jane remembered and sang a spiritual about the "breath of the Spirit." This song had touched her deeply early on her life and she chose to sing it in her session. Jane was quite surprised that she did this because she had never sung for anyone before, but she said it "just felt right."

Jane continued in this empowerment, self-awareness and self-regulation process. After three weeks of this work, her blood pressure, which had initially been 160/100, dropped to 126/84 and stabilized at that level. After eight weeks of this treatment, her physician discontinued her antihypertensive medication. Jane's migraines, which had been occuring two to three times per week, began to occur only periodically (once every few weeks). Jane recognized that one migraine occured after an experience in which she had difficulty expressing herself with someone, and had been made to feel guilty and selfish. Because of those feelings she had not taken care of herself in that particular situation.

Jane continued to work with imagery, her wellness plan, her assertiveness skills, and her self-awareness and self-regulation. In addition, the therapist began to introduce imagery of working with Jane's inner child. This included getting in touch with an inner image of herself as a child and getting to know, understand and acknowledge that child's needs. Jane worked with establishing an ongoing relationship with this part of her self and a sensitivity to self-nurturing. Through this work, Jane was free of a migraine headache for eight weeks, and when she did experience one, she was able to significantly reduce its intensity and duration.

Jane's focus is now on continuing to learn the language of the body-mind and how she can continue to learn to integrate these body-mind messages into a more healthful way of life. Jane was seen for a total of fifteen sessions over a period of nine months. Her willingness to take what she learned in sessions and actively incorporate them in her life was a key factor in the success of her treatment. The last few sessions focused on developing new patterns and rituals to integrate into her life. These included her reconnection with her creativity through walking, gardening, nature-focused meditation, and imagery work.

This case demonstrates how biofeedback technology can act as a facilitator of imagery work. The technology helps to engage the client by reinforcing the fact that internal images and thoughts have direct impact on physiological functions. This helps in building the client's motivation to then follow through in the practice of self-regulation and self-healing techniques. Jane used the biofeedback machines and the liquid crystal bio-square to develop and affirm her ability to vasodilate and create deep states of relaxation. The biofeedback "training wheels" were no longer needed as she developed her own self awareness, sense of balance, and sensitivity to her internal images.

Imagery approaches are invaluable for the practitioner working from a bio-psycho-social-spiritual framework. This holistic nursing model includes sensitivity to and awareness of cross-cultural issues, incorporates clients' strengths and their inherent drive towards wholeness, recognizes the transpersonal dimension of human experience, and integrates an understanding of the mind-body connection. Using imagery and biofeedback approaches within this model, one becomes aware of the healing, intuitive interaction between the practitioner and the client. This interaction illustrates the importance of the caring relationship, referred to in nursing theory as "the carative tradition." The healing qualities of empathy, faith, trust, hope and safety can be evoked within this therapeutic relationship. The skillful, sensitive and creative use of imagery can be the foundation for the work of drawing these qualities out, a process that constitutes the heart of healing.

REFERENCES

Assagioli, R. (1965). *Psychosynthesis*. New York: Penguin.
Beck, C. M., Rawlins, R. P. and Williams, S. R. (1984). *Mental Health – Psychiatric Nursing: A Holistic Life-cycle Approach*. St. Louis: C.V. Mosby.
Sheikh, A. A., Sheikh, K. S. and Moleski, L. M. (1986). Techniques to enhance imaging ability. In A. A. Sheikh (Ed.), *Anthology of Imagery Techniques*. Milwaukee: American Imagery Institute.

IMAGERY IN SPORT: AN HISTORICAL AND CURRENT OVERVIEW

Dan Smith, Ph.D.

Department of Physical Education and Sport
State University of New York
Brockport, NY 14420

The subject of imagery is receiving a great deal of attention in applied sport psychology. The purpose of this overview is to trace the development of the field of imagery, synthesize theories explaining how it affects performance, and then relate how it may best be used today. In the first section imagery is defined and the history of its use discussed, followed by explanations for how imagery affects physical and psychological skills. The use of imagery in sport is then described, and the scientific literature pertaining to the effectiveness of imagery in developing physical and psychological skills is examined.

ELEMENTS OF IMAGERY

Imagery Defined

Contemporary writers refer to "movies of the mind," "seeing with the mind's eye," and "visualization" when discussing the phenomenon of imagery. Richardson (1969) defined imagery as:

> (a) all those quasi-sensory or quasi-perceptual experiences of which (b) we are all self-consciously aware, and which (c) exist for us in the absence of those stimulus conditions that are known to produce their genuine sensory or perceptual counterparts, and which (d) may be expected to have different consequences from their sensory or perceptual counterparts. (pp. 2-3)

Martens (1982) defines imagery simply as "an experience similar to a sensory experience but arising in the absence of the usual external stimuli" (p. 3).

Imagery is a general term describing many related internal processes. Richardson (1969) identified four types of imagery: afterimagery, eidetic imagery, memory imagery, and imagination imagery. An afterimage can be obtained by looking at some object and then closing the eyes and mentally reconstructing the image of that object. The afterimage usually occurs without conscious control and rarely lasts for more than 10 seconds. Eidetic imagery is a form of precept-like imagery differing from afterimagery by persisting longer and not requiring a fixed gaze for its formation. It is sometimes referred to as "photographic memory" due to the clarity of detail and because it is viewed in the same sense as it is perceived. For example, if the object is seen, it will be imagined in the visual mode; if it is heard, it will be imagined in the auditory mode. Memory imagery is the relatively familiar imagery of recording everyday life that is voluntarily controlled and usually refers to specific events with personal reference. Imagination images tend to be novel, substantial, and vividly colored in the visual mode and to involve concentrated and quasihypnotic attention with inhibition of associations (Richardson, 1969).

Mental Imagery, Edited by R.G. Kunzendorf
Plenum Press, New York, 1990

Historical and Current Overview

Although once considered an irrational pursuit of mystics and shamans, imagery is today being used by physicians, psychotherapists, artists, business people, teachers, and athletes. European psychologists, particularly clinicians, were the first to emphasize imagery in psychotherapy (Skeikh & Jordan, 1983). Janet (1898) was probably the first European to employ imagery in therapeutic work. He discovered that substituting one image for another was helpful in overcoming the "idea fixes" of hysterical patients (Sheikh & Jordan, 1983). Although, unknown to most, Freud's use of imagery was extensive prior to 1900; in fact, he ultimately abandoned the use of hypnosis in favor of an imagery procedure more under the patient's conscious control (Sheikh & Jordan, 1983).

These early uses of imagery declined sharply in the beginning of the twentieth century as the study of imagery fell into disrepute. From 1920 to 1960, with the emergence of behaviorism, a "moratorium" occurred in North American psychology on inner experience, including imagery (Klinger, 1971).

Renewed interest in imagery during the 1960s and 1970s was brought about chiefly by developments outside the mainstream of psychology (Holt, 1964; Watkins, 1976). Fields such as engineering psychology, sensory or perceptual deprivation studies, biochemical and neuropsychological research, and research on sleep and inactivity all contributed to the imagery Zeitgeist currently in vogue. Maltz's (1960) work in psychocybernetics helped imagery resurface as a topic on inquiry. By the 1970s imagery had become a major topic of research (Singer & Pope, 1978).

Numerous psychological therapies now use imagery as a component of their treatment program. Solutions rehearsed at the imaginal level during therapy appear to generalize outside the therapy situation (Klinger, 1980; Richardson, 1969). Therapies such as autogenic training, systematic desensitization, implosive therapy, covert modeling, stress inoculation, thought stopping, induced anxiety, self-control desenitization, systematic rational restructuring, and hypnosis all involve imagery. Meichenbaum (1978) proposes three psychological processes to explain the effectiveness of most imagery-based therapies: (a) the feeling of control that the client gains as a result of the monitoring and rehearsing of various images; (b) the modified meaning or changed internal dialogue that precedes, attends, and succeeds examples of maladaptive behavior; and (c) the mental rehearsal of alternative responses that leads to the enhancement of coping skills. Imagery appears to affect behavior for a variety of reasons.

HOW IMAGERY AFFECTS BEHAVIOR

Behavioral scientists' understanding of how imagery affects behavior is far from complete although some progress has been achieved. In this section the theories and research pertaining to how imagery influences behavior will be reviewed, first for physical skills and then for psychological skills. The following explanations of how imagery affects behavior apply to many skills, including sport. These will be followed by a review of research specific to sport.

Physical Skills

The typical imagery experimental paradigm consists of two groups. One group practices a skill using only physical practice, and another group uses only imagery. In some studies a third group uses a combination of imagery and physical practice. Some plausible explanations of how imagery influences skill acquisition and performance have emerged based on this research.

It is thought that actual physical performance appears in a mental scenario during imagery. This mental scenario may be perceived in about the same way as actual physical experience. Finke (1980) and Hebb (1968) believe that imaging is functionally equivalent to perceiving real stimuli at certain levels of the nervous system. Because of this equivalence, hallucinations, dreams, hypnagogic fantasy, and other vivid forms of imagery may be mistaken for reality, and many imagery techniques in therapy rely on this principle when substituting imaged events for actual stressful situations (Cautella & Baron, 1977; Kazdin & Smith, 1979; Sheikh & Panagiotou, 1975). Klinger reitrerates this theory of perceptual similarity in his 1980 statement: "Experiencing something in imagery can be considered to be in many essential ways psychologically equivalent to experiencing the thing in actuality" (p. 5). Marks (1977) concurs: "Imagined stimuli and perceptual or real stimuli have a qualitatively similar status in our conscious mental life" (p. 285).

Nodal activation theory. Three major theories explain this equivalence: McKay's (1981) "nodal activation theory," Hebb's (1968) "cell assemblies theory," and Eccles' (1972) "neuronal hypothesis of learning." McKay's (1981) theory hypothesizes that imagery affecting the higher order mental nodes in the central nervous system has a priming effect on the muscular movement nodes:

> Activating the lowest level movement nodes results in muscle movement, but activating a higher level node primes or partially activates the subordinate nodes connected to it, and this priming effect remains subthreshold until the triggering mechanism is applied. Only the mental nodes are activated during mental practice whereas both mental and muscle movement nodes are activated during physical practice. Response time in the mental practice condition therefore measures in part the time to activate the mental nodes...As a consequence of a faster rate of priming, practiced or repeatedly activated nodes at any level in the system can be speeded up as a function of high level practice. This explains why mental and physical practice have equivalent effects. (p. 281)

Imagery and physical practice seem to have perceptual similarity, and perceiving information from the environment must be an important step in skill acquisition. Therefore, it seems logical to assume that skill can be acquired or refined through imagery.

Cell assemblies theory. In Hebb's (1968) view, imagery is a reinstatement of perception in which some type of cell assemblies in the synapses of the nervous system are reactivated in the absence of the original stimulus pattern on which they were based. This assembly of cells may lower the threshold needed by future impulses to travel along that nerve. This threshold may lower even to the extent that some muscle innervation occurs during imagined performance. Therefore, vividly imagined events should produce similar neuromuscular responses to those produced by actual experience although with less intensity.

Jacobson (1930, 1931, 1932) found support for this hypothesis. He reported that the imagined movement of bending the arm was associated with small but measurable contractions in the flexor muscles of the arm. Arnold (1946) observed that when a person is told to imagine falling forward or backward, slight movement was made in the imagined direction. Another study by Suinn (1980) used electromyography on the leg of an alpine skier as he imagined a downhill run. He found slight muscular action in exactly the same sequence as during the actual event.

Neuronal hypothesis of learning. Eccles (1958) also found support for such hypotheses. Slight firings of neural pathways occurred during imagery of motor responses, establishing what he termed a "mental blueprint" that helps the individual execute that movement at a later time. Eccles (1972) later explained this movement through his "neuronal hypothesis of learning." He believes that the effectiveness of a synapse increases with use and that given sufficient repetition of this activation, the synapse becomes "plastic," which facilitates future bridging. The activation that leads to this plasticity can be either actual or imagined.

The theories of McKay (1981), Hebb (1968), and Eccles (1972) are similar in their explanation: imagined events cause some event to occur at the synapse in the central nervous system. Easier conductivity occurs either because low-level nodes are primed and the synapse becomes more plastic, or because an essembly of cells facilitates this conductivity. One or all of these events facilitating motor performance have been hypothesized to occur during imagery.

Feltz and Landers (1983) question whether the effects of imagined practice on actual skilled performance are due to low-gain innervation of muscles, because of the minimal magnitude of the muscle innvervation. They cite methodological problems with studies supporting the effects of low-gain muscular innervation during imagery. Most research showing that muscle innvervation is localized to the muscles used in that overt movement place electrodes only in one location, so they can measure movements only in that specific muscle. They argue, however, that there is generalized activation of the entire motor system, not specific muscle action related to the skill being imagined. In addition, after subjects practiced overt movements involved with squeezing a hand dynamometer, singing, and playing a wind instrument, Shaw (1938) found an increase in numerous muscular action potentials from nearly all the various muscle groups tested during the imagining of these tasks.

Conceivably, therefore, imagery does not facilitate motor performance through low-gain innervation of muscles that are used to perform the motor skill. Nevertheless, the innervation at the muscular level may be only a by-product of what takes place in the central nervous system. If so, the theories by McKay, Hebb, and Eccles may indeed explain why imagery facilitates motor performance, and evidence suggests that the sequence of muscular movements may be the important variable in skill acquisition. The studies by Jacobson (1930, 1931, 1932), Arnold (1946), and Suinn (1980) all have shown the sequence of imagined muscular movement to be similar to the movements during the actual task. Because the acquisition of skill involves the refinement of the sequence of muscular contraction and because the sequence of muscular contraction is similar whether the skill is practiced mentally or physically, it seems to follow that at least some skill acquisition and refinement can occur during mental practice even though only low-gain innervation of many muscle groups occurs.

This perceptual similarity between imagined and real stimuli is not likely to be a complete explanation for how imagery affects behavior. However, other learning theories offer additional insight and support the notion that imagery facilitates the learning and performance of the sequences of skilled movements.

Symbolic learning theory. Sackett (1934) explains the effects of imagery through a "symbolic learning" theory. This theory posits that imagery of a task gives the performer a rehearsal in the sequence of movements as symbolic components of the task. Imagery thus facilitates motor performance only to the extent that cognitive factors are inherent in the activity. This theory would especially apply to sports skills requiring the athlete to think through each sequence of the task. By practicing through imagery the performer "can think about what kinds of things might be tried, the consequences of each action can be predicted to some extent based on previous experiences with similar skills, and the learner can perhaps rule out inappropriate courses of action" (Schmidt, 1982, p. 520).

Symbolic perceptual hypothesis. Sage (1977) explains the benefit of mental practice through the "symbolic perceptual hypotheses." According to this theory mental practice allows the subject to gain perceptual insights into the movement pattern by practicing the sequence of these patterns in the mind. The new insights result in reduced errors and improved performance because these imagined general factors transfer to actual motor skill execution.

Consolidation memory theory. Sage (1977) also explains the benefits of mental practice through the "consolidation memory theory." He writes:

> Information requires rehearsal to ultimately achieve long-term storage. The rehearsal may take the form of overt movements or, apparently, may take the form of covert rehearsal; in other words, covert rehearsal my have some of the same characteristics of activating and maintaining short-term memory processed as overt practice, and in so doing bring about a more robust long-term memory. (p. 409)

This notion hypothesizes that mental practice activates many of the neural components in the brain that are responsible for actual direction of skill execution, which is similar to the previous explanations by McKay, Hebb, and Eccles.

Many studies have shown imagery to be effective in improving performance on tasks that are predominantly cognitive in the their orientation. Ryan and Simons (1981) found that imagery significantly improved performance on a cognitive dial-a-maze task but had no effect on the highly motor task of stabilometer balancing. In a meta-analysis of imagery, Feltz and Landers (1983) found evidence that imagery facilitates performance of cognitive tasks to a greater extent than it does for motor tasks.

The "symbolic learning" theory (emphasizing cognitive aspects of learning sequential movements), however, also does not seem to be a complete answer because of the abundance of investigations showing significant effects of imagery on predominantly motor tasks. For example, Vandell, Davis, and Clugston (1943) found imagery to improve performance on basketball shooting and dart throwing. Twining (1949) found similar improvement on a ring toss. Clark (1960) found improvement for basketball free throw shooting, Gorbin (1967) for juggling, Kellner (1976) for basketball shooting, and Ryan and Simmons (1982) for stabilometer balancing. Although the causal mechanism remains undetermined, performance in both cognitive and motor tasks has been reported to improve through imagery. An examination of the motivational aspects of imagery training may therefore help explain reported performance improvement.

Hawthorne effect. The Hawthorne effect contributes to the relationship of imagery and behavior. McKay (1981) explains improved performance from mental practice partly as a consequence of giving special treatment to and expending more time and effort with this group than with those who do not practice mentally. Improved commitment also increases motivation to succeed. Feltz and Landers (1983) believe that the mental practice group becomes more "ego-involved" when asked to mentally rehearse a task. Sheikh and Jordan (1983) contend that because images are capable of representing situations, these pleasurable situations act as motivators for future behavior. If athletes believe imagery will help, they gain confidence in their ability to perform the skill. Confidence breeds less anxiety and may alleviate other psychological barriers to successful performance. This cycle may be especially evident with elite athletes or persons possessing well-learned skills because the mental blueprint is well established.

In summary, a single, comprehensive explanation of how imagery affects physical skill development is not available although a variety of hypotheses appear plausible. Whether the effect is explained by the priming of lower level nodes, reactivating cell assemblies, or enhancing synapse plasticity, evidence indicates that some activity is taking place in the synapse of the central nervous system that makes future conducting of these specific impulses easier. Mental practice also seems to give the subject perceptual experience with the sequence of a movement pattern. This imagined experience may especially facilitate learning and refining the sequence of the task, and this view is supported by research indicating that imagery facilitates the performance of more cognitively based motor tasks. Nevertheless, other evidence contradicts this interpretation and suggests that imagery does more than simply aid the subject in learning the sequence of a task. For instance, imagery may function as a means of rehearsal, or it may act to motivate the performer. Regardless of how one presents the case, however, imagery appears to aid the performer in the development and refining of physical skills.

Psychological Skill Development

Psychotherapy research accounts for many of the explanations for facilitating psychological skill development:

> Many of the classical emotions and feelings such as happiness, love, fear, anger, sadness, hope, and sexual arousal are accompanied by imagined scenes and situations in our fantasy world. Deliberate attempts to control or heighten these emotions are becoming an important part of modern cognitive behavior modification in which imagery plays a central role. To the extent that imagery techniques such as covert conditioning bring about generalized changes in overt behavior, we have further evidence of functional equivalence between imagery and perception (Marks, 1983, p. 105).

Most athletes learn to handle stress and anxiety through successful experience with stressful situations. An athlete who imagines successfully combating stressful situations may therefore have more experience to draw from when similar situations occur in a game. When stressful situations occur the athlete simply remembers his or her successful performance during the previously-imagined stressful situation. According to Cautella and McCullough (1978):

> Problem behaviors, overt as well as covert, are assumed to be subject to learning principles, and therapeutic improvement depends upon systematically manipulating specially constructed imagery according to learning principles to increase adaptive behaviors and to decrease those that are maladaptive. (p. 228)

Because adaptive behaviors can be learned by visualizing them in imagined stressful situations, imagery seems capable of building a reservoir of coping experiences that can be drawn upon during anxious times.

Psychotherapy techniques use imagery for the reduction of anxiety. Wolpe (1958) legitimatized the investigation of covert processes within a behavioristic framework with systematic desensitization. In this program overt as well as covert problem behaviors are assumed to be learned, and therapeutic improvement depends upon systematically manipulating specially constructed imagery to replace the maladaptive behaviors with more adaptive behaviors (Cautella & McCullough, 1978). Using a sport example, choking in critical situations may be a learned behavior. By systematically manipulating specially constructed imagery, the athlete may replace negative thinking with increased concentration and determination in these critical situations. The maladaptive behavior of choking in critical situations thus becomes extinct.

Imagery for the development of psychological skills in sport has not been studied as much as the use of imagery for the development of physical skills. However, a few researchers have found imagery helpful in anxiety and stress reduction in sport. Somatic functions, like heart rate, tend to increase as competition nears (Smith, 1982). Evidence from bioelectric measurement shows that imagery can help an individual control his or her autonomic nervous functions and thus decrease somatic anxiety (Lang, 1977). Sheikh and Shaffer (1979) found imagery helpful in the reduction of blood pressure, oxygen consumption, and heart rate, and it also accounted for changes in gastrointestinal activity and body temperature. Suinn (1972) found Visuomotor Behavior Rehearsal (VMBR), a sport imagery and relaxation program, effective in reducing test anxiety for a Ph.D. student. He found that VMBR aided the student in his examination performance by simulating stress conditions, developing skills to cope with emotional blocks and anxiety, and establishing feelings of competency and confidence through imagery.

Imagery may also be a valuable tool for psychological skill development in the area of self-confidence. Maltz (1960) calls our brain and nervous systems a highly complex servomechanism that acts as a goal-setting machine, steering the way to a goal using feedback and stored information. The servomechanism automatically corrects the course when necessary. Maltz suggests programming that servomechanism by imagining the goal and then letting the servomechanism take over in guidance toward the goal. Maltz gives no viable explanation of exactly what a servomechanism involves, but because positive reinforcement of a behavior strengthens the possibility of the recurrence of that behavior, the servomechansim may simply suffice as a term to describe some type of mental set for motivating the individual toward a goal for obtaining positive reinforcement. This concept has not been tested in the field.

Goal attainment through imagery may be a method to help athletes break out of the vicious cycle--playing poorly, experiencing the negative reinforcement of losing, lowering self-confidence, and mounting anxiety--that leads to increased incidents of poor play. According to the theories of Marks (1983) and Cautella and McCullough (1978), successful completion of difficult skills in a person's mind, accompanied by the positive emotions for being successful, may lead to improvement in two areas: confidence gained in one's imagined ability to perform these skills and the increased determination to experience these imagined positive emotions again in actual game situations. This idea of imagined success may be similar to Maltz's programming of the servomechanism. Poor psychological skills seem to lead to poor performance, and poor performance may lead to decreased psychological skills.

An interrelationship is likely to exist between imagery for the development of these psychological skills and imagery for the development of physical skills. Imagery for the development of physical skills may constantly improve motor performance, and imagery for the development of psychological skills may be especially beneficial during performance for handling psychological roadblocks such as stress, anxiety, fear, and lack of self-confidence.

IMAGERY IN SPORT

The ability to image the execution of complex sport skills has been reported to aid the performance of numerous successful athletes. High jumper Dwight Stones, miler Dick Burkel, golfer Jack Nicklaus, tennis star Chris Evert Lloyd, professional football player Bill Glass, and skier Jean Claude Killy all acknowledge using imagery in their training (Martens, & Burton, 1984; Suinne, 1983). Athletes apparently learn of imagery's benefits through trial and error because few coaches have taught imagery methods to athletes.

Although many athletes use imagery to some extent, few appear to develop this skill to its potential. In a questionnaire administered to Olympic gymnasts (Smith, Martens Burton, Vealey, & Bump, 1982) 92% professed using imagery in varing degrees to practice skills and strategies of their sport, to recall and control emotions, to improve concentration, and to set goals. These athletes used imagery less frequently to relive pain or to improve interpersonal relations. An interesting result of the survey is that 42% of the gymnastic coaches did not encourage imagery and may have stood in the way of athletes utilizing a systematic approach for the development of imagery skills. Most coaches do not emphasize imagery because they do not know enough about it to effectively train their athletes. This is a key problem hindering the application of psychological skills training programs in sport.

Imagery for Physical Skill Development

Imagery has been used to help develop physical skills through the symbolic rehearsal of motor tasks. This symbolic rehearsal is termed motor imagery. Motor imagery has been found to be helpful in learning laboratory and sport skill tasks in various environmental conditions using many methods with different types and numbers of subjects. Most of this motor imagery research is included in three reviews, which will now be cited, emphasizing task, environmental, subject, and methodological variables. Specific studies will be given detailed discussion within the appropriate variable sections.

The three major reviews were done by Richardson (1967), Martens (1982) and Feltz and Landers (1983), who jointly have surveyed most of the past motor imagery research. Richardson (1967) found that 19 of the 20 subject groups in various studies improved their performance through motor imagery on various physical tasks. Fourteen of these 20 studies used novel tasks in a laboratory environment. Only two of them investigated performance improvements with experienced athletes, and none of these studies investigated the effects of motor imagery on psychological variables like self-confidence. Eleven of the 20 studies used statistical analysis whereas the others simply cited the percent of performance improvement.

In Martens' (1982) review, 30 studies were cited in which motor imagery improved some aspect of physical performance whereas 4 studies showed no improvement. Ten of these investigations studied athletes in their competitive sport, and five used a field study approach. Three of the 30 studies found that motor imagery decreased state anxiety or negative thoughts.

Feltz and Landers (1983) found that 112 imagery groups benefited from motor imagery, compared to 32 groups that showed no improvement. Only 17 of 144 groups consisted of experienced performers, and all but three of the experienced groups showed improved performance through motor imagery. Laboratory tasks were used by 84 of the groups, and 26 of those found no benefit from motor imagery.

Most motor imagery research uses laboratory tasks or sport tasks in a controlled environment. Researchers seem to prefer the precision of measurement obtainable in a controlled setting because they do not have to accommodate a constantly changing environment. The learning of a variety of laboratory tasks has been found to be augmented through motor imagery. For example, Vandell, Davis, and Clugston (1943) found a 4% improvement for a junior high school group that used motor imagery for dart throwing compared to a 2% decrement for a matched group that did not use motor imagery practice. In a group of college freshmen they found a 23% improvement for a group using motor imagery on dart throwing and no improvement for a matched group that did not use the imagery practice. Using a ring toss task, Twining (1949) found that a group of college men using motor imagery improved 36.2% compared to the no-motor imagery group, which improved only 4.3%. Kohl and Roenker (1980) discovered that, for a pursuit rotor task, a motor imagery group of 21-year-old males improved significantly more than a matched control group. Ryan and Simons (1982) used a stabilometer task and found that a group of California highway patrolmen using motor imagery improved significantly more than a matched control group. Zecker (1982) found that a group of undergraduate psychology students using motor imagery improved significantly more than a matched control group on a bean bag toss task. These studies are typical of the general trend in past motor imagery research.

These controlled laboratory findings, which often involve novel tasks and inexperienced performers, may not generalize to the real world of sport competition. Studying intact athletic teams to determine the actual effects of imagery on physical performance is now necessary because, even when studying actual sport skills like free throw shooting, the laboratory environment cannot duplicate the actual stresses of the competitive situation. Partly because of the difficulty of creating realistic, stressful sport situations in the laboratory, most previous research has dealt with the use of imagery for the development of physical skills without attending to psychological factors.

Imagery for Psychological Skill Development

In comparison with motor imagery literature, far less research exists on the role of imagery in psychological skill development within sport. Weinberg, Seabourne, and Jackson (1981) found that long-term (6 weeks for 20 minutes per day) motor imagery and relaxation training significantly decreased competitive state anxiety and improved karate performance for a group of collegiate karate club subjects compared to a matched control group. Performance improvement was judged by experts viewing specific skills in a controlled setting and in an intersquad sparring tournament. It seems doubtful, however, that state anxiety is maximized in a controlled environment or even in an intersquad competition. Would this same relaxation and motor imagery training be beneficial in a major national tournament in front of thousands of screaming fans? A few other investigations have studied elite athletes in a field setting.

DeWitt (1980) implemented biofeedback and imagery training with two groups of intercollegiate athletes. The first group consisted of 6 football players who were rated by their coaches as having high levels of stress during competition. They attended 12 biweekly, 1-hour sessions consisting of EMG biofeedback, relaxation, and imagery training. The dependent variable was subjective coaching staff ratings of game performance for each athlete before and after the treatment. Statistically significant improvement was shown by 4 of the 6 athletes. With an N of only 6 and only 4 of those showing performance improvement, methodological problems may exist especially because no control group was used for comparison.

In a second study by DeWitt (1980), 12 basketball players also used EMG biofeedback and imagery training to promote relaxation. Again using a two-factor repeated measures ANOVA, performance improvement between pre- and posttest was significant. But this time the dependent variable measured by subjective performance evaluations was completed by two team managers, not by coaches, and again no control group was used for comparison. Because team managers are usually students and rarely basketball experts, this performance measure may be suspect.

Meyers and Schleser (1980) used relaxation and imagery training to aid an intercollegiate basketball player with concentration and confidence problems. The athlete received seven sessions. He showed significant improvement in field goal percentage, and his overall performance improved significantly more than that of three of his teammates. This study attempted to use a control group from the same team for comparison. However, a problem of validity may arise due to the fact that an intercollegiate basketball team spends so much time together on and off the court that the control subjects were likely to be familiar with the intervention techniques used with the treatment subject. They may have used some of these strategies on their own. Another problem involves the number of treatment sessions. Seven sessions may not be enough to alter firmly engrained cognitions.

In a follow-up study Meyers, Schleser, and Okwumabua (1982) used imagery and relaxation training with two collegiate women basketball players. One woman experienced concentration problems on free throw shooting and the other on field goals. The methodology was similar to that employed in the previous study, except that the intervention was evaluated in a modified multiple baseline design with a reversal on one of the athletes. Also, the number of treatment sessions increased to 23 for 1 subject and 15 for the other. The subject who received intervention for free throw shooting shot 41.3% during baseline, 54.8% during the treatment, and 28.6% during the return to baseline. The subject who received intervention for field goal shooting shot 36.7% during the baseline period and 52.2% during the treatment period.

Gravel, Lemieux, and Ladouceur (1980) found that a group of cross-country skiers using relaxation and imagery displayed significantly fewer negative self-reports than a placebo group from the same team viewing a silent movie on cross-country skiing. Questionnaire results and subjective reports from the athletes showed significant decrease in intensity of the experimental group's maladaptive cognitive pattern between pretest and follow-up and posttest and follow-up. Again, treatment subjects may have contaminated the control subjects inasmuch as they were from the same team. Nevertheless, this study is unique in that it investigated cognitive improvements instead of performance change. What may be a vital need is research that probes both cognitive and performance improvements.

As is evident from the more recent investigations reviewed, a trend may be emerging toward more research in the use of imagery for the development of psychological skills for improvement of sport performance. Most have some methodological limitations, but at least the external validity of sport imagery training is improving.

REFERENCES

Arnold, M. (1946). On the mechanisms of suggestion and hynosis. *Journal of Abnormal and Social Psychology*, 41, 107-128.

Cautella, J., and Baron, M. (1977). Covert conditioning: A theoretical analysis. *Behavior Modification*, 1, 351-368.

Cautella, J., & McGullough, L. (1978). Covert conditioning: A learning theory persepctive on imagery. In J. Singer & K. Pope (Eds.),*The power of human imagination*. New York: Plenum Press.

Clark, L. (1960). Effect of mental practice on the development of a certain motor skill. *Research Quarterly*, 31, 560-569.

Corbin, C. (1967a). The effects of covert rehearsal on the development of a complex motor skill. *The Journal of General Psychology*, 76, 143-150.

DeWitt, D. (1980). Cognitive and biofeedback training for stress reduction with university athletes. *Journal of Sport Psychology*, 2, No. 4, 288-294.

Eccles, J. (1958). The physiology of imagination. *Scientific American*, 199, 135.

Eccles, J. (1972). Possible synaptic mechanisms subserving learning. In A. Karyman & J. Eccles (Eds.), *Brain and human behavior*. New York: Springer-Verlag.

Feltz, D., & Landers, D. (1983). The effects of mental practice on motor skill learning and performance: A meta-analysis. *Journal of Sport Psychology*, 5, No. 1, 25-57.

Finke, R. (1980). Levels of equivalence in imagery and perception. *Psychological Review*, 87, 113-132.

Gravel, R., Lemieux, G., & Ladouceur, R. (1980). Effectiveness of a cognitive behavioral treatment package for cross-country ski racing. *Cognitive Therapy and Research*, 4, No. 1, 83-89.

Hebb, D. (1968). Concerning imagery. *Psychological Review*, 75, 466-477.

Holt, R. (1964). Imagery: The return of the ostracized. *American Psychologist*, 19, 254-264.

Jacobson, E. (1930). Electrical measurements of neuromuscular states during mental activities. I. Imagination of movement involving skeletal muscles. *American Journal of Physiology*, 91, 547-608.

Jacobson, E. (1931). Electrical measurements of neuromuscular states during mental activities. V. Variation of specific muscles contracting during imagination. *American Journal of Physiology*, 96, 115-121.

Jacobson, E. (1932). Electrophysiology of mental activities. *American Journal of Psychology*, 44, 677-694.

Janet P. (1898). *Nervoses et idees fixes*. Paris: Alcan.

Kazdin, A., & Smith, G. (1979). Covert conditioning: A review and evaluation. *Advances in Behavior Research and Therapy*, 2, 57-96.

Kellner, S. (1976). Psycho-cybernetics, mental practice makes perfect. *Scholastic Coach*, Feb., 40-45.

Klinger, E. (1971). *The structure and function of fantasy*. New York: Wiley.

Klinger, E. (1980). Therapy and the flow of thought. In J. Shorr, G. Sobel, P. Robin, & J, Connella (Eds.), *Imagery: It's many dimensions and applications*. New York: Plenum.

Kohl, R., & Roenker, D. (1980). Bitalteral transfer as a function of mental imagery. *Journal of Motor Behavior*, 12, No. 3, 197-206.

Lang, P. (1977). Imagery in therapy: An information processing analysis of fear. *Behavior Therapy*, 8, 862-886.

Maltz, M. (1960). *Psycho-cybernetics: A new way to get more living out of life*. NJ: Prentice-Hall.

Marks, D. (1977). Imagery and consciousness: A theoretical review from an individual differences perspective. *Journal of Mental Imagery*, 2, 275-290.

Marks, D. (1983). Mental imagery and consciousness: A theoretical review. In A. Sheikh (Ed.), *Imagery: Current theory, research, and application*. New York: Wiley.

Martens, R. (1982, September). *Imagery in sport*. Paper presented at the VII Commonwealth and International Conference on Sport, Physical Education, Recreation, and Dance, Brisbane, Australia.

Martens, R. & Burton, D. (1984). *Psychological skills training*. Unpublished manuscript.

McKay, D. (1981). The problem of rehearsal or mental practice. *Journal of Motor Behavior*, 13, 274-285.

Meichenbaum, D. (1978). Why does using imagery in psychotherapy lead to change? In J. Singer, & K. Pope (Eds.), *The power of human imagination*. New York: Plenum.

Meyers, A., & Schleser, R. (1980). A cognitive behavioral intervention for improving basketball performance. *Journal of Sport Psychology*, 2, No. 1, 69-73.

Meyers, A., Schleser, R., & Okwumabua, T. (1982). A cognitive behavioral intervention for improving basketball performance. *Research Quarterly*, 53, No. 4, 344-347.

Richardson, A. (1967). Mental practice: A review and discussion. *Research Quarterly*, 38, 95-107 & 262-273.

Richardson, A. (1969). *Mental imagery*. New York: Springer.

Ryan, E. & Simons, J. (1981). Cognitive demand, imagery, and frequency of mental rehearsal as factors influencing acquistion of motor skills. *Journal of Sport Psychology*, 3, No. 1, 35-45.

Ryan, E. & Simons, J. (1982). Efficacy of mental imagery in enhancing mental rehearsal of motor skills. *Journal of Sport Psychology*, 4, No. 1, 41-51.

Sackett, R. (1934). The influences of symbolic rehearsal upon the retention of a maze habit. *Journal of General Psychology*, 10, 376-395.

Sage, G. (1977). *Introduction to motor behavior: A neuro-psychological approach*. (2nd ed.). Boston, MA: Addison-Wesley.

Schmidt, R. (1982). *Motor control and learning: a behavioral emphasis*. Champaign, IL: Human Kinetics.

Shaw, W. (1938). The distribution of muscular action potentials during imaging. *The Psychological Record*, 2, 195-216.

Sheikh, A., & Jordon, C. (1983). Clinical uses of mental imagery. In A. Sheikh (Ed.), *Imagery: Current theory, research, and application*. New York: John Wiley & Sons.

Sheikh, A., & Panagiotou, N. (1975). Use of mental imagery in psychotherapy: A critical review. *Perceptual and Motor Skills*, 41, 555-585.

Sheikh, A., & Shaffer, J. (1979). *The potential of fantasy and imagination*. New York: Brandon House.

Singer, J., & Pope, K. (1978). *The power of human imagination*. New York: Plenum.

Smith, D., Martens, R., Burton, D., Vealey, R., & Bump, L. (1982). *Psychological testing of the gymnastic teams at the National Sports Festival*, Unpublished manuscript.

Suinn, R. (1972). Behavioural rehearsal training in ski racers. *Behavior Therapy*, 3, 519-520.

Suinn, R. (1980). *Psychology in sports: Methods and applications*. Minneapolis: Burgess.

Suinn, R. (1983). Imagery and sports. In A. Sheikh (Ed.), *Imagery: Current theory, research, and application*. New York: Wiley.

Twining, W. (1949). Mental practice and physical practice in learning a motor skill. *Research Quarterly*, 20, 432-435.

Vandell, R., Davis, R., & Clugston, H. (1943). The function of mental practice in the acquisition of motor skills. *Journal of General Psychology*, 29, 243-250.

Watkins, M. (1976). *Waking Dreams*. New York: Harper.

Weinberg, R., Seabourne, T., & Jackson, A. (1981). Effects of visuo-motor behavior rehearsal, relaxation, and imagery on karate performance. *Journal of Sport Psychology*, 3, 228-238.

Wolpe, J. (1958). *Psychotherapy by reciprocal inhibition* . Stanford, CA: Stanford University Press.

Zecker, S. (1982). Mental practice and knowledge of results in the learning of a perceptual motor skill. *Journal of Sport Psychology*, 4, No. 1, 52-63.

SYMBOLIC IMAGES IN PSYCHOPATHOLOGY AND PSYCHOTHERAPY

REPAIRING NARCISSISTIC DEFICITS THROUGH THE USE OF IMAGERY

Jerold R. Gold, Ph.D.

Ferkauf Graduate School of Psychology
Yeshiva University
Bronx, NY 10461

INTRODUCTION

In this presentation I will describe a method for utilizing imagery techniques within the context of dynamic psychotherapy specifically as a means for the repair of deficits in the structure of the self. Imagery procedures are viewed as measures through which to promote corrective internalization, thus providing the narcissistically impaired patient with the necessary experiences for advantageous developmental progression.

The presentation will begin with a review of psychoanalytic approaches to self disorders, to be followed by a discussion of the rationale for, and methodology of, an imagery enhanced therapy and then by several case examples. Some hypotheses about the reasons underlying the observed potency of imagery techniques for promoting internalization will be considered in conclusion.

CURRENT APPROACHES TO DISORDERS OF THE SELF

In the last three decades the attention of a significant portion of the psychotherapeutic community has moved from the study and treatment of the neuroses to another group of disorders, which are known under such names as *narcissistic personality disorder* (Kohut, 1971), *schizoid personality* (Fairbairn, 1952), and *self disorder* (Newirth, 1989). Other labels have been suggested as well, but all of these terms essentially refer to a shared set of symptoms, experiences, and behaviors which are centered around the constructs of the *self* and the *ego*. These constructs refer to the patient's experience of himself or herself in relation to others and to themselves (the self), and to the patient's adaptive and coping capacities (the ego.) Persons with narcissistic psychopathology are described as suffering from a variety of disturbances in the realm of relatedness and self experience, including an inability to experience the self in an authentic, playful, and openly expressive way (Mitchell, 1989); from deficits in the ongoing regulation of self esteem and in the capacity to soothe oneself when distressed and from an impaired capacity to internally represent the self as separate or autonomous in relation to others (Kohut, 1971); and from a defective capacity to integrate contradictory images of the self or of others into a single, consistent representation (Kernberg, 1975).

Defects in ego functions which are associated with narcissistic pathology include poor frustration tolerance, an inability to delay gratification, an absence or excess of signal anxiety, and impaired cognitive functioning, in particular, weaknesses in differentiating fantasy and wishful psychic activity from concrete, external experience. These and all of the other manifestations of this type of psychopathology are believed to reflect early and severe warps and compromises of psychological development.

Despite ongoing debates about etiology, there exists some consensus that such psychopathology requires intensive psychotherapeutic intervention. Most psychoanalytic work

Mental Imagery, Edited by R.G. Kunzendorf
Plenum Press, New York, 1990

with narcissistic disorders is based on a critical assumption: deficits in the self can be ameliorated only when these deficits and their effect on the patient's relatedness and adaptive capacities are expressed in, and come to dominate, the transference relationship. Equally important is the idea that a full "cure" of warps in ego and self is possible only if the developmental compromises which caused the condition to evolve are re-experienced and resolved in the transference relationship as well. Most importantly, out of these experiences in the transference relationship come new, benign, and progressive experiences which are internalized and become the stuff of a newly structured and completed ego and self which are capable of the relational and adaptive tasks of adulthood.

RATIONALE FOR AN IMAGERY ENHANCED PSYCHOTHERAPY OF THE SELF

It is an unfortunate paradox that many of those individuals who suffer from narcissistic disorders are prevented by the effects of that pathology from undertaking or completing the intensive psychotherapy which was described above. Such psychotherapies require a commitment of three to five therapy hours weekly in order to generate the affective and interpersonal intensity necessary for deep regression and the emergence of the desired infantile transferences. This commitment of time, money, and psychic pain is difficult for many people for pragmatic reasons, but such a commitment often is impossible for narcissistically impaired persons due to the specific nature of their pathology: difficulties in relatedness which make a frequent, intense, regressive and painful therapeutic relationship intolerable at the outset of treatment, and for many patients, for a considerable time thereafter.

As a result, it is necessary to develop therapeutic approaches to deficits in the self which are appropriate for, and which provide significant therapeutic benefits within, the limits of once or twice weekly therapy sessions with a group of patients who cannot or will not tolerate the regressive and passive stance required in psychoanalysis. In particular, what seems crucially necessary are methods for the rapid and efficient promotion of benign experiences which can be internalized and thus serve as the building blocks of new self structures. The remainder of this presentation is concerned with the use of imagery techniques as a potent and direct intervention to be used to promote internalization.

TRANSLATING SELF AND EGO DEFICITS INTO VISUAL IMAGES

Experiences based on visualization and on the manipulation of visual images may be effectively introduced into psychotherapy when the patient or the therapist recognizes the effects of psychological processes reflective of a presumed defect in the structure of the patient's self or ego. For example, to select a number of common self deficits for illustration, such processes will be most evident in the patient's descriptions of interpersonal or intrapsychic events in which the patient is unable to soothe himself or herself when troubled, or cannot sort out what his or her thoughts, feelings, and motives are, or to whom those experiences belong. Such data allow the therapist to infer that this is a person who lacks a nurturing internal object, and who has difficulties in experiencing himself or herself as separate and autonomous in relationship to another person. Similarly, when the patient describes having experienced someone as a different being when that person evokes in the patient an affect or perception contrary to the patient's preferred image of that person, that patient is unwittingly reporting a defect in the ability to maintain a consistent representation of another person. These are only a few of the many types of potential self defects.

Ego deficits are expressed in reports of difficulties in controlling oneself when it is necessary to do so, in displaying an inability to detect and to respond to impending physical or mental dangers when they exist, or in an impairment in using the awareness of the long term consequences of one's actions to guide and to inform immediate decision making.

Once these and other self defects are identified, anoperational definition of the deficit and a potential corrective experience is formulated by the therapist in terms of an image or series of images for the patient to use, in session and in daily life, when situations and relationships evoke the deficit. Suggestions for imagery tasks can be offered to the patient with or without interpretations of the underlying structural warps upon which the images are based. The decision to use imagery in tandem with interpretation is an empirical decision which evolves out of work with each individual. Some patients are better able to use imagery experiences when they understand the intent and the meaning of the therapist's suggestion, while many others require and benefit from interpretation only *after* they have found the imagery to be helpful. The state of the therapeutic relationship and the temporal location of the use of imagery also influence the need for, and utility of, insight in conjunction with these active techniques.

CASES STUDIES

Several cases will be presented which illustrate the operational definition of self and ego deficits into visual images and the utilization of those images in a reparative manner. Imagery techniques are introduced on the assumption that such techniques promote the internalization of new self and object representations, and ego structures, more effectively than would be possible through the use of interpretation alone. Some theoretical arguments for this assumption will be discussed following the case examples.

Case 1

In the example which follows the patient's dysphoria is understood to reflect the absence of a soothing and protective parental representation. A concrete interpersonal interaction is transformed into a image of the missing psychic component on the basis of this inference, and the use of this image over time leads to internalization and to an enhanced ability on the part of the patient to provide herself with the necessary psychological functions.

A young woman entered a session in a state of panic, reporting that an upcoming oral presentation at work was the source of her upset. The patient was a conscientious and extremely capable worker who was well prepared for this event. Exploration of her distress led to the understanding that the anticipation of the presentation was causing her to feel entirely alone, and separate from, all of the important people in her life. As she put it, "I am the only member of the Jello Head family (an often used description of her parents and siblings) to have a job where a brain is necessary. They would have no idea what I'm saying or why this is so important to me. Every time I think of speaking to the group, I feel as if every one at home has melted away. When I'm here it feels better. If only you could come with me, maybe I wouldn't feel so abandoned."

The therapist seized on this last statement and suggested that the patient envision the therapist having shrunken down to the size of a wallet or card, and that while preparing for and making her presentation, the patient could imagine the therapist to be in her pocket, holding her hand. Though initially skeptical, the patient agreed to this suggestion. This technique enabled the patient to complete her presentation with greatly diminished discomfort. This image, and a series of related and expanded images, were used repeatedly by the patient in situations where the intellectual demands exposed her impaired internal representations of approving parents, until these deficits were corrected by new internalizations: "I don't have to use the images any longer because it feels like you're with me all of the time now."

Case 2

This examples illustrates the corrective effect of imagery for a patient who suffered from an almost total inability to spontaneously experience himself as alive, vital, and expressive, reflecting the dissociation of the true or creative self (Winnicott, 1971) from his ongoing state of awareness. This schizoid state was linked to an inner experience of isolation which seemed to be based on an absence of internalized others, similar to the patient described above. The imagery task was designed to counter this inner estrangement by the gradual introduction of the spontaneous self into the patient's deadened experience, and by the development of benevolent representations of other people which could serve as inner supports and buffers against loneliness.

A young man spent the greater portion of his time in therapy sitting quietly and unresponsively, unable to speak spontaneously or to answer questions with more than brief responses. After many sessions he was able to say that at times when he was quiet he saw himself in an empty, gray room which he linked to the state of his internal life. A suggestion was made that he might prefer that the room be furnished or decorated in a more lively and stimulating way. He agreed, and over the course of many sessions the patient discussed his image of the room as he attempted to envision the room in a modified and more enlivened version of the empty, grey original image.

The patient commenced work by attempting to add to the image a single item, such as a piece of furniture, a painting on the wall, or an ornamental rug. As the individual items became permanent features of the image, the patient would then go on to add another, until after several months of work the room was fully furnished and decorated. The patient reported that the modified image elicited affects and feelings of vitality and energy rather than the deadly emptiness and isolation of the original vision. He also stated that he was able to generate this image whenever his interactions with other people made him anxious, and that this use of the image greatly limited the extent and severity of his interpersonal withdrawal. In describing the specific features of the furniture and decorations in the image, the patient mentioned that he had based these items on the decor of the therapist's office, and on memories of rooms in which he had spent joyful times with a childhood friend and a beloved uncle. As he said, "those decorations make me safe and warm. When I can see them I feel like you're all with me."

A final phase of the therapeutic use of the room imagery involved populating that chamber with people, with whom the patient could imagine interacting pleasurably and comfortably. As the image was expanded in this way, the patient reported that his real dealings with others had increased in frequency and in enjoyment, and had become more emotionally open.

As the image became multicolored and filled with objects and signs of human habitation and life, the patient became more able to talk to the therapist and to other people. His awareness of his own spontaneity and vitality gradually emerged and became a major issue for exploration as a result of the extended use of the image of the room.

Case 3

In this example two images were used sequentially; first, to assist the patient to establish an autonomous and separate self representation, and secondly, to help her to integrate dissociated assertive aspects of her experience.

A successful businesswoman sought therapy for a severe depression. Exploration revealed that the patient was unable to retire from work because of her inability to distance herself from the financial anxieties with which her husband was afflicted, despite their solid economic status. In the patient's words, "Whenever my husband or my mother were or are anxious, I catch it like the flu. It's as if we become the same person and I can't use my own ideas or information." During one session the patient recalled that during her spouse's past hospitalization his isolation in intensive care allowed her a period of time in which she felt free of his "infectious" anxiety. An image of herself in protective quarantine was developed for the patient to envision whenever she had difficulty maintaining a state of psychic independence. The patient used an image of an isolation room filled with entrance barriers whenever her husband's anxieties made her doubt or forget her own opinion of their finances, until she was able to forgo the use of the imagery and to retire from active employment.

Imagery was used again in this therapy when the patient's depressogenic difficulties in behaving assertively with her family was found to reflect her association of assertiveness with a "bad" and dissociated self image. In order to promote the integration of this aspect of the self into her ongoing experience, an image of "badness" was connected with scenes of pleasure and triumph: the patient envisioned herself gleefully spending all of her family's savings on jewelry, clothing, and lavish vacations, while she deposited spouse and children in a Victorian poorhouse. She particularly enjoyed picturing her family "begging for gruel" while she gorged herself at restaurants. The patient used this image to fortify and to hold onto the "bad" assertive part of herself whenever she was faced with a demand by a family member which she did not want to meet. The repeated use of such imagery allowed the patient to enjoy and to integrate self protective and assertive behavior into a more realistic and complete self image.

Case 4

This case illustrates the therapeutic use of imagery to correct a deficit in experiencing appropriate signal anxiety when the patient was faced with very real dangers. The therapeutic images were selected to counter the maladaptive effects of the patient's existing grandiose self images, which interfered with his judgment and with the ability to make informed decisions.

A patient casually said that he had received an IRS letter, requesting his income tax returns for the three previous years. The patient stated that he had never filed an income tax return, and that he would not respond to the letter. When his lack of anxiety was explored, there emerged an image of himself as a ancient Greek hero. This image was often present during his interactions with others, causing him to feel invulnerable to the commoners with whom he deigned to consort. As the reality of his tax situation made the patient more painfully aware of the destructive influence of this self image, he began to desire a way to rid himself of that image. A scenario was developed in which the patient imagined himself as Achilles, vulnerable only in one area of his body. The patient visually expanded the areas of his body which could be injured until the envisioned Achilles was as vulnerable, and prone to the experience of fear and impending danger, as were the "commoners" in his image. The patient evoked the modified Achilles image in a variety of assigned situations as a way of opening himself to potential internal warning signals, thus building his capacities for appropriate signal anxiety, and judgment, until those functions operated more automatically.

THEORETICAL CONSIDERATIONS ABOUT IMAGERY AND INTERNALIZATION

Imagery has been presented herein as a potent and rapid methodology for the establishment of new psychological structures through the internalization of corrective and benign experiences. Images and imagery techniques can be understood to be suited uniquely to this task for a number of theoretical reasons. Internalization is believed to occur under certain conditions: in affectively charged interactions which are emotionally gratifying and in which the rules of reality and rationality are suspended. At such times, the person's rational, linguistically based, cognitive structures and defense mechanisms are elastic, and/or are more easily bypassed, thereby allowing more direct access to more developmentally primitive and vital levels of experience. It is in these levels of experience that the narcissistic injuries can be imagined to exist, rather than in the spheres of the personality which are closer to, and more involved with, the secondary processes of language, cognition, and reality testing. As a result, therapeutic procedures which are composed of the same or similar stuff as the areas to be cured are more likely to be helpful immediately than are techniques which are based on, and operate in, more distant psychic realms. Narcissistic injuries are remnants of early, painful life experiences which are present in the adult mind in fantastic, inchoate, and largely unconscious forms. A methodology that can work fantastically and creatively seems to touch these remnants very directly, as portrayed in the preceding clinical examples.

Winnicott (1971) described internalization as occurring during the mother-child interaction in "transitional space" through the "transitional experience" of play, with transitional referring to a type of experience which is both real and not real simultaneously. Imagery seems to be located in transitional space as an active and playful experience that is affectively charged. Patient and therapist suspend the rules of reality and develop a game in which the content and process of their activities are aimed at the deeper levels of the patient's psyche. Because linguistic, reality oriented aspects of the self are ignored and bypassed in constructing and practicing images, the internal effects of the images and the associated affects appear to touch the patient in a deep and moving way. The visual nature of images, and the level of activity involved in constructing and using images seems to move the experience closer to early development experiences which were based on action and on visual input, rather than on later developed verbal processes. Certainly, the discussion of imaginary pictures and events is closer to play than is most conversation, in and out of therapy. As therapist and patient play together by generating and tossing around images, they may be recreating and repairing unconsciously an early developmental scenario wherein play went awry and led to the establishment of insufficient or maladaptive self and object representation.

Mitchell (1989) suggested that narcissistic pathology is based upon an inability to approach the world, and especially one's own inner life from a flexible and playful point of view, resulting in a rigid, concrete, and grim approach to the self, one's thoughts, emotions, and needs. The playful and flexible attitude toward psychological processes inherent in imaginal experiences and activities can elicit changes in the patient's relationship to his or her psychology, thus enabling the patient to interact with himself or herself in a kinder, joyous, and flexible way.

Imagery also may promote internalization because of the symptomatic relief which often is obtained through such active interventions. Patients whose representations of others are marked by an absence of benevolent others will be prone to identify with, and to internalize, the therapist who offers a comforting and helpful technique. The self image and self esteem of narcissistically impaired persons will be affected positively when the individual experiences himself or herself as altering problem behaviors and internal events. The patient may internalize a new, effective, and self regulating self image which is based on the observation of the self acting in a comforting, effective manner.

REFERENCES

Fairbairn, W.R.D. (1952). *An object relations theory of the personality*. New York: Basic Books.

Kernberg, O. (1975). *Borderline conditions and pathological narcissism*. New York: Jason Aronson.

Kohut, H. (1971). *The analysis of the self*. New York: International Universities Press.

Mitchell, S. (1989). *Relational concepts in psychoanalysis*. Cambridge, MA.: Harvard University Press.

Newirth, J. (1989). *Disorders of the self*. Paper presented at spring meeting of APA Division of Psychoanalysis, Boston.

Winnicott, D.W. (1971). *Playing and reality*. New York: Basic Books.

THE RECOVERY OF TRAUMATIC MEMORIES: THE ETIOLOGICAL SOURCE OF PSYCHOPATHOLOGY

Donald J. Levis, Ph.D.

Department of Psychology
State University of New York
Binghamton, NY 13901

The diversity and range of the unusual and puzzling behavior emitted by persons who are labeled as neurotic or psychotic have created conceptual chaos in the mental health field. Over 400 different psychotherapy approaches exist representing divergent theoretical orientations and treatment techniques (Karosu, 1986). This disarray has been fostered largely by the field's failure to reach a consensus on issues of etiology, symptom maintenance and treatment. Problematic to obtaining a solution to the above issues, is the inherent difficulty in isolating the antecedent conditions responsible for psychopathology development. This paper outlines an imagery technique that provides a "window" to the past, reactivating, in incredible detail, stored memories of past traumatic learning experiences. The affective component embedded in the avoided traumatic memory is believed to be the primary motivational source for maintaining psychopathology. Clinical observations obtained from using this procedure, with a wide range of clinical nosologies, has resulted in a number of the discoveries that challenge many currently held beliefs (Levis, 1988, 1990). These findings ocurred following the incorporation of minor changes in the author's use of the technique of Implosive Therapy. A brief overview of this approach will be provided first, followed by a discussion of the alterations made and resulting observations.

THE IMAGERY TECHNIQUE OF IMPLOSIVE THERAPY

The theory and technique of Implosive Therapy (IT) was first conceptualized and developed by Thomas G. Stampfl (Stampfl and Levis, 1967). The therapy represents a dynamic behavioral approach to the treatment of psychopathology originally intended to integrate into one technique the basic findings of Freud (1936) and Pavlov (1927). The theoretical rationale underlying the technique is based on an extension of Mowrer's (1947, 1960) two-factor theory of avoidance learning and Solomon and Wynne's (1954) conservation of anxiety hypothesis (see Levis, 1985, 1989; Stampfl and Levis, 1967, 1975). The theory is unique in its ability to integrate areas of psychology, in its resolution of the neurotic paradox, and its ability to reduce complex behavior to basic principles of experimental psychology. The theory has resulted in the development of new areas of research and has been supported empirically by both infrahuman and human research (see Levis, 1989, 1990).

According to this approach, maladaptive behavior is viewed as a learned response that is considered to be an end product of antecedent aversive conditioning involving specific experiences of punishment and pain. These conditioning events remain stored in long-term memory, encoded with a strong affective component possessing motivational or energizing effects. The motivational component associated with these memories is capable of secondarily conditioning new sets of stimuli. Avoidance behavior in the form of symptoms and defense

Mental Imagery, Edited by R.G. Kunzendorf
Plenum Press, New York, 1990

mechanisms are learned in an attempt to avoid experiencing the full emotional impact of a given traumatic memory (Freud, 1936; Stampfl and Levis, 1967; Wolpe, 1958). Such behavior is strengthened by the resulting reduction in affect from reduced exposure to these "dangerous", anxiety-eliciting signals.

Although symptomatic behavior is nonfunctional in that no inherently aversive stimulation follows the absence of symptom occurrence, it serves a functional purpose in that it provides an immediate reduction in conditioned stress. Repeated exposure to the eliciting stimulus does produce a weakening or extinction effect but the patient's defensive maneuvers prevent full CS exposure retarding the extinction process. Further, the traumatic conditioning that occurred to most patients usually included numerous conditioning sequences comprising a variety of stimuli both external and internal. The resulting affectively encoded memories are believed to be ordered in a serial or sequential arrangement in terms of accessibility, with the most intense conditioning experiences being least accessible to conscious awareness. With the reactivation of each new memory in the sequence, the aversive affective level increases and produces a secondarily reconditioning effect, strengthening old or resulting in new defensive maneuvers (see Levis and Boyd, 1979; Stampfl, 1987). This process of secondary reconditioning, which occurs intermittently, is the primary principle responsible for symptoms maintenance (Levis, 1985; Stampfl, 1970).

The therapeutic change agent is based on the well-established pinciple of Pavlovian extinction. This principle states that repeated presentation of the conditioned stimulus (CS) in the absence of a biologically harmful unconditioned stimulus (UCS) leads to a reduction and eventual extinction of the conditioned properties associated to the CS. To achieve this objective in therapy one must represent, reinstate, or symbolically reproduce the conditioned cue patterns associated with the symptomatology. Since many of the conditioned cues capable of eliciting anxiety are believed to include neural representation of past specific events involving the experience of pain and punishment, the therapist's usual strategy is to attempt to reproduce the avoided cues through the use of an imagery technique, rather than by simple verbal statements or complete reliance on *in vivo* presentations. The use of imagery not only facilitates a fuller presentation of the CS complex by permitting the elicitation of the visual, auditory, and odoriferous sensory modalities but represents the medium originally encoded in the neural engram. Through verbal instructions to imagine, scenes are developed by the therapist and presented to the patient. The scenes are designed to include various stimuli and sensory modalities hypothesized to be presently motivating the patient's maladaptive behavior or present during the original conditioning events. Complete accuracy in reconstructing the original conditioning events is not essential since some effect, through the principle of generalization of extinction, would be expected when an approximation is presented.

The technique has the distinct advantage of being a feedback procedure which operationally determines the merits of a given scene presentation. If the material presented elicits a strong emotional response and/or defensive reaction, support for the relevance of the cues introduced is obtained. Images function solely as CSs and any affective component attached to an image reflects prior learning. The stronger the emotional affect elicited, the greater the unlearning or extinction effect. Scenes are repeated until emotional extinction occurs. New scenes then are introduced and the process is continued until symptom removal is obtained. By focusing on the patient's reported associations to the stimuli presented and incorporating them into imagery scenes, a chain of associations is produced that not only adds new unexposed fear cues but also appears to reflect the decoding of an actual traumatic memory. Repetition of the scenes is critical and patients are taught the technique and assigned "homework" to facilitate the extinction process.

The technique has been used successfully to treat a wide range of clinical symptoms including phobic behavior, obsessive-compulsive behavior, depression, pervasive anxiety, hysteria, hypochrondriasis, psychopathy, hallucinations and delusions and other types of maladaptive behavior that occur in patients labeled neurotic or psychotic. Further, the techniuqe has been in use for over 30 years and its "safety" has been established firmly (Boudewyns and Shipley, 1983; Levis, 1985; Shipley and Boudewyns, 1980). Because the experience of high levels of anxiety in the context of this technique leads to an overall reduction in anxiety, patients typically require only a 5 to 10 minute rest period following a given scene to return to a baseline level of affect. Details of the treatment procedure and its implementation can be found in several references (Levis, 1980; 1985; Stampfl, 1970; Stampfl and Levis, 1967, 1969, 1973, 1976). Research support for the underlying principles of the theory also has been established (Levis, 1985, 1989, 1990; Levis and Boyd, 1979), as has been the treatment evaluation of outcome research (Boudewyns and Shipley, 1983; Levis and Hare, 1977; Levis and Boyd, 1985).

MEMORY REACTIVATION

Stampfl (Stampfl and Levis, 1967) recognized early in the development of the IT procedure, that the technique was capable of eliciting previously non-reportable memories that apparently were not in conscious awareness. These newly recovered memories were reported to occur during or after a scene presentation. The technique's emphasis on presenting context cues (e.g., description of the patient's childhood bedroom) and imaging multiple stimulus sensations (e.g., visual, auditory, tactile, odoriferous and taste) represent the key variables believed to enhance memory reactivation. The principles employed are similar to those used to demonstrate memory recovery (Spear, 1978). But the primary focus of the technique was to eliminate the patient's reported symptoms. To achieve this objective, Stampfl (1970) recommended that the therapist follow a four-fold cue category. The first category referred to as *symptom contingent cues* emphasized the presentation of those environmental cues correlated with symptom onset. The second category consisted of *reportable, internally elicited cues* experienced from exposure to the first cue category. These cues involved thoughts, feelings, and physical sensations which the patient reportedly experienced while imagining or engaging in their problematic behavior. The third category, *unreportable cues hypothesized to be related to reportable internally related cues*, represented the therapist's hypotheses concerning the patient's "bottom-line" fear. Examples of cues in this category include losing control, death, sexual acting out, rage, or external damnation in hell. The final category, *hypothesized dynamic cues* incorporated the presentation of unresolved childhood conflicts involving Oedipal conflicts, death wishes, castration and a variety of primary process material. Considerable symptom reduction usually is reported within one to fifteen sessions and in many cases requires only the presentation of the first two cue categories. Therapy is usually stopped when symptom elimination is achieved. Thus, complete memory reactivation of the avoided traumatic experience is not obtained nor the primary objective.

ENHANCING THE MEMORIAL COMPONENT

Over the course of some 30 years experience using the IT technique, I occasionally noted the reporting of strange and puzzling associations during scene presentations. These cues which appeared to be irrelevant and without meaning were largely ignored until about five years ago when I had a patient focus solely on them. This strategy produced some interesting associations which led to other associations which eventually resulted in the recovery of a traumatic memory. For example, one patient reported seeing a field of white. By focusing on the white, a white table appeared. This was followed by a white hallway and a brown bottle on the table. Eventually, the full traumatic memory was recovered which involved an alcoholic uncle inserting a beer bottle into the patient's vagina. The event took place when the patient was four or five years of age in a summer cottage which she visited for many years. Apparently the patient had no conscious memory of this cottage prior to presenting the scene. Further, the patient started to reveal a number of other fears and symptoms which were not reported during the initial intake. The extent of a patient's pathology is rarely revealed at first no matter how thorough the intake and may be missed completely with the use of short-term symptom reduction techniques.

Once the memorial process is started and facilitated by the therapist having the patient focus on the cues reported, more and more traumatic memories surface. The memories appeared to have their own directional course with one memory leading to another more anxiety provoking memory. The therapist's role in participating in scene presentation becomes less and less with each new memory. Following the application of this procedure to other cases, which represented a fair cross section of nosologies, it became clear to me that a large number of painful experiences were being avoided in the vast majority of cases treated. Once the conditioning history is discovered, the connection between the past and present symptomatology becomes abundantly clear. The memory reactivation process frequently is accompanied by a very intense emotional reaction. Through repetition of this material, an orderly process of emotional extinction is obtained which, in turn, is accompanid by the reporting of greater detail and the elicitation of new traumatic experiences in need of extinction. The process produces a series of events covering different age periods and involving different conflicts and stimulus situations. In case after case, the principles of stimulus and response generalization appear to be the key variables in linking one association to the next.

For the last six years I have been able to uncover the conditioning histories of a number of cases representing different nosologies. At first I questioned the reality of these findings, searching, and when possible, clinically testing other interpretations. The reported traumatic memories appeared beyond belief and human endurance. They involved severe physical torture and pain usually accompanied with extensive sexual abuse. They freuqently start at an early age, before two, and continue until age 14 or 15. They also are present in cases which provided no history of such abuse and in which I never suspected such material existed. The frequency and variety of cases in which this material is found is disconcerting.

The memorial reactivation appears lawful in that the decoding process is similar within and across patients. Some documentation of the realities of these events has been forthcoming from significant others, hospital records, and existing bodily scars. But the most compelling evidence comes from the high degree of internal consistency from one repetition to the next of the material elicited; from the unbelievable level of emotional reactivity elicited by the material; from the correlation of current symptomatology to the content of the past traumatic memory; and from the substantial positive changes in symptom behavior and personality structure following the emotional deconditioning of the trauma.

OBSERVATIONS AND CONCLUSIONS

As a result of my experience with this type of material, a number of important discoveries about psychopathology have emeged. I have become clinically convinced of the reliability and validity of these findings but it is not my intent to argue for their scientific validity. Case material does not represent nor can it be a substitute for experimental validation. Rather, the intent is to alert the field so the appropriate research can be conducted. Many of these conclusions are quite contrary to currently held beliefs. They are outlined briefly as follows:

(1) The vast majority of patients seeking treatment for clinical symptoms have "blocked out" or avoided memories of traumatic conditioning events involving the experience of severe pain which frequently included sexual abuse. These events are encoded in long term memory complete with the resulting affective component. It is this conditioned affect which provides the motivation for symptom development and maintenance. The existing psychopathology is primarily a result or end product of the patient's attempt to avoid conditioned aversive stimuli (internal and external) that have been associated to, or are part of the original traumatic events.

(2) Cognitive defenses, as well as behavioral symptoms, play a major role in preventing the deconditioning and reactivation of these traumatic memories. The defenses of denial and especially disassociation appear to have been used regularly as coping mechanisms during the experience of the actual trauma. For example, patients frequently report during the process of memory recovery that the father or mother administering the pain is not the parent but a devil, witch, or some other monstrous or faceless figure. Depersonalization during the trauma frequently is reported with "mind out of body" experiences being common. Once "outside the body" the patient reports complete cessation of pain. The disassociation appears to be learned, elicited by the patient's focusing on an object like curtains, wallpaper, crack in the ceiling or some color. Patients often report having split or multiple personalities which appear effective in reducing the emotional impact during and following the traumatic experience.

(3) The type of defense pattern developd also appers to play a major role in determining later symptom development and whether or not the patient will be diagnosed as neurotic or psychotic. Individuals who are labeled psychotic appear to have retreated inward, using fantasy as a form of escape. Neurotics tend to fight their abusers more frequently, learning defense mechanisms which keep them more reality oriented. Contrary to what I previously believed, the seriousness of the patient's presenting problems does not necessarily reflect the extent and severity of the traumatic conditioning. I have found in what initially appeared to be relatively mild cases of psychopathology an unbelievable series of severe traumatic conditioning events that typically have previously been reported only for cases of multiple personality. The severity of the initially reported psychopathology appears to be a function of a failure in the defense structure rather than necessarily a sign of the severity of earlier conditioning experiences.

(4) Clinical psychopathology is not easily learned and appears to require a whole series of traumatic conditioning events. The abuse usually starts early in life and continues for years. Hundreds of encoded memories can be present and at times the process of uncovering seems endless. Fortunately, cinical gains are obtained when each memory is deconditioned. The abuse usually stops in early adolescence and in most of my cases involving women patients, pregnancy occurred with the patient being exposed to an abortion usually performed at home or the killing of the baby usually by a parent.

(5) In cases where a complete amnesic reaction to the abuse occurs, the process of memory avoidance appears to follow an event where the patient tells an adult of the abuse, is found out by

the abuser, and is severely beaten and threatened. The threats not only involve the life of the patient but may be leveled toward a sibling. Most of the patients I have treated have 'escaped' death a number of times. I believe the development of complete amnesia relates not only to the severity of the traumatic event but to the inability of other defenses to work. The patient feels no other options are available and starts to accept the abuser's "lie" that it is partly their fault. At this point, a large part of the spirit of the fighting child is lost and the most defended against emotion becomes the direct expression of anger toward the abuser. The battle for control beween the abuser and the patient is over.

(6) One of the most fascinating findings, which is commonly associated with traumatic memory reactivation, is the appearance of a physical symptom. These memory-reactivated symptoms are physical in nature such as feeling of a weight on the chest, pain in various bodily areas, the appearance of black and blue marks on the body, bumps on the genital area, burning sensations or blood discharge from the vagina, and involuntary spasms or breathing difficulties. These symptoms represent that part of the body injured during the trauma and they quickly disappear once the complete memory is recovered and the affective component extinguished. They occur in all cases so far treated and some appear initially not to be psychological in nature. Apparently, the brain in some way affects the patient's immune system producing the physical symptom. It may well turn out that many physical and medical problems are elicited, in part, by partial release of these encoded traumatic memories. Much more research needs to be conducted in this area (see Dyck, Greenberg and Osachuk, 1986).

(7) The content of the traumatic memories represent a series of unbelievable horrifying events that defy acceptance. Violent beatings, severe deprivation, knives, hair brushes, and other objects being placed in the patient's vagina or anus to insure compliance are commonly reported. Ritualistic ceremonies with religious overtones are also recalled with the patient being tied to a cross, tortured, or forced to witness sacrifices usually involving animals. Being burned by cigarettes or placed in boiling water are frequent occurrences, as is the exposure to a variety of sadistic sexual acts. The list goes on and on to the point where the normal human brain has difficulty accepting that such horrors could occur and in such frequency. At one level, despite being exposed to hundreds of these memories, I still have difficulty believing they are real. But the details reported, with the accompanying intense affective component and the internal consistency in the memories decoded, defy an alternative explanation. One only has to have contact with a social worker who has worked with abused chilren or a judge who deals with these types of cases, to realize the frequency and extent to which young children are subjected to this kind of physical and sexual abuse. Many chilren die from it and I suspect those that survive do so because of their ability to disassociate these events from memory. If my observations about psychopathology are accurate, despite the recent media attention to this problem, the extent and frequency of abuse of children is one of our country's most closely guarded secrets.

(8) The content of the material being recovered appears to be completely unmodifiable by suggestion from or expectation of the therapist. Numerous attempts have been made by me to control the content of the material being recovered, all without success. It seems that once the patient starts the recovery process, it appears to have a life of its own. The therapist's input becomes minimal except occasionally to help the patient through a defended or difficult area. Despite extensive experience in having patients imagine bizarre primary process scenes, the material forthcoming frequently extends beyond my own restrictive conceptual ability.

(9) As noted earlier, the content of these memories typically involves severe physical pain and sexual abuse combined with a variety of emotional conflicts. The emotion attached to these memorial events includes feelings of intense fear, rage, loss of control, guilt, humiliation and fear of abandonment and rejection. The etiology of the patient's current maladaptive behavior can be traced directly once the traumatic memories are recovered. The mystery of why a given symptom or maladaptive behavior develops is completely removed. The whole process fits together in a completely logical sequence. Repeated exposure to the stimulus complex associated with these conflicts results in a number of positive changes in the patient's current behavior including the complete removal of the maladaptive behavior. Cognitive discussion, interpretation, or the expression of emotional empathy and support by the therapist appear to have little direct effect (other than motivation) on altering the patient's behavior or removing the conflict. If this conclusion is correct, the field's recent emphasis on cognitive therapy is a misdirected and misguided expenditure of effort.

(10) The process involved in the recovery of these memories appears to be very lawful across patients. Typically, the recovery process is reproduced in stages, with sensory feeling being reported first (e.g., a feeling, sensation, or physical symptom), followed by the reactivation of part of the contextual stimuli (e.g., a color, an object such as a knife, a sound, a

taste or smell), which in turn is followed by short flash-backs of segments of the traumatic event. Focusing on each of these elicited cues leads to additional cues until complete recovery. Repetition is a critical ingredient in the recovery process and the therapist should guard against assuming a memory is completed before full emotional extinction is obtained. It is important to elicit the complete memory including the beginning, the end, and the past trauma behavior. It is not uncommon to discover with repetition that embedded within a given traumatic memory are "hidden" or undetected cues encoded with extremely high levels of conditioned affect (see Levis, 1988, 1990). These memories appear to be encoded completely, in that, upon full reactivation, they elicit incredible details of the events including objects in the room, clothing and words spoken along with the accompanying conditioned affect. Loss of memory is believed to be minimal because of infrequent rehearsal. The patient seems to be reliving the events as they originally occurred. Voice and language changes are common and appear to correlate with the age period of the memory. Physical pain in the body area which was injured frequently occurs. The recovery of each new memory leads to the next with each succeeding memory being more aversive in terms of content uncovered and the emotional reaction elicited. During the initial activation of a given memory it also appears at times that a memory associated with the post-trauma events may also be currently activated. The patient may report feelings of guilt, anger or depression between sessions. A sense of abandonment or rejection also may be present. These emotions can be reduced by extending the patient's feelings and placing them in a post-trauma context (e.g., crying in you room or cleaning yourself in the bathroom). This diversion actually facilitates the recovery process of the trauma *per se*. Remember a memory is not completed until the beginning, middle,end and post-trauma memories are recovered completely and deconditioned of its emotional component.

(11) Many areas of the patient's adult life appear to represent a reinactment, at a lower level of intensity, of avoided childhood conflicts. It seems as if part of the brain is attempting to decondition the stored affect associated with the encoded memories and another part is attempting to inhibit or protect the patient from these painful experiences. One gets the impression that the patient's life is like a needle stuck in the groove of a record, playing a given segment over and over again.

(12) The final observation to be reported centers on the abuser's behavior which appears to be dominated by an overwhelming sense to control. Sex does not appear to be the key motivating source but rather it is hypothesized that the abuser is projecting onto the child those sadistic and torturous experiences that the abuser was exposed to historically. By engaging in the act of abusing others, the abuser can avoid the pain associated with their own buried traumatic experiences and at the same time release some of their repressed anger and frustration.

EPILOGUE

The above observations and conclusions are a direct result of my own experience in working through hundreds of traumatic memories. Although others I have trained are confirming these results clinically, I do not expect the reader to accept them. Clearly, there is a danger in only briefly outlining this material without providing full documentation and clinical transcripts. However, this is not the place for such a presentation. I realize it is hard for the normal human brain to conceptualize that such horrors could occur and in such frequency. But research suggests millions of children have been and are currently being physically and sexually abused with the number affected being increased dramatically with each new report. For years, the mental health field has avoided dealing with this issue dismissing the clinical data provided as hysterical fantasy. If what I have observed is fantasy, then I am at a loss to explain the high level of affect and the internal consistency noted in the reporting of this type of material. If it is fantasy then we need a new theory of psychology. If it is actual memories, as I suspect, then we need to take responsibility in therapeutically dealing with this type of material and working to prevent further abuse. In either case, fact or fantasy, patients report major reductions in symptomatology and positive changes in personality structure following the decoding of the emotional affect attached to the material produced.

Finally, it should be emphasized that my therapeutic experience clearly supports the contention that the initial recovery of a traumatic memory does not, in itself, necessarily reduce symptom behavior. Self-understanding or insight, which frequently is correlated with partial memory decoding, also does not appear to be responsible for symptom reduction. Rather self and empathetic understanding appears to be important primarily in helping to motivate the patient to continue the process of memory recovery. Significant therapeutic changes appear to occur only when the emotional encoded affect associated with the memorial cues undergoes extinction through repeated repetiton of the stimuli eliciting the strong affect. This conclusion was reached in 1893 by Freud and unfortunately since forgotten. In his words:

> The discovery that we made, at first to our own great surprise, was that when we had succeeded in bringing the exciting event to clear recollection, and had also succeeded in arousing with it the accompanying affect, and when the patient had related the occurrence in as detailed a manner as possible and had expressed his feeling in regard to it in words, the various hysterical symptoms disappeared at once never to return. *Recollection without affect is nearly always quite ineffective; the original physical process must be repeated as vividly as possible*, brought into *statum noscendi* and then 'talked out'. (Freud, 1959, Volume 1, p. 28; italics added).

REFERENCES

Boudewyns, P.A., & Shipley, R. H. (1983).*Flooding and implosive therapy*. New York: Plenum.

Dyck, D. G., Greenberg, A. H., & Osachuk, T. A. G. (1986). Tolerance to drug-induced (Poly I:C) natural killer cell activation: Congruence with a Pavlovian conditioning model. *Journal of Experimental Psychology: Animal Behavior Processes*, 12, 25-31.

Freud, S. (1936). *The problem of anxiety* (Trans. by H. A. Bunker). New York: Psychoanalytic Quarterly Press and W. W. Norton.

Freud, S. (1959). *Collected papers, Volume 1* (Trans. by J. Riviere). New York:Basic Books.

Karasu, T. B. (1986). The specificity versus nonspecificity dilemma: Toward identifying therapeutic change agents. *Journal of Psychiatry*, 143, 687-695.

Levis, D. J.(1980a). Implementing the technique of implosive therapy. In A. Goldstein & E. B. Foa (Eds.), *Handbook of behavioral interventions: A clinical guide*. New York: John Wiley & Sons.

Levis, D. J.(1985). Implosive theory: A comprehensive extension of conditioning theory of fear/anxiety to psychopathology. In S. Reiss & R. R. Bootzin (Eds.), *Theoretical issues in behavior therapy*. New York: Academic Press.

Levis, D. J.(1988). Observation and experience from clinical practice: A critical ingredient in advancing behavioral theory and therapy, *The Behavior Therapist*, 11, 95-99.

Levis, D. J. (1989). The case for a return to a two-factor theory of avoidance: The failure of non-fear interpretations. In S. B. Klein & R. R. Mowrer (Eds.), *Contemporary learning theories, Pavlovian conditioning and the status of traditional learning theory*. Hillsdale, NJ: Lawrence Erlbaum Associates.

Levis, D. J. (1990). A clinician's plea for a return to the development of nonhuman models of psychopathology: New clinical observations in need of laboratory study. In M. R. Denny (Ed.), *Aversive stimuli and behavior*. Hillsdale, NJ: Lawrence Erlbaum Associates.

Levis, D. J., & Boyd, T. L. (1979). Symptom maintenance: An infrahuman analysis and extension of the conservation of anxiety principle, *Journal of Abnormal Psychology*, 88, 107-120.

Levis, D. J., & Boyd, T. L. (1985). The CS exposure approach of implosive therapy. In R. McMillan Turner & L. M. Ascher (Eds.), *Evaluation of behavior therapy outcomes*. New York: Springer.

Levis, D. J., & Hare, N. (1977). A review of the theoretical rationale and empirical support for the extinction approach of implosive (flooding) therapy. In R. M. Eisler & P. M. Miller (Eds.), *Progress in behavior modification IV*. New York: Academic Press.

Mowrer, O. H. (1947). On the dual nature of learning - A re-interpretation of "conditioning" and "problem-solving", *Harvard Educational Review*, 17, 102-148.

Mowrer, O. H. (1960). *Learning Theory and Behavior*," New Yori: Wiley.

Pavlov, I. P. (1927). *Conditioned reflexes*, Oxford: Oxford University Press.

Shipley, R. H., & Boudewyns, P. A. (1980). Flooding and implosive therapy: Are they harmful?, *Behaviour Therapy*, 11, 503-508.

Solomon, R. L., & Wynne, L. C. (1954). Traumatic avoidance learning: The principle of anxiety conservation and partial irreversibility, *Psychological Review*, 61, 353-385.

Spear, N. E. (1978). *The Processing of Memories, Forgetting and Retention*, Hillsdale, NJ: Lawrence Erlbaum Associates.

Stalmpfl, T. G. (1970). Implosive therapy: An emphasis on covert stimulation. In D. J. Levis (Ed.), *Learning approaches to therapeutic behavior change*. Chicago: Aldine.

Stampfl, T. G. (1987). Theoretical implications of the neurotic paradox as a problem in behavior theory: An experimental resolution, *The Behavior Analyst*, 10, 161-173.

Stampfl, T. G., & Levis, D. J. (1967a). The essentials of implosive therapy: A learning-theory-based psychodynamic behavioral therapy, *Journal of Abnormal Psychology*, 72, 496-503.

Stampfl, T. G., & Levis, D. J. (1969). Learning theory: One aid to dynamic therapeutic practice. In L. D. Eron and R. Callahan (Eds.), *Relationship of theory to practice in psychotherapy*. Chicago: Aldine.

Stampfl, T. G., & Levis, D. J. (1973). Implosive therapy. In R. M. Jurjevich (Ed.), *The International handbook of direct psychotherapy. Vol. 1: Twenty-eight American originals*. Coral Gables: University of Miami Press.

Stampfl, T. G., & Levis, D. J. (1976). Implosive therapy: A behavioral therapy. In R. C. Carson & J. W. Thibaut (Eds.), *Behavioral approaches to therapy*. Morristown: General Learning Press.

Wolpe, J. (1958). *Psychotherapy by reciprocal inhibition*. Stanford: Stanford University Press.

WHEN EVIL APPEARS IN IMAGERY

Lewis E. Mehl, M.D., Ph.D.

University of Arizona
P.O. Box 42721
Tucson, AZ 85733

> Lange Nas' und spitzes Kinn,
> Da sitzt der Satan leibhaft drin.
> --Sprichwort

In the clinical practice of imagery, frightening, powerful, spontaneous images occur which hold a foreboding quality. They send chills down the therapist's back. They engender a cold sweat, hyper-alertness, a kind of fear response. We are not tempted to help our client lovingly embrace these images. As therapists, we may want to flee from them as rapidly as possible. Great therapeutic potential can be lost when we succomb to that fear.

What are these images? From where do they come? Given the title of this paper, one might suspect that I believe these images represent evil. If so, what is evil? From where does it come? Is evil an ethical abstraction or does it have form and substance? Do these images come from within the client or do they represent the genuine appearance of an "other" temporarily internalized by the client?

We can begin to consider these questions through a phenomenological description of our experience of their moment of appearance and verbalization. I speak of the images accompanied by a cold sweat, perhaps in both therapist and client. Suddenly the room is colder. We become restless. We want to change the subject or invoke a nicer image. We feel threatened or fearful, and may consciously or unconsciously invoke rituals of protection--rubbing a rabbit's foot, lighting a pipe, sprinkling corn meal in the room. Personal experience can best illustrate this concept.

Tanice was in her 50's and from Dallas. She had suffered for years from environmental allergies. She came for an intensive residential therapeutic experience (Mehl, 1990). Within that process, she spent time alone with herself. One night as we sat together, she had become particularly angry with me. It is not uncommon for patients to become angry during the therapeutic process because of its intensity. Tanice was angry that I had not come when she had perceived I should. (Part of the therapeutic process involves distorting the client's usual perception of time by not scheduling on a clock when the therapist will come since the client is presumed to be engaged in the process continually.) Tanice became progressively more enraged. Her face changed. It appeared demonic, as if it were part of the old Christian image of the devil sneering, with horns and fangs. Her face appeared triangular, even pointy, like the face described in the proverb with which this essay began. She screamed at me. I threw cornmeal on the floor, and invited her to go ahead and "go for it." She became engulfed by this creature. I was scared. A point came when I rose from my chair and demanded that the creature be gone. Tanice sank back into her couch exhausted. She moved to the massage table, and I immediately felt the need to cleanse the energy of the room. I was shaking. I felt a coldness up my spine. I burned sage in all the corners of the room and lit candles. (These are means of addressing and dispersing evil from my Native American tradition.) Slowly the room began to warm. I re-enacted an ancient ritual I had learned from an elder. I placed crystals in the appropriate positions, offered tobacco to the spirits, and cleaned the energy of Tanice's body and spirit. The next morning, the room was still full of the odors of sage, sweetgrass and tobacco.

The following morning we discussed the night's occurrences. That was no ordinary event, was it?" asked Tanice. "It was like something was inside me, something alien and frightening that takes me over. I'm like a viscious beast. I would have attacked you, clawed your face, torn you to pieces. Is that why you reacted so differently to me?"

"Exactly," I said. "I was scared. I caught the glimpse of something truly evil inside you. Your face changed. Your chin became sharp and pointed and your eyes glowed an evil green."

"I'm aware how dramatically my voice changes when that happens," Tanice said. "I scare even me. What's more horrible is that I've turned into that thing around my daughter. I've terrified and tormented her with that voice, the same voice my mother used to torment me."

I intuitively sensed a connection between Tanice's disease and this evil "other" inside her. During my week with her, I learned that she could suddenly and without warning become this vicious and attacking creature with the slightest provocation, in contradistinction to her usual whining and somewhat helpless demeanor. We worked on her disgust at having terrorized her daughter through her excursions into this mode for the 14 years since the divorce from her husband. I sensed that this evil fed on helpless hatred and rage, remaining from her upbringing with her mother and later activated by a similar relationship with her husband. Tanice had stayed connected with her mother, now in a caretaking role. To her, she reported, her mother was the essense of that evil. Her mother was demented in a nursing home, cursing Tanice when she came to see her, invoking all of Tanice's guilt that she had not done enough. Guiltily Tanice admitted praying that her mother would die to release her from the torment of calling on her almost daily.

Nothing in Tanice's secular Judaism came close to helping her cope with this evil presence. During the week together we came close to agreeing to a kind of exorcism ceremony to help her remove the evil. Tanice drew pictures of the evil within her, left the drawings for me to consider, and then promptly retracted them, embarassed that she could draw such venomous pictures. She made a foreboding doll of the evil which we used in a ceremony to request protection for her. She is still debating continuing our work with a more formal exorcism. Since Tanice is a "doctor-shopper," she vacillates. Immediately after her retreat with me, she went on a week long retreat with a healer who advocated only love, and suggested that she make the evil go away by simply not believing in it. Tanice wanted to call me and argue philosophy, which I would not do. There are many roads to the truth, I told her. Pick the one that gets you there fastest.

WHAT IS EVIL?

Tanice is a good example of a common enough client for whom images of evil spontaneously erupt during the therapy. Jung would have called this an archetypal complex. In keeping with my Native American heritage, I prefer to see it as an evil "other" actually residing within the person. This view makes treatment more straightforward as we will see in a case to be presented at the end of this paper.

Before proceeding further we should define evil. I am not concerned about the so-called relative evils. Within this view, being eaten by a lion is evil for a lamb but not for the lion. Whatever nature does is not evil in my view. I reserve evil for a deliberate malevolence aiming to hurt and make others suffer, even murderous, taking pleasure from that stance. With this definition I have only observed evil in humans or animals who have been so severely abused that they have lost their natural restraints. In the wild, a lion will not kill when not hungry. This so-called relative evil is part of the cycles of nature, all of which are self-regulatory. Without the predator, the deer would rage out of control and would starve themselves to death from overgrazing. Similarly arctic wolves thin out the sick and dying caribou from the herd, making sure there is food for all and a strong breeding stock. (And one could argue, protecting the caribou from a death of greater suffering through starvation or exclusion from the herd). In the remarks that follow, I am interested in what seems to me to be an absolute evil, a sinister, intentionally harmful presence which takes pleasure, evil delight, in the unnecessary suffering of others.

Having not had a Christian upbringing, I have not been trained to see the earth as man's workshop. My Native American heritage and teachings were closer to the views of the ancient Greeks who saw nature as perfect and beautiful as it is. My view tends to see man as one of many guests upon the earth, our future to be determined by our actions. From the earth's point of view, we are expendable. For the Native American, the earth is a conscious being to whom we pray and relate. God is never separately omnipotent as in the Judeo-Christian point of view. So I am concerned with what humans can do to each other and to nature, and about the energies and spirits we create when we do evil. We will not really consider the question in this paper of why there exists evil in the first place. Rather we will accept it as a given.

One theological theme states that the potential for evil is always an outgrowth of creation. When God creates the world, it is less than perfect, because God is less than perfect. Perfection does not appear. In the Lakota view, we are an experiment in producing a being more able to consciously serve the Creator. We were never imagined to be perfect, for the gods were not either. Perfection is an ideal for which we and the gods (and the Creator) strive, but were we or God to achieve perfection, the Universe would stagnate and die. Evolution must proceed to the creation of higher and higher structures (Prigogine's dissipative structures) or entropy supercedes and decay ensues. Therefore a discontent is established in the act of creation. We the created become aware of an evolutionary process. There are obstacles to the achievement of the aims of evolution. The Hebrews called these obstacles satans. When objects exist, temptation arises to skip the process, to blast through these obstacles with nuclear force. Evil enters through the participation in this personal fantasy of omnipotence. Even God does not omnipotently dictate. God, or the Creator, does not say, "Here, Joe, you've been a good boy, so now I'm going to reward you by making you a U.S. Senator." It seems more likely that God, in a sense, officiates over a participatory process of change by mutual consensus. (Barring "miracles" in which personal faith is so great and the inertial drag of consensus demands sufficiently weak, that an instantaneous, quantum change can occur in a situation. Nevertheless, even here God does not command the change over and against the will of the supplicant and his or her family, but in answer to their prayers, desires, and faith.)

Before further considering evil and its appearance in imagery therapy, I wish to review some images from evil as they appear in other cultures.

IMAGES FROM THE NEAR EAST

Some of our most ancient images of evil come from the Near East. In their ancient traditions evil usually appeared as a monster, often a dragon. Evil there was encountered as a cosmic principle of hostility toward the divine (Widengren, 1967, p.21) Within ancient Middle Eastern traditions, sin brought one into the dominion of demons which resulted in sickness. "Consequently one who is gravely ill...describes his condition ... in purely mythical colors. He is in the realm of death, the waters of the underworld are crashing over his head. Or [he is] surrounded by voracious demonic beasts...threatening to devour him." (Widengren, 1967, pp.22-23) The person who suffered from a prolonged illness already imagined himself as lying in the realm of death and demons.

In Iran the figure of the dragon played a prominent role as the image of evil throughout its religious history (Oldenberg, 1917, pp133-141; Burchardt, 1945; Rohde, 1946; Widengren, 1955; Benveniste-Renou, 1945). This dragon was the Ahi Dahaka of the Pahlavi books (writings from the so-called Middle Iranian time). who drove out Yim(a), the first man and first king, and had him sawed into pieces by his executioners, taking Yim(a)'s two sisters as his wives (Widengren, 1967, pp.29-30). Among the Zoroastrians, black was always the evil, demonic color (Widengren, 1950, Chap. 1; Widengren, 1938, pp.342-349).

MIDDLE EASTERN IMAGERY OF THE BATTLE OF GOOD AND EVIL

In Iranian imagery, evil is often associated with being dark and foul-smelling. It is a constant battle which appears in the imagery. In Zervanism, Zervan is the god of unlimited time and of the time of the long rule. He sacrificed for 1000 years so that a son would be born to him who would create the heavens and the earth. When he stopped to wonder if his efforts would be in vain, two sons were conceived to him, Ormizd and Ahriman: Ormizd in consequence of his sacrifices, and Ahriman in consequence of his doubt. Ahriman was dark and foul-smelling. Ormizd was luminous and fragrant (Eznik of Kolbe, 1938, p.8; Schmidt, 1900, pp.88-93). Ahriman was said to have entered the world in the form of a fly; hence the influence upon the Christian name for the devil--Beelzebub, or Lord of the Flies (Sanford, 1982, p.17). Ahriman sought to destroy the moral fiber of the soul, and was pitted in a desparate struggle to win power over all the Universe (Sanford, 1982, p.19). From the Bundahisn (one of the Pahlavi books), we read:

Then Ohrmazd, in his omniscience, knew that if he did not fix a time for battle against him, Ahriman could do unto his creation even as he had threatened; and the struggle and the mixture would be everlasting; and the Ahriman could settle in the mixed state of creation, and take it to himself. Thus even now, in the mixed state, there are many men who work unrighteousness more than righteousness--that is, they work chiefly the will of the Evil Spirit. And Ohrmazd said to the Evil Spirit, "Fix a time so that by this pact we may extend the battle for nine thousand years." For he knew that if a time were fixed in this wise the Evil Spirit would be made powerless. Then the Evil Spirit, not seeing the end, agreed to that treaty, just as two men who fight a dual fix a term, "Let us on such a day do battle until night falls." (Zaehner, 1955, p.279 and 314).

To the Zervanists, the appearance of evil was that of a frog. To the Zoroastrians, the frog was a symbol of the repulsive aspects of the evil power. The frog was a symbol of fertility in Indian and Indo-Iranian mythology in general (Widengren, 1967, p.48) (also in Native American). The tendency was to believe that Ahriman--himself loathesomely ugly--created women and sexual desire as a means of seduction of the good toward the evil (Widengren, 1967, p.50) Native Americans did not share this denigrating view of women.

Everything connected with Ahriman was foul-smelling, diametrically opposed to the fragrance of the celestial beings (Widengren, 1967, p.49).

Dragons appear elsewhere. In the Gnostic "Song of the Pearl," the Redeemer defeats the hissing dragon (Widengren, 1952, pp.97-114). In the Jewish prayer of Cyriacus, the hero fights the terrible dragon, the Snake King (Reitzenstein, 1921, pp.77). This theme, the fight with the dragon, appeared in epic form in the wall paintings of Pianjikent in Sogdia (Arts Asiatigues, 1958, 177f). Early Judaism took up this motif of the fight with the dragon and passed it on to early Christians (Bousset-Gressman, 1926, p 516f; Merkelbach, 1919, p.238ff).

Plutarch tells us at length how in Zervanism a sacrifice was offered to Ahriman (Hades) and to darkness (Plutarch, 1960, Chapter 46). Having experienced the terrible power of evil, men sought to appease the evil ruler of this world by rites and sacrifices.

Nearby, in ancient India, evil was often visualized as a water dragon, Ahi, who governed the waters and withheld water from the land. Evil connoted one "who encompasses or offers resistance, the adversary" (Widengren, 1967, p.21).

BIBLICAL IMAGES OF THE CONFLICT OF GOOD AND EVIL

In Zachariah 3.11ff we see Satan as an evil being who seeks to destroy Joshua's soul, standing in opposition to the angel who defends him. Satan is also presented as an accuser in Psalm 109:6. In 1 Chronicles 21:1 we read about Satan as an evil power working on a man to influence him to break the law of God for destructive purposes. This passage is most similar to the Native American view of evil spirits, for evil must usually work through a person's own choices and cannot directly influence except through persuasion.

In another book of Job, Satan is represented as dwelling in God's court with Him. Job's torment comes from God to satisfy an argument begun by Satan that Job is faithful only because God showers him with gifts.

Sanford (1982, pp.26-27) points out that the ancient Hebrews believed Yahweh to be the originator of both good and evil. He cites Amos 3:6: "...shall there be evil in a city, and the Lord hath not done it?"; Isaiah 45:5-7:"I am the Lord, and there is none else.... I form the light, and create darkness. I make peace and create evil; I the Lord do all these things."; and Isaiah 54:16: "I create the blacksmith, who builds a fire and forges weapons. I also create the soldier, who uses the weapons to kill."

In a Christian text describing the martyrdom of the barbarian Christopher, the following description of the battle between good and evil occurs which is typical of these battles and can be traced backwards to the Zoroastrian concept of the two forces, good and evil, battling each other for dominance:

In the middle of the city market place I saw a man of tall stature and beautiful mien; his face and raiment shone like the sun; he wore a wreath of wonderful glory on his head, and several warriors who were with him were also resplendent as light.

But I also saw another man who was deep black, surrounded by a large band of men like him. His hair coiled like the links in a coat of mail, and ghastly with his armor.

The radiant one began the fight but the dark one defeated him, killed his heroes, and for a time deported himself upon his throne. But the radiant one returned in terrible anger, split the heads of the enemy warriors, defeated the leader, and chained him with fiery chains, destroyed his palace, and shattered his camp. (Reitzenstein, 1924, p.135)

EGYPTIAN IMAGES OF EVIL

Set was the evil god, the eternal adversary of good, a personification of the arid desert, the bringer of darkness and drought. From him came everything destructive and inimical to human life (Sanford, 1982, p.16). Set built a beautiful chest just the right size for his good brother, Osiris. He invited Osiris to a feast and offered the chest to whomever it would fit. Unsuspecting, Osiris entered the box. Set and his accomplices rushed upon it, nailed it shut, and cast the chest into the sea. When the body was found and rescued, Set happened upon his brother's remains, and divided them into 14 pieces, scattering them about the earth to ensure eternal destruction.

NATIVE AMERICAN IMAGES OF EVIL

In another essay, I have considered the Lakota conception of evil (Mehl, 1990b). For Lakota society evil could assume many guises. The base image for evil was the demon, Gnaski, his son, Gnas, and Ibom, the cyclone. Iktomi, the image of perverted wisdom, appears later in the cosmology. These images combined grotesque aspects of various animals to produce a frightening creature, in size or shape. Gnas, on the other hand, could assume a pleasant shape, and in the cosmology, takes on the appearance of wisdom, to become Ksapela, or false wisdom. At this point it becomes very difficult to tell wisdom from folly. There are several stories of the fall of the original god of wisdom, Ksa, to torment people since no one would listen to him anyway. Other stories tell of Iktomi, a trickster and shapeshifter, who is born from Wakinyan, the Thunderspirit, and Inyan, the rock, and consequently has a queer shape which commands honor by being laughed at. Iktomi vows to humilitate all who laugh at him (at his original shape), which means anyone who honors him in the proper heyokah manner (in which laughter means its opposite, respect). Since evil can be present in the most pleasant image, a covenent is made with the Creator that evil will depart whenever music is made, a fire burns, or when it encounters the smoke of sage.

Other tribes present other images. The Algoquins' hero god, Gluskap, had his evil wolf-brother, Malsum, who made rocks, thickets, swamps, and poisonous and unpleasant animals. In the Lakota cosmology, similarly Gnas and Gnaski make poisonous animals and plants, since whatever they touch becomes ill. Malsum tries to treacherously kill Glaskup through the only plant (the mistletoe) able to harm his good brother. Interestingly, the evil Norse god Loki killed his good brother Baldur with the mistletoe (Sanford, 1982, p. 20). Similar to the Egyptian and the Middle Eastern stories is the battle of the good and the evil brother. Lakota stories are less direct. Evil appears as the offspring of Unkh, the rejected passion of the Earth (Maka). These offspring set out to oppose creation almost on principle. They say they are trying to honor Unkh, their mother, who becomes ruler of the underseas, yet even she rejects their deeds.

Another common image of Eastern Native Americans is that of the rolling head. In the Natchez Indian version one of two brothers die, but his head lives on, rolling toward the other brother, persecuting the surviving brother and wife, until it can be defeated.

IMAGERY FROM AIDS PATIENTS

In my own practice of imagery therapy with AIDS patients, I have encountered a consistent image of evil embodied within AIDS. A videotape (Mehl, 1990c) sold with my book, *The Language of Healing* (Mehl and Peterson, 1990), clearly portrays the emergence of this image.

In the typical situation we begin to sense an ominous grayness, a dark blotch, a malevolent darkness. One patient encountered a large, shadowy, man-like figure, covered by hat and overcoat, forever cloaked in darkness. He voraciously fed on life, draining the life energy from whomever he encountered and had the opportunity to feed upon. The image of the vampire is called to mind, particularly the imagery of Wilhelm Murnau's film, *Nosfertu*. Wherever this gaunt, baldheaded old vampire appears, people succumb to pestilence and death. Schlappner

(1967, pp. 131-133) writes about this film in a manner analogous to the imagery of the appearance of the AIDS virus (perhaps this imagery is a propos to any epidemic):

> He [Nosfertu] arrives in a begabled little city by the sea in a coffin stowed away in the hold of a ship. Invisible hands open the coffin. Nosfertu rises from the boards and vanishes through doors which open of their own accord. Behind him scurry enormous rats, which swarm over the ship and over the city: the plague....
>
> Monotonous, crumbling brick house-fronts line a long narrow street; on a height dominating the city huddles the vampire's castle, fraught with menace....The vampire's approach is announced by crashing waves...and a frosty wind from another world grips our hearts....
>
> Thin men in shabby swallowtails and greasy top hats stride stiffly as they carry the rough-hewn coffins of the plague victims....The vampire strides slowly through the ship, his silhouette falls obliquely across the deck. With awe-inspiring slowness Nosfertu approaches along the long narrow street, gliding upwards from its deep canyon....
>
> Slowly [a] door opens.... We see the young man who has taken refuge on the bed...and the vampire's shadow, blown up to gigantic proportions. We see the eerie shadow coming toward us...with the terrified eyes of the young man on the bed.

Schlappner's description captures exactly the feeling tone of the imagery of these AIDS patients. One patient visualized a mishapen darkness hiding in the corners of his body, like Nosfertu entombed in the coffin. It engulfed whatever light was near it, absorbing light until only death remained. It represented a shadowy vacuum from which there was no escape, like Nosfertu's slow, terror-filled approach toward the young man on the bed. Tracing the origins of this image backwards in time led to a violent, abusive sexual encounter with a dark, mysterious man of the night. My patient remembered burning candles, muttered incantations, the drawing of symbols, followed by a brutal sexual encounter with this anonymous man of darkness. The sex left him feeling defiled, invaded, beaten and used. He felt the darkness enter his body through the semen of this night-man. Our clinical work led to a distillation and a crystallization of that image to one which had boundaries and could be seen sufficiently clearly for expulsion. The release of this energy was associated with an improvement in his physical health.

IMAGERY AND CHRONIC FATIGUE

In my book, *Healing Ceremonies* (Mehl, 1990d, Chapter 6), I tell the story of a patient with chronic fatigue syndrome. We discover an image of her dead husband from the last year of his severely alcoholic life. She describes his wild gazes, his urinating in his shoes, his threatening her with knives, her fear of his rage. As we dialogue through the imagery process, she begins to sense a ghoulish, green, malevolence behind his eyes, in the knife's gleam, in the pain of the back-handed slaps he throws across her face. Then she holds an image of her husband before he fell prey to alcoholism. We progress timewise through his decline. I suggest that she see the presence slowly overtaking him until only the presence remains. His eyes are empty. The windows of his soul reveal only the ghoulish evil of the alcoholism spirit. By the last year of his life he is only a shell for that malevolence. Slowly, the image of this presence "solidifies," crystallizes. We shudder. Its presence frightens us. The image of alcoholism stands before us. It has consumed her husband, beaten her, and abused their daughter.

This woman makes a doll to represent this evil. Its nose is a shriveled red pepper, like the rosaceous nose of the alcoholic. It holds a knife in one gnarled shrubbery hand; cocaine and alcohol vials in the other. It sweats malevolence. We do a ceremony to purge its presence from her life. The chronic fatigue improves and her estranged daughter (angry at her mother for allowing the abuse to happen) calls her after four years of silence for reconciliation.

EUROPEAN IMAGES OF EVIL

The evil in fairy tales relevant to this essay comes from figures who derive pleasure from destruction and murder for its own sake. A Norwegian fairy tale (*Nordische Volksmarchen*, 119ff) describes a wicked giant who is invulnerable because his heart is not in his body. The giant has turned to stone the king's six sons and their brides-to-be. The youngest, seventh son has gone to search for them. (Seven is also the completion number in Native American lore; the number of principle directions to which one prays.) The young prince helps various injured animals on his way--a raven, a salmon, and a wolf--who promise to help him in return. Von Franz (1967, p.100) interestingly has observed that "Though...all attempts to deduce a fairy tale morality end in utter paradox, there is one exception: Anyone who earns the gratitude of animals, or whom they help for any reason, invariably wins out. This is the only unfailing rule I have found."

When the young prince reaches the house of the wicked giant, he finds a princess who falls in love with him and tricks the giant into revealing the location of his heart. With the help of his animal friends, the prince finds the heart, commands the giant to release the spell upon his brothers and their brides, and then destroys the giant. In other tales, the giant is replaced by an old man (Deutsche Marchen, 1951), Koschchei the Deathless (*Russische Marchen*, p. 160) or the Devil himself (von Franz, 1967).

The Ukrainian forest king, Och (Russische Marchen, 1934, p. 29), is a similar demon with the appearance of a wrinkled, old, green-bearded man who teaches a peasant lad magic and as his reward demands that the lad stay forever with him in the underworld. Everything in his "world under the earth" is green. The souls of the children who have died without baptism serve him.

Von Franz (1967) notes that this evil figure is often a troll in northern Europe. In one German tale, he is an old man of the mountains, who possesses an altar upon which lies a prickly fish. She notes that:

He is a personification of a partly evil god or nature spirit, which regularly tries to take possession of a man and make him the instrument of his own evil designs. In states of cold madness characteristic of certain psychopaths I suspect that such a spirit is at work--the madman is justifiably said to be "possessed by the Devil," wholly assimilated by a dark, divine (i.e. overwhelming) power. (p.101)

Her description is similar to what I have described for the alcoholic consumed by alcohol (or the drug addict or perhaps the professional killer). The essence of the evil with which I am concerned is represented by the view into the eyes of my client's deranged, dying alcoholic husband. It is the cold, calculating, possessive force behind alcoholism. Yet as von Franz (1967, p.102) also notes, "This evil principle has a weak point, though it is hard to find. The madman does have a heart, or a 'death' only...it is hidden somewhere far away." Unfortunately this truth kept my client living with her madman to the sad detriment of her daughter.

Regarding animals, von Franz (pp.102-103) provides an example of an Irish fairy tale (*Irische Marchen*) in which the hero plays a one-sided game of hide-and-seek with a king assisted by a magician. On the advice of his helpful, white, talking horse, the hero hides in all sorts of places, but the king always finds him, aided by the wicked magician who sees where the hero hides in a book he carries. The hero finally saves himself by hiding under the tail of his horse where the magician is powerless to find him.

"Animals, says Jung, are more obedient to God than is man; they live out their foreordained lives without doubt and without deviating from their inner patterns....As a non-canonical saying of Jesus has it: 'Ye ask me who will lead you to the kingdom of heaven...:the birds of heaven and that which is under the earth and the fishes of the sea--they will lead you to the kingdom of Heaven and the Kingdom is within you." (James, 1945, p. 26). In the I Ching, the 'firm lines' that the wild goose follows in its flight are a guiding symbol recommended to the perfect man (I Ching, 1951,No. 53,Gradual Progress).

Breaking the trust of a spirit, animal, or helper can have disastrous consequences. In Grimm's tale of the Two Brothers, a witch is able to turn one of the heroes to stone because, at her request, he has touched his helpful animals with her magic wand. The second brother refuses to hurt his animals and overcomes her without difficulty (von Franz, 1967, pp.101-102). These views are consistent with Native American views of animals as closer to the original intentions of creation.

Within the confines of what I would consider European are modern fantasy novels. The series of novels which best portray the evil with which I struggle to define are those of Stephen R. Donaldson, representing two sets of trilogies of Thomas Covenent. Covenent is a modern day leper, living in a rural American community, a writer by trade, abandoned by his wife and child when the leprosy is diagnosed. He falls unconscious and awakens in another land which he first refuses to accept as real. He comes to be called Ur-Lord, Unbeliever, and White Gold Wielder, since his wedding ring apparently has magical power within this reality. The strength of the books lies in their depiction of the struggle with evil, represented by Lord Foul, the

Despiser. The depictions of Foul are dramatic and potent, as Foul struggles to taint even the noblest of intentions with despair, doubt, and destruction. After a seeming victory over Foul at the end of the first trilogy, he emerges in the beginning of the second, stronger than ever, having learned how to wreck evil, even over nature, with an unnatural pestilence called the sunbane. The key ingredient is that he is evil for its own sake and for his own pleasure, taking pride and enjoyment from the torment of others.

Therapeutic imagery often involves finding the weakness (discovering the hidden heart) of the evil presence. This is marked in the Donaldson books and also in the approach I will describe in the next section which I utilized with Lori.

IMAGERY THERAPY WITH EMERGENT EVIL

Frey-Robin notes that "The seductive and destructive power of evil is rightly feared; for it possesses a secret attraction, which is all the greater the more one resists it." In speaking about evil as an entity (an archetype in her terms), she states that "the archetypal shadow is [often] the only possible access to the lost levels of the soul, for one of its essential possibilities is to lead the individual back to his buried possibilities." As in the vision from Christ's 40 days in the desert wilderness, evil promises quick access to wealth and power. It promises "power over" as opposed to "power in participation," which is the power of Creation. The Navajo tell that evil entered the world when Blue Heron was sent back to the underworld to get the medicine bundle which provided the power to obtain quick wealth. Evil seduces because its promises are more palpable and quickly realizable than the promises of co-creation in a cooperative process. To command and demand is quicker than engaging in a participatory process with another, in which a shared mutual experience is created, in which each is satisfied. Rape is a quicker way to achieve sex than developing a meaningful relationship. Incest can be more satisfying than undertaking the work of rehabilitating a frustratingly dead marriage. Drug trafficking (with the implicit participation in the murder and brutalization of others on the route from field to sale) is a quicker route to wealth than developing an honest business.

This paper is more concerned with the appearance of evil in the imagery of the victim than with the seductiveness of evil in the perpetrator. Yet, if we consider sexual abuse, we find an inevitable loyalty to the perpetrator when that person is a family member. Equally important is the identification of the victim with the power of evil. "I got fucked, so now I'm going to fuck on you." This variation of a common movie line displays the mentality of courting evil power. The victim becomes obsessed with revenge. For this reason, I will recommend an approach which externalizes the evil in a cooperative, co-creation process of healing.

The current popularity of Satanism in some aspects of our society may point to the way in which modern society has lost contact with the richness of being. Because evil has been avoided by polite society, it alone retains the power of immediate contact with primordial imagery in which the image is immediately made manifest. Satanism, for example, retains an original connection with the age-old paths of nature even if that connection is twisted and perverted. Satanism is the closest many modern people have seen to shamanic ecstasy. Satanism preserves the passion of spirit possession in a society which has sanitized everything. In Native American inspired imagery therapy, we recover the power of positive connectedness with nature, of shamanic ecstasy without perversion.

The story of the monk Medardus (Hoffman, 1824) gives us some insight into the seductiveness of evil and the treatment of its effects. Intoxicated by his own eloquence and his lust for power, Medardus is tempted to increase his effectiveness by taking a drink out of the Devil's own elixir. By drinking from the Devil's bottle, he gains the secret of rejuvenation, but falls into the Devil's power. His greed and overwhelming materialist desires overpower him and place him on a path toward self-destructiveness. It is only in the twilight zone between life and death, that he experiences a reconciliation of his divided self, a unification of soul and nature, seeing that transmutation as the pure beam of eternal love. Similarly in shamanic therapies, the shaman takes the patient to the spirit world, to the twilight zone, and allows a re-experience of the healing powers of primordial nature. This allows a rebirth through imagery to the power of spirit, to the love of Creator and Nature. In this process, healing occurs almost epiphenomenally.

Lori's story provides an example of these principles at work. Lori came with both physical (a disease called lupus erythematosis, an auto-immune disease in which the patient's own antibodies attack the self) and emotional suffering. She imagined that she had forgiven those from her past who had abused her, yet still craved an end to her physical existence. She didn't understand this desire for the release of death, since her life had been proceeding smoothly and easily for the past few years.

Lori was an attractive, thin woman in her late thirties with large, owl-brown eyes. Her movements were quick, bordering on frenetic. An underlying pathos of despair clung to her.

Lori had a car accident on the way to our first appointment. She called in tears saying she couldn't come even though she was only a few blocks away. I drove to where she waited. We followed the tow truck to the garage, and I waited until her tire was replaced and the fender banged out to make room for the tire to turn without scraping. A sledge hammer finally finished the bashing of the fender necessary to liberate the tire. We made plans to meet again the next day.

Our next appointment came and I struggled to learn what really bothered Lori. What contributed to her ennui with life? Her story emerged attractively packaged, well-rehearsed. I never trust a neatly tied package in therapy, one which lacks the unrestrained wildness of newly discovered material. Yesterday's insights and worked-over truths are as unsatisfying as old croissants. Lori's words carried that hardened crust of denial.

We began with imagery. I wanted to reach a deeper layer of the self, to find an entry to the dark cave of pain I sensed beneath the overly calm surface. I encouraged relaxation with a permissive style of induction, asking Lori to set aside the concerns of her daily life, the mental lists of tasks yet to complete, the critical, rational intellect, and to simply let the images come, to let the deeper structures of consciousness send what they would.

We seemed to be making good progress until a series of almost convulsive shakes rocked Lori's body. She had an image of driving an empty bus and of an evil energy sitting in the back of the bus. It had seeped upward and into the bus through the rear tires. A foreboding presence lurked invisibly behind her, terrifying her. She wanted to stop the bus, get out and run, but the ground outside was unstable. Her body continued to jerk spasmodically. I encouraged her to give in to the energy and let her self discover its source. Instead she fought her way back to full consciousness, saying that she didn't trust me enough to let herself go through the process, for she knew tears would soon burst forth. She feared my negative judgment of her crying. If she really let go, she said, I might find her weak or unpleasant. Being a psychiatrist, Lori was ingrained through her residency training with the wish for physician approval. She feared feeling silly and ridiculous if she were to let go.

Lori had seen a notice that I was conducting a Native American sweat lodge ceremony that weekend. She asked to come, saying that she felt the desire to experience purification. No matter how hard she tried, she felt an intrinsic, inner dirtiness. She linked this to her Roman Catholic upbringing, to having learned a distrust of the body, even a repugnance toward the body. I agreed she could attend.

When we met Friday night to prepare for the sweat lodge, Lori was surprised by the apparently expected intensity of the experience by others there. "I thought we would go into a lodge for about an hour and a few beads of sweat would appear on my upper lip and that would be all," she later confessed.

The sweat lodge ceremony is powerfully evocative of imagery through the traditional Native American songs, prayers, and procedures. The heat can be intense, and the lodge Lori attended lasted for 5 hours.

After the lodge we sat together in a traditional Lakota talking circle, sharing our dreams and experiences. Besides the sheer, physical struggle to tolerate the heat, Lori was most affected by the imagery of the transformation of the water into the blood of the earth during the ceremony. As she drank the sanctified water, she tested earth essence, felt the water, now earth medicine, filling her body, flowing through the rivers and tributaries of her arteries and veins, opening and purifying the old wounds and pains.

In our next session, Lori was eagerly ready to work. I began with my usual body-centered induction (Mehl and Peterson, 1990). As time progressed, I departed toward imagery of birds singing in her brain and flowers growing in her heart. These images allowed her consciousness to move toward deeper levels. In time Lori could go no further, so I told her a story:

> Once upon a time many years ago, a village suffered from the effects of evil. The rains had ceased. Crops wilted and died. Animals scarcely roamed within hunting distance. The people had grown weak and disconsolate. The rain clouds sat steadily atop Thunder Mountain to the West. Rain fell there, but nowhere else. The village diviner had seen an Evil Spirit atop that mountain, controlling the rain, keeping it only for himself. The people suffered from the effects of this evil.
>
> One young man and woman spoke urgently between themselves of this crisis. The people had grown passive and disheartened. They were content to let the evil consume

them. Afterall, who could lift a finger against such a powerful Evil Spirit. The young man had resolved to conquer that Evil or die with honor and dignity in the battle. He had gone to the Chief of the village who had been too lethargic to properly receive him or even bless his journey. "Do as you will," the Chief had laconically offered. "Your wanderings are no affair of mine."

The young woman wanted to be part of this quest. She sensed the footsteps of Death closing in upon the village. The horror of their predicament inspired desparate action. The man refused her offer to accompany him. His pride and sense for the duties and constraints of the hero precluded feminine company and help, at least until the quest succeeded.

The time came for the journey to commence. As the night of the New Moon approached, Laughing Deer gathered his supplies. The woman, Snow Bird, assisted in the making of prayer arrows which they hoped would draw the power needed for success and protection. They followed the old and elaborate preparation rituals ignored now by the morally weakened tribal members. He would rest throughout the next day and begin his journey in the night of the New Moon as tradition dictated.

Snow Bird begged her leave. She said it would be too heart-breaking to watch him leave in the night. She would fain part sooner, without having to watch him walk away into the darkness. Laughing Deer reluctantly agreed and left for the prayer lodge in which his arrows rested. He would doze and pray there all day.

Snow Bird quickly gathered her secret cache of supplies and set out upon the path toward Thunder Mountain. She would show him who could leave her behind. Beneath her sweet exterior lay a will comparable to that of the Great Buffalo himself. She was tired when Laughing Deer finally overtook her near dawn. The path was illuminated only by the faint light of the Morning Star. Laughing Deer's arrow was drawn upon his bow as if he meant to sneak up upon her, though she had been aware of his presence for some time. Perhaps he imagined her to be the Evil Spirit for his easy conquest. Snow Bird began to giggle, disarming the great warrior.

"Snow Bird!" he stamped his feet. "You shouldn't be here."

"Says who?" she retorted.

"Says all who know better!" he replied huffily.

"Who?" she demanded.

"The people..." he began.

"The people are sleeping, even when they should be awake," she interrupted. "It is only you and your silly pride. You can stop me only by knocking me senseless or tying me to a tree."

"That would be too dangerous," he replied, as if he had considered both these possibilities. "And there's not enough time to take you back to the village. I would lose an entire day's journey." His tone was pensive.

"More than that," retorted the hot-tempered Snow Bird. "I would fight you every step. Perhaps I would knock you senseless."

"Perhaps," mused Laughing Deer, rubbing a scar he got from fighting with Snow Bird as a child.

"Come," she announced. "Time is wasting." Snow Bird strode off determined, and Laughing Deer humbly followed her.

The cycles of sun and moon blurred for the two as they trudged toward distant Thunder Mountain. They knew only motion and the ache of incessant, arduous travel. They slept as briefly and as little as possible to sustain the speed of their mission.

As the sun set one evening, an eerie green glow filled the Westerm sky. The malevolent glow reminded them of pus dripping from a wound. When the wind picked up, a foul, acridly nauseating smell assaulted their noses.

"I'm afraid of what's there," Snow Bird whispered. They were very close to the base of Thunder Mountain. Laughing Deer pulled a special arrow from his quiver and placed it upon his bow.

"I'll be ready," he growled, grimly determined. Snow Bird was not so sure.

The beast assailed them when they crested the next hill. It was more hideous than Snow Bird could have imagined. Glowing, green pus dripped from every pore. It held the stature of a buffalo. but walked on 2 legs. Atop its trunk swayed the venemous head of rattlesnake, eyes glowing in the night. It prepared to charge. Laughing Deer dropped to one knee on the hard ground to steady himself to fire his arrow. Snow Bird sensed the futility of his bravery.

"Thunder Beings," she cried out. Using the ancient formula, she canted, "We don't need your help, especially not now. You're too weak to help us against this monster over here. We curse the ground upon which you walk. We laugh at the queerness of your shape, and mock your powerless state, so afraid you cover yourself with a black cloud so none can see your shamefulness. You could never help us against such a magnificent beast such as this here...."

Snow Bird continued as the beast charged. Laughing Deer fired his arrow which melted before ever reaching the beast. As he grabbed another arrow, a dark cloud appeared. Instantly lightning shot forth from the cloud, striking the beast. Bolt after bolt flew from the cloud, bringing the beast to its knees as it slowly began to melt. A river of green pus and decaying, burning matter ran down the hillside beneath the deafening din of the thunder. When only a small, slimy puddle remained, the cloud began to drift away. A swallow flew down from it and approached the two. "The Thunder Spirits bid me congratulate you for knowing the ancient way of calling." The swallow addressed Snow Bird. It then rumbled at Laughing Deer. "Within your pride is your ruin. Had not the female accompanied you and called for help, your mission would be nought." Laughing Deer hung his head in sheepish shame. "Remember the first lesson," said the swallow. "Help will not be provided unless requested. Don't forget to ask." Leaning toward Snow Bird, the swallow seemed to materialize a beautiful, long-shafted arrow. "We offer you this gift with which to defeat the Evil Spirit. Its feathers are the swallow's. Its aim is ever true. Its head is lightning and it will cut any material, even stone. Use it at the right moment; it will not fail you."

Snow Bird bowed in thanks as she accepted the gift. The swallow flew onward to catch the departed cloud and the pair turned to face Thunder Mountain. They continued until they reached a sheer stone wall. Their path upwards was blocked in all directions. "The Evil Spirit guards himself well," Snow Bird remarked. Laughing Deer grimly faced the cliff and started to climb. "Wait," Snow Bird commanded. "Didn't you learn anything from the swallow? First we must pray for help from the Spirit of the Mountain." Snow Bird promptly sat down and removed her sage and crystal from the medicine bag hanging by her waist. She took out her fire starter and gathered sticks and twigs to light. When a little fire burned brightly, she lit the sage and blessed herself, then offered tobacco to the Spirit of the Mountain. Snow Bird sang the spirit gathering song and asked the Mountain for help.

When she finished her song, the earth moved before them. A mole stuck its head through the ground. "Follow me," it called out. "The Mountain has heard your prayer. I have been sent to make a path for you to follow." It disappeared, leaving a hole just large enough for them to squeeze through. Crawling snake-like behind the mole, they humbled themselves to the Spirit of the Mountain. The mole wound its way toward the innermost chamber of the mountain. The mole's tunnel merged with a wider, pre-existing, well-traveled passageway. Its stone was smoothed from frequent use. A light caught their eyes up ahead. They climbed fearfully and carefully to the edge of the tunnel, to behold a great crystalline chamber, a frantically hot fire covering its floor. They drew backwards in shock at the sudden blast of heat and vertigo.

"The fires are maintained with the blood of the beasts," stated the mole. "Whosoever would desire the beasts' aid, let him quench this fire." Suddenly their attention was drawn by a roar behind them. A wall of flame was torrentially rushing down the tunnel toward them.

Snow Bird grabbed her crystal and placed it on the earth. "Mother," she cried. "Send us your water, the life blood of the rock for our protection. Save us and the beasts with your grace." A spring arose from the stone, flowing toward the onrushing flame. Where it touched, the fire burned no more. Laughing Deer held out his pouch to collect water bubbling forth from the stone. He ran to the entrance to the great, crystalline chamber and threw the water upon the fire. Immediately it burned less brightly. With several trips the flame was transformed to a fountain and water began to rise in the chamber. While the pair and the mole panted in relief, a spider emerged from the spring.

"I have been sent by the Mother," the spider said, "to assist you on your way. I will ride behind the ear of the female and will alert you to danger when it is near." With that, they gathered their things, climbed into the chamber, waded across the developing pool of the fountain, and climbed the oppsite wall to a tunnel opening. The spider whispered to Snow Bird, "Soon you will reach the home of the Evil One. Tell your companion to prepare his lightning arrow."

Not long thereafter they entered a huge, domed cavern with a boulder-strewn floor and high overarching stone ceilings. A large, ponderous stone lodge sat at the center of the rocky plateau. Snow Bird instructed Laughing Deer to fire his arrow into the stone dwelling. On impact, it split apart, the two halves falling away, splintering and breaking apart to either side. "Tell him to challenge the demon," urged the spider. Following Snow Bird's instructions, Laughing Deer called out to the Evil One. The green-glowing monster was enraged. It roared and roared, bellowing its hatred. It approached them menacingly, an enlarged version of the beast previously met on the trail. Its visage was mishapen and distorted, a huge nose hanging from its face as if sewn on, one nostril narrow and oval; the other, a gaping abyss into which whole war parties could disappear. Its snake eyes burned green flame and were asymmetrically placed upon its face. Everything about it was out of harmony.

The demon responded, "Take the first challenge; pull the tree from the stone by its roots." It pointed toward two trees--a thin, brittle dead one, and a large, towering oak. "You choose first."

"Pick the large one," hissed the spider. "All is opposite here to what is natural. The large tree is dead and has no roots. The smaller tree is rooted tenaciously to stone."

Laughing Deer strode over to the large tree and easily lifted its hollow trunk from its base. Its thin layer of bark crumbled in his hands. The demon cursed and strained but could not uproot the smaller tree. Finally it gave up, the greenish-fire of its eyes, flickering red.

"Now," it said. "We will run a race around this cavern." The spider told Snow Bird to expect a hole and to jump inside as soon as it appeared. Then the spider vanished. The demon gestured toward the starting mark. Ready, set, go. It was quickly lengths ahead of them when the hole appeared, steam billowing from its nostrils. The pair jumped into that hole, rapidly circling down and around the cavern until they were spewed out on the other side at the finish line, steps ahead of the demon. Mole crouched behind a rock obviously proud of his handiwork. The spider climbed up Snow Bird back to her place behind the ear.

"It's your turn to challenge," said the spider. "Tell the demon to follow you to the room of fire. You will both have to cross the pool of water to the other side. The winner will prevail. You will dive into the water and walk across on the bottom where we will make a tunnel of air for your sustenance."

Snow Bird announced their challenge. The demon followed them quietly toward the pool. The water had risen to almost the floor of the tunnel. A fire burned on its surface.

"Be brave," the spider whispered. "Trust us. The air will be there. Do not attempt the fire. Dive straight to the bottom."

Snow Bird whispered the spider's instructions to Laughing Deer. "We will go first," she announced to the demon who was suddenly full of glee and devilry.

"Be my guest," rolled its unctious voice.

The pair dove into the water, down and down. When their lungs were about ready to burst they reached the bottom. A corridor of air awaited them and guided them across the moat. On the other side, they swam upwards along the wall to emerge into the tunnel.

The demon laughed. "Fire is my ally," it bragged. It obeys me completely. My time will be quicker than yours." It jumped into the water to swim across the fire. At first it gained brightness and illumination in the fire. Then it began to burn. Horror and pain crossed its face. It dove to escape, but the fire was unquenchable. The demon surfaced and writhed in agony as it burned and disappeared. The spider spoke: "The Mother Earth has blessed you," it said. "Go forth and speak to your people, for the touch of evil has been removed. They will need your courage and guidance."

The mole led the two out of the mountain and they returned to their people to do as the spider had instructed. Of course, they married, and lived happily ever after.

During our next session, I explored Lori's experience of the imagery of the story. She had vividly seen and participated in the images, sometimes before they were spoken by me. We returned to review the abuse of her life. She saw the demon behind the eyes of her father and her uncle who had sexually abused her. We distilled and crystallized this image of evil through her own similarly visualized journeys with the help of animals who aided her. She made a doll to embody the evil in her father and uncle. Ceremonially we implored the evil that had been left in her by that spirit to depart from her body into the doll. During a ceremony we burned the doll and prayed for the spirits to take the evil from the doll to the lodge of the Creator to be transformed into goodness. At the conclusion of our work, Lori was at more peace. Her disease had greatly improved and she wanted to live. Today, one year later, she is completely healthy and vibrantly alive.

I conclude with these ancient words from the I Ching, which says that evil, living on negation, is not destructive to the good alone, but inevitably destroys itself in the end (I Ching, 1951, No. 23, Nine at the Top and No. 36, Six at the Top). Imagery is the therapy which can best concretely deal with the problem of the effects of evil in the world, and one method of doing so has been presented.

REFERENCES

Arts Asiatiques V. (1958).

Benveniste-Renou. (1945). *Vrtra et VrOragna*. Paris.

Bousset-Gressmann. (1926). *Die Religion des Judentums*. 3rd ed. Tubungen.

Burchardt. (1945). *Vrtra*. Copenhagen.

Deutsche Marchen seit Grimm, I . (1951). Von Mann ohne Herz, No. 15.

Eznik of Kolb. (1938). *Against the sects II*, I.

Hoffman, E.T.A (Amadeus). (1824) *The devil's elixir*. Edinburgh.

I-Ching, The book of changes . (1951). Princeton: Princeton University Press.

Irische Marchen. (1954). Der Vogel mit dem lieblichen Gesang, No. 28.

James, M.R. (1945). *The Apocryphal New Testament*. Oxford: Oxford University Press.

Mehl, L.E. (1990a). *Intensive psychotherapy for the physically ill*. Manuscript under editorial review.

Mehl, L.E. (1990b). Native American Concepts of Evil. In *VIIth International Conference on Shamanism*. (U.C. Berkeley Dept. of Asian Studies). San Rafael, CA: in press.

Mehl, L.E.(1990c). *Using hypnosis with AIDS: A training videocasette*. New York: Irvington Publishers.

Mehl, L.E. (1990d). *Healing ceremonies: Bridging native American spirituality with the modern world*. New York: Irvington Publishers, in press.

Mehl, L.E. and Peterson, G.H. (1990). *The language of healing*. New York: Irvington Publishers.

Merkelbach. (1919). *Reallexikon fur Antike und Christentum*. Drache, IV.

Nordische Volksmarchen, II. (1948). Von dem Reisen, der sein Herz nicht bei sich hatte, No. 23.

Oldenberg. (1917). *Die Religion des Veda*. 2nd printing.

Plutarch. (1960). New York: Doubleday.

Reitzenstein. (1921). *Das iranische Erlosungsmysterium* . Bonn.

Reitzenstein. (1924). *Weltuntergangsvorstellungen* . Kyrkohistorisk Arsskrift.

Rohde. (1946). *Delivery us from evil*.

Russische Marchen . (1934). No. 6.

Russische Marchen . (1957). No. 29.

Sanford, J.A. (1982). *Evil: The shadow side of reality*. New York: Crossroad.

Schmidt. (1900). *Des Wardepet Eznik von Kolbs Wider die Sekten* . Vienna.

Schlappner, M. (1967). The Cinema. In the Curators of the C.G. Jung Institute (eds.), *Evil* . Evanston, IL: Northwestern University Press.

Von Franz, M.-L. (1967). Fairy Tales. In the Curators of the C.G. Jung Institute (eds.), *Evil*. Evanston, IL: Northwestern University Press.

Widengren, G. (1938). *Hoch gottglaube im alten Iran* . Uppsula Universitets Arsskrift VI.

Widengren, G. (1950). *Feudalismus im alten Iran* .

Widengren, G. (1952). *Zeitschrift fur Religions und Geistesgeschichte, IV*.

Widengren, G. (1955). *Stand und Aufgaben der iranischen Religionngeschichte* . Leiden.

Widengren, G. (1967). The principle of evil in the eastern religions. In the Curators of the C.G. Jung Institute, Zurich (eds), *Evil* . Evanston, IL: Northwestern University Press.

Zaehner. (1955). *Zurvan*. Oxford, 1955.

GOD IMAGES

Nicholas E. Brink, Ph.D.

Clinical psychologist, private practice
202 S. Second Street
Lewisburg, PA 17837

Several years ago while in a therapy session I asked a client to imagine God. This request produced a very interesting response and I have since asked that question many times. The purpose of this brief paper is simply to present a number of brief case studies about how each individual responded to that question.

This first case is a middle aged woman with generalized anxiety. She is married and has a teenage son. She continues to be close to her parents and two brothers. She and her one sister have been in conflict and the sister has become much more distant.

She is a very religious person and talked about her religious beliefs freely. When I asked her to imagine God, she saw God as a man wearing a white robe, standing on a cloud with arms outstretched. The expression on His face was loving and caring. He was looking down on earth, but earth and its inhabitants were small and He was unable to recognize her or relate to her specifically. She felt that she was insignificant in God's eyes and that God did not know her. This image was threatening to her because, rationally, she believed in a personal God.

In pursuing this image further, she related this image of God to her feelings of not being loved by her parents. She felt that her parents did not specifically love her. If her parents did not love her, how could God love her? Her parents frequently praised her brothers but never complemented her. She felt that they loved her brothers more. She had an opportunity to mention this therapy experience to her brothers and they related to her how her parents had often praised her. This experience provided a turning point in her therapy.

A second person, a woman 24 years of age and a college graduate, suffering with cerebral palsy, was asked to imagine God. She saw God again as a man looking down on her, but God did see her and had offered her many good things. Yet, God was not paying attention to what she wanted or needed. God, though good and aware of her, was unaware of her needs and wishes. Again this example reflected this woman's relationship with her mother. Her mother cared for her invalid daughter and had constantly pushed this daughter to be independent. The mother did not take the time to realize the pain and rejection the daughter was feeling in being pushed to be independent. What the daughter needed and wanted was to be listened to and understood.

A third case was of a man who was trying to quit smoking. He was a construction worker. When asked to imagine God, he stated that he was an atheist and could not imagine God. I then asked him to describe the God that others might visualize. He described an angry God of wrath and vengeance. He then was able to describe the way he had been abused by his father and his own need to be defiant. One act of defiance to get even with his father was to smoke.

Another woman when asked to imagine God, saw ocean waves breaking on the shore. This image was beautiful but powerful, something over which she had no control. She felt inadequate while watching the waves. This feeling of inadequacy and lack of control became a major issue in therapy.

Another man saw a blinding light when asked to imagine God. His experience was one of being blind, confused and lost in this light. He was an individual who was having an

Mental Imagery, Edited by R.G. Kunzendorf
Plenum Press, New York, 1990

extramarital affair, excited but very confused by the affair and struggling with what to do about his life.

This last year I was invited as a local professional to lead the adult Sunday school class at a rural Lutheran Church. I was to chose my own topic. I chose to explore the use of this imagery of God. I began this imagery experience with the use of an imagery technique to aid in building trust between the members of the class by asking them to look around the room at the others in the class and acknowledge to themselves what these other people meant to each person. This exercise was followed with asking them to imagine God.

Two of this group's images stood out in my mind. First, the local physician saw God as the God of creation in the fresco of the ceiling of the Cystine Chapel in Rome. God was reaching out with his finger, touching the finger of man, giving him life. The other image was that of the Pastor of the church. He imagined God as the picture of Jesus sitting on a rock surrounded by children, holding some, touching others and talking with them. In both cases the images reflected their position in life, first as a healing physician and second as a Pastor.

One thought, in preparing for teaching the Sunday school class, was that God has many aspects and for each individual, only a few aspects may predominate. I felt that with the members of the class sharing their images, each might have an experience as to how their own image of God was limited which could open a door to personal growth. Meeting this goal was limited because the class was very restrained.

One client I am seeing for pain because of a back injury talked of believing in a personal, loving God, yet her image of God was at a distance, and, as hard as she tried, she was unable to bring that image closer.

In questioning myself as to my own image of God, I realized that I could not visualize God because I experienced God being somewhere behind me over my left shoulder, as a more impersonal source of strength. I am perplexed as to why the experience of God is to my left.

One image of God that I have appreciated in my reading is in the *Eagle's Gift* by Carlos Castaneda (1981). God is imaged as an Eagle with its emanations as the source of power that is available to anyone who is open to receiving it. That God is impersonal and does not have human characteristics of loving, caring, being angry, etc. God is only a source of energy and strength.

These images of God suggest several dimensions that can provide useful information in therapy. These dimensions may include the dimension of power and authority, of trust, compassion and love, of the nature of parental relationships, and of personal striving. God, as a personal internal archetype, reflects how an individual relates to these and other dimensions. Even when the belief in a God is denied there still exists an internalized image of God.

REFERENCE

Castaneda, C. (1981). *The Eagle's Gift*. New York: Pocket Books.

USING SOUND TO DEEPEN AND ENLIVEN IMAGERY WORK

Archa Mati, B.A.

Ontario Association for the Study of Mental Imagery
c/o The Sahaj Yoga Centre
745 Markham Street
Toronto, Ontario, Canada M6G 2M4

"Every illness is a musical problem ..." (Novalis)

As sound is the essence of verbal communication, and tone fundamental to the expression of emotion, the use of sound combined with imagery is a powerful therapeutic tool. From my work I have found that the addition of sound to imagery helps the imagery to work faster.

It is well established that images are less likely to be censored through conscious evaluation. Similarly, sounds based on the alphabet have a neutrality that enables access to the underlying emotion without judgment. Drawing from the psycholinguistic traditions of Yoga and Mantra, I combine the use of sound, imagery and breath in my private work with clients.

HISTORICAL BACKGROUND

The healing of psychological disorders by means of musical sounds is centuries old stretching back through all cultures. The major task of the medicine man and shaman was to provide the patient with healing chants.

The Ancient Greeks believed it possible to cure sciatica by blowing notes of the Phrygian mode against the affected parts of the body. Pythagoras used songs to cure bodily pains, to soothe the pangs of bereavements, to calm anger and to still desire (Hamel, p.165). Singing or rhythmical speech is a creative act. Sound is a component of many of the early creation myths of Africa and Asia which speak of an unfathomable sound as the mother of the worlds' creator.

In more recent times the use of music for healing in the late 19th century, documented by Aleks Pontvik, includes the use of an orchestra to treat nervous cases. He writes of the foundation of a mental institution near Naples in which musicians were employed in a curative capacity (Hamel, 1979).

INFLUENCE OF SOUND ON BODY:
DEVELOPMENTS IN THE SOVIET UNION AND EUROPE

The interrelationship of sound and body vibration has been established by U. Berdiyen, a Soviet scientist who has shown that notes of various pitches, volumes and tones have a discernible effect on the cardiovascular system. He uses an image (long known in the Yoga Tradition) that man's nervous system is like a string and the rhythmic processes of the organism can be strengthened by the use of music.

Some references of music therapy that bear directly on my use of flowing sound with imagery come from the work of Dr. Ilse Middendorf of the Berlin Institute for Breath Therapy and Instruction, West Berlin. Dr. Middendorf works with imagining the inward speaking of the vowels which open specific inner regions of the body to the breath. Drawing from the Leser-Lasario school the following correspondences are given which link specific sounds and their influence on definite areas of the body:

I (EE)	-head, mouth
E (Eh)	-throat, larynx, upper chest, sides of body
AE (Air)	-pharynx, apex of lungs
A (Ah)	-upper chest and also the body as a whole
OA	-mid lungs
O	-heart, abdomen as far as the navel
OE (Er)	-diaphragm, liver, stomach
U (OO)	-lower body and pelvis
UI	-kidneys, rectum.

The vowels can be sounded, sung out or silently thought (Hamel, p.125, pp.180-181). The breath-suffused body is an instrument which will resonate to every sound, every note, every word in which a person can experience and recognize himself just as he does in his movements. This approach is subtle and gentle with attention steadily observing the breath - when it comes in, when it goes out, whether it is regular or restricted.

The most important consideration for Dr. Middendorf is "self-recollection" conscious presence in those parts of the body in which the flowing of the breath is to be experienced. She emphasizes the following:

> Once one has learnt to detect this breath movement and is at the same time "present" throughout one's body, one has a chance to become aware of the primal rhythmic movement of the breath without altering it. The unselfconscious breathing function enters our consciousness ... Through the procedure mentioned we create for ourselves a state of breathing which is under our control and yet whose rhythm is undisturbed by our will ...Out of this comes awareness of hitherto unconsciously followed paths, bodily as well as spiritual, whose energies can now be transformed [my italics]. (Hamel, 1979, pp.178-179)

PSYCHOLINGUISTIC TRADITIONS OF YOGA AND MANTRA

The experience of breath linking sounds has been for centuries part of the investigation and experience of the psycholinguistic traditions of Yoga and Mantra. Very simply - I invite you to a small experiment: simultaneously inhale and say your full name. You will find that you are unable to do this on the inhale as you need the force of the exhalation to emit the sound and enunciation of your name. Since the mouth is open while talking we do not usually associate it with breathing. From a yoga perspective each exhalation is an expressing out of an individual's energy. This can account for the drained feeling one gets when much of the day has been spent in speaking engagements or long, drawn-out conversations. Breath, sound, eyes and mind are powerfully interrelated in the psychology of meditation and mantra.

Teachers of Sanskrit linguistics called the letters - aksharas, literally "the undestroyables", "immutables" or "imperishables". It was recognized that each syllable of the alphabet is attuned to particular powers, faculties and attributes of the mind. Each syllable has a different effect on one's mental energy. The syllable or phoneme is regarded as an eternal vibration that dwells in the knowledge of the superconscious and when uttered, it vanishes from the audibility scale, but as knowledge, it never disappears; it is never lost. This parallels the recycling (or rebirthing) of energy from one form to another - a basic formulation of physics. No fresh form of energy can ever be created nor can it ever be destroyed.

MANTRAS PRODUCE MENTAL EFFECTS

Mantras are considered sounds that vibrate out from inner energy flows, which are within the electromagnetic nature of each one of us. The word man/tra derives from the Sanskrit verb root *man* from the word *manas* meaning to think, to contemplate, to meditate and *tra* which relates to the word *transcend*. Mantra is thinking in order to transcend, the subtle process of cleansing subconscious impulses and emotions through sound so that one transcends random thinking and experiences the complete fulfillment of pure Consciousness.

For example, the mantra Om was not figured out by three rishis sitting on a mountain top deciding what letters should become the sacred sound. The sound of Om is heard spontaneously in deep meditation when the life force (prana) is deeply vibrating at the forehead centre or "third eye centre" known in yoga as the ajna chakra and related to the pituitary gland.

Sanskrit is considered one of the revealed languages due to the process of sphota or bursting forth where different concentrations of energy at different levels of personality, such as the chakras, burst forth as various syllables into the mind (Arya, p.107). This happens spontaneously, naturally and effortlessly (a "sahaj" experience). Concentration of specific sounds and mantras leads to a reawakening of relevant energies. An extensive presentation of mantric and tantric sound practices and theories is documented by Pandit Usharbudh Arya (1981).

In the Western concept of time, words are linear - they begin at one point and end at another; however, mantras and I would add sustained sound express a vibration of the infinite consciousness which has no beginning and no end. The sound penetrates all levels of being-- physical, emotional, mental and spiritual--in a wholistic way to resolve and reestablish the individual in his or her extended primary state of pure undisturbed consciousness.

The mantras sound up inside of the individual in an advanced meditative state from an energy source that is potentiated within each one of us. This is slowly coming to be recognized in Western psychology as genuine Kundalini experiences are researched (Sannella, 1976).

All sounds produce a mental effect. Certain words through the sounds of the syllables produce an impact in the mind that is related directly to their meaning. For example, the word *thud!* in its very sound carries an impression of strength and loudness while the word *lull* conveys a softer intonation correlated with the intent of its meaning.

MY USE OF SOUND COMBINED WITH IMAGERY

Through eighteen years of working with sound and meditation, I noticed the profound ability of certain sounds to free and open up the physical body and release emotional blocks. During this time I developed a meditative process based on the neutrality of alphabet sounds. Individual letters or syllables are free of associated beliefs and judgment systems. This allowed individuals to explore the effects of a variety of sounds within their own bodies. The one sound would be repeated over and over and become a continuous sound for several minutes and then another sound would be explored.

Individuals blocked emotionally will eventually arrive at a plateau in meditation. Realizing that feelings have a "hum" inside of us, I began bringing sound work into my private counselling practice. I have found that as clients express the varying sound syllables, they experience spontaneous changes in both body sensations and their imagery. This often results in a greater sense of aliveness and a feeling of fusion with their innate self. This treatment mode is well suited for working with depressed individuals, people with "frozen" areas within their body and psychosomatic disorders.

As I work with clients I put an emphasis on breathing and teach them a technique to open the throat called ujjiya breathing. Wilhelm Reich observed that psychological resistances and defenses use the mechanism of restricting the breathing. Grof in his holotropic breathing therapy notes that increasing the rate and depth of breathing typically loosens the psychological defenses and leads to a release or emergence of unconscious and superconscious material (Grof, 1988).

SOUND AS A THERAPEUTIC TECHNIQUE

Emotions have a distinctive charge or "hum" in the body. I guide the client to tune into this feeling and invite an image or let an animal emerge from the area of focus. As the client interacts with the image I either have them ask the animal what sound it feels like making or, as they deeply connect with the image, have them sense the charged feeling in their body and go ahead and verbally express it. As the therapist you sense these "feeling sounds" building in your client. I often get a sense of one or two sounds and ask my client whether they are feeling sounds like an "ahhh" or "ehhh" or a "wurr" for example. Often the client knows exactly the sound and then I suggest he or she make the sound and let the sound organically change as it wants to and to notice the imagery that arises with the sound.

259

As I want the client to feel comfortable in this new exploration and not to have the sense of being watched, I tell them that I will join in on the sound and let myself go with the sounds and expand the sound. I stay with the core of the original sound told to me and vary the pitch, rhythm and tone. Once the client is into the sound and has less need for the encouragement of my sounding, I go a little quieter and also pick up on some of the sounds that are being expressed. I maintain my sounding for as long as the client continues. At first there can be hesitancy so I just keep the sound going and invite the client to start again.

The pure sound helps free old emotions and gives them expression without judgment. The sound and imagery combined intensifies and deepens the process of self-awareness. The power and repetition of the sound becomes a wave of energy that enables the client to move through psychological defenses, let go of long-held anger, rage and shame and finally reclaim their energy and aliveness.

The vibration of the sound floods the brain and reaches the deepest levels of the mind. The sound resounds throughout the brain, filling the skull and bringing a sense of lightness and expansion throughout the body.

I check for energy residues and any holding sensations in the body and work with them. At any one session the work feels completed when the individual experiences an expanded aliveness through his or her whole body. There is a feeling often of total calm, a natural smile, a sense of well-being and an inquisitive appreciation of one's extended self.

CLIENT EXPERIENCES

In one session with a Legal Aid Assistant who experienced a profound waiting anxiety, we worked with several images and then brought in sound. The fear she felt in waiting was linked with a sense of having done something wrong, which related to watching her parents fight and waiting until it was over.

The client experienced a tightness in her stomach and noticed her breathing was irregular. She stayed with the tightness and got an image of a wooden square box that was like a jewel box, however it was closed. She felt she was not living her purpose and was isolating herself. She decided to change the box and add carved hearts and flowers and to paint it with bright colours. Then she put hinges on the top of the box so it could remain open on its own. She also put a purple lining in and made various sections for rings and necklaces. She had a sense of filling the void. She had recently felt an emptiness in her career goals.

As she focussed back into the tightness in the stomach, another image arose of a straight-back chair. It was brown wood with white upholstery and was seen as a symbol of authority. The chair began to change to an ornate chair of the 17th century and the client did not seem to be happy with the chair.

This image dissolved and in her stomach she felt an emptiness. I invited her to let the emptiness become friendly and have the stomach give her a sound. Her stomach was a dark cavern that gave her the "mmm" sound. She started expressing the "mmm" sound and then noticed the cavern was beginning to brighten up and she saw another chair, old, more comfortable with hand rests and well-upholstered arms. She sat in the chair - continued with the "mmm" sound - I noticed her breath deepening and her stomach moving. She related she was feeling more relaxed, lighter and fuller. She continued a bit longer with the sound and her stomach became "a lot more relaxed". I then had her anchor the "mmm" sound and suggested she silently do the "mmm" sound when waiting and also do it out loud at home when she needed, jazzing it up as she felt inclined. We continued to work through the areas related to authority figures and gradually the waiting anxiety was reduced.

In working with sound, it shifts the client from a passive position to an active one. Sustained sound coming organically from within the texture of feeling is emotionally expressive and cathartic. The use of sound can mitigate the fear of anger and rage, considered by the client as uncontrollable and overwhelming. One releases the charge of anger and its festering hold within the body, then the client is more open to deal with the emotional issues supporting the anger or rage. After the use of sound, these issues become accessible as clearer images and feelings that can be owned and revealed often for the first time.

Any image can be used to elicit a sound. The easiest sound to begin with is the "ah" sound. One client, a Ph.D. Computer Research Analyst had high blood pressure and although brilliant in the walled privacy of his computerized office had a very soft voice and said, "I just stand around till someone takes over." His face had a boyish smile. He continued, "It's hard for me to do anything loudly. It's like I don't want to be heard." This related back to the disturbed relationship with his father. In one session, he tuned into the anger towards his father with the "ah" sound being repeated, drawn out and growled. He said after the sound work that "This feels good. It feels interesting. It feels good to own my own sound."

It is well known that certain sounds can generate memories, a certain tune can remind us of a past event. With one client a particularly traumatic incident where she was spanked in school before the whole class came up as she returned to university. She found her linguistic professor reminded her of both her previous teacher and her father.

The shame she felt from this incident was so great that she remembered saying, "I will never be myself again, I am dead." She decided to put her emotions into her painting. She said how she tried not to remember this incident, that she felt blocked in her life and blocked in her breathing. As we worked through this incident she got into saying and screaming the "ah" sound while seeing an image of the teacher from twenty-five years before. Each time she got into the "ah" sound, she would throw a pillow out.

As a client gets into the sound, I invite them to say whatever else they want to say. It can be other alphabet sounds, single words or sentences. With this particular client as she vented her rage the image of the teacher moved further and further away from her until she vanished. My client's words were, "I'm casting her out." She admitted that from this incident, "Something had closed up inside of me--everything stopped there. I've been so impersonal."

At the end of this session - she felt calm, cleansed out and in a warm place. She related, "In meditation, I've had this hug."

SOUNDS CAN STIMULATE EXPANDED STATES OF BEING

Working with sound is powerful, exciting and expansive both for my clients and myself. Some of the sound tones I have used with clients and in workshops are:

Ahh	EEE	III	Da Da Da
Hu Hu Hu	Ba Ba Ba	Va Va Va	Ma Ma Ma
	ZZZ	Ooh Ooh	

Ha Ha Ha -   will eventually bring out spontaneous laughter
Na Na Na -   gradually becomes No No No
Ya Ya Ya - Yi Yi Yi -   gradually becomes Yes Yes Yes

I invite clients and participants to notice the direction of inwardly perceived vibrations as a specific sound continues. Sometimes colours are perceived and an extended state of consciousness develops bringing deep feelings of peace, inner unity and self-appreciation. As Abhinavagupta, an eleventh-century Kashmiri teacher relates, "... the state of bliss is like that of putting down a burden; the manifestation of the Light is like the acquiring of a lost treasure, the domain of universal non-duality."

CONCLUSION

The potential of using sound combined with imagery is vast. It is a method that is simple and organic as the sounds emerge from the individual. I find the general application of sound to be very effective in enhancing the process of imagery as a therapeutic technique. At once it is playful and profound; for many, a first real beginning to owning their own organic voice.

REFERENCES

Arya, P. U. (1981). *Mantra and meditation*. Honesdale, PA: The Himalayan Institute.
Grof, S. (1988).*The adventure of self-discovery*. Albany, NY: State Univ. of New York Press.
Hamel, P. M. (1979). *Through music to the self*. Boulder, CO: Shambala Publications Inc.
Sannella, L. (1976). *Kundalini: Psychosis or transcendence*. San Francisco, CA: H.R. Dakin.

PSYCHODRAMA: AN INTRODUCTION TO IMAGERY IN ACTION

Daniel Tomasulo, Ph.D.

Clinical psychologist, private practice
21 White Street
Shrewsbury, NJ 07701

Psychodrama is a deep-action method of psychotherapy founded by Jacob L. Moreno. A variety of sources credit Jacob Moreno with having founded group therapy (Blatner 1988; Fox, 1987) and, moreover, as having coined the phrase. According to Moreno, group therapy was an outgrowth of his work in developing psychodrama; and not, as is popularly misconstrued, the other way around (Fox, 1987). As such the understanding of psychodrama may provide a historically advantageous foundation for group psychotherapy.

A psychodramatic session emerges in three stages: a warm-up stage, an enactment stage, and a sharing stage. In training groups and in technical demonstrations, an analysis or processing stage may follow. The contextual arrangements for the setting of a psychodramatic session may influence the process and content. As an example, a psychodramatically-oriented group held in a hospital environment may influence the patients in a very different way than a psychodramatic group held in a school setting. Alternately, a psychodrama session held for the purpose of a demonstration at a conference, with the entire life of the group lasting only the length of a single session, will influence its members in a way that will have a direct impact on the process and content of the group.

Similiar in many ways yet different from psychodrama is sociodrama (Moreno, 1951, 1953; Hale, 1985). Psychodrama refers to an individual's life. That is to say, a member in the group may be talking about "her" husband or "her" daughter; and consequently the roles played in that person's psychodrama will be tailored to the specifics of the people in their lives. Whereas in sociodrama, the scenes enacted portray a "collective" role where "a" mother and "a" child are designated; and it is in this collective role that we focus on the encounter. Thus, a sociodrama is closer to the idea of "roleplaying". Whereas, psychodrama is tailored more specifically to deeper action aimed at unveiling the particulars of one's life.

THREE STAGES OF PSYCHODRAMA

The three stages of psychodrama--warm-up, enactment, and sharing--are inherent experiences each time the group functions. The three stages of a psychodrama can now be elaborated.

Warm-Up

The warming-up process in psychodrama may involve the facilitator (called a "director" in psychodrama) being responsible for initiating the warm-up process. This may be achieved through a formal warm-up which may employ any variety of techniques designed to focus the group's thinking. The group may also begin by simply allowing for a general go-around with each of the members relating a piece of information from the previous week's psychodrama (if it is an on-going group) or some information about their current life experience. In groups which meet only one time, either a prepared warm-up by the director or a question concerning the

Mental Imagery, Edited by R.G. Kunzendorf
Plenum Press, New York, 1990

warm-up of each individual to the group is helpful. The warm-up engages the group members into a readiness state for action. The primary purpose of the warm-up is to move the group into the enactment stage.

Enactment

In this stage some action element of the group is prescribed by the director. Enactment employs a variety of psychodramatic techniques which enable members to enhance their participation in the group through action. Usually the action part of the psychodrama is initiated by a sociometric measure. Sociometry assesses the interconnectedness between people on a variety of questions (e.g. "After hearing people in the group speak who do you feel you could learn something from if they did their psychodrama tonight?"; "Who reminds you of a family member?"; "Who do you have unresolved issues with?")

The measure of a group's sociometry will direct the focus of the group. Indeed it has been said that if dreams are the royal road to the unconscious, then sociometry is the jet stream (Blatner, 1988). As such the sociometry of the group helps to establish the best use of the group's energy. The enactment usually allows for a series of encounters between some or all of the group members.

Sharing

The sharing phase is a time when the people who played a role during the enactment phase share with the group and with the protagonist their experiences in the role that they played. They then may share from their own lives what experiences related to the drama. Those who did not play a role (the "audience") may share their thoughts and feelings as the enactment stage was taking place. The primary means of the sharing phase is to have members in the group connect with the enactment by finding something from their lives which relates to the enactment. In addition to helping the protagonist, sharing is one way in which the co-unconscious of the group can be made manifest, and where the future dramas in an on-going group may blossom.

THE PSYCHODRAMATIC PROCESS

A typical psychodramtic process might emerge in the following way, manifesting the three stages just described:

A warm-up (a general go-around, reading of a poem, processing comments from the previous week, issues relevant to the particular group, etc.).

Following the warm-up (or as part of it) there is a sociometric measure. There are many techniques for this and the reader is referred to Blatner (1988) and Hale (1985) for a further discussion of sociometric process and techniques. An example of some questions which might be asked include: "Who's pain do you feel drawn to tonight?"; "Who do you feel would be easy to talk to tonight?"; "Whose issue is most closely related to your own?"; "Who could you learn the most from this evening?".

The warm-up and sociometric questions are designed to produce either a protagonist or an action experience for the group. If a protagonist is chosen, then the protagonist would be allowed to set the scene or stage for their psychodrama. If a theme is chosen (e.g., each person to present their "shadow" side in a metaphorical way) then the group's partipation in the event is facilitated. The director works toward some degree of closure, clarification, or point for termination following the production of the drama.

Following the enactment the group goes back to sharing, where each member talks about their experience in playing a role within the psychodrama and then relates that to their personal life. (This inhibits the usually strong tendency to give advice.) In closing, the director may encourage those who have not shared to speak. The group is then brought to a close.

As would be expected, transference in psychodrama plays a part in the interactional features between group members. The "tele", however, provides an explanation for the real encounter, the genuine condition of attraction, repulsion or neutrality that occurs between two people. Transference and tele then provide varying proportions of an experience we have during a meeting with another person. As an example, if a person in the group reminds you of your sister, and you notice characteristics and behaviors that cause you to respond or react to this member in a way similar to how you may respond to your sister, then this part of the relationship may be termed transferential. However, there is another important component in the relationship which involves the difference that exists by definition since the person you're interacting with is not your sister. This real encounter then is tele, which involves a *mutality* and reciprocity between the two members. To continue the example, if you have a negative transference to a member in the group because they remind you of your sister, you may be aware of this transference and yet react to them as they are, as a real person regardless of their transferential status. They in turn may respond to you with their own transferential elements as well as their own tele reactions.

THE DEVELOPMENT OF TECHNIQUES

Moreno provides for a theory of psychodrama which is developmental in nature. He postulates three levels of development: the double, which is essentially the sense of being understood; the mirror, which is how we are perceived by the outside world; and role reversal, the completion of the process of encounter with another person. It is through the role reversal that we gain empathy and understanding of another's perspective. Through the use of various techniques these developmental principles are employed within the psychodramatic format.

Doubling is a technique where another member (or members) or the director stands behind the protagonist and expresses the thoughts and feelings experienced in the moment by the portagonist. The double has several purposes. It can provide emotional support, give emotional expression, and reorganize perceptions. The process and techniques used in doubling include: speaking the unspoken; exaggeration, minimization, introducing alternatives, restatement, amplification, verbalizing the resistance, and induction of paradoxes. The double(s) may enter the process by way of a volunteer or they may be chosen by the director or the protagonist. Doubles may be singles, in pairs, or multiples.

At a theoretical and technique level, it is difficult to introduce the mirror (how one is viewed by others) when the person has not been adequately doubled. If a person does not feel understood by at least one other person, it may be very difficult for them to cope with information from the mirror.

Role reversal provides an opportunity for empathy to be gained by experiencing another person's perspective. The greater the distance between the perceptions of those involved in the encounter, the more difficult the role reversal.

OVERVIEW

The five main components of psychodrama are: the *protagonist*, the individual working during the enactment phase; the *audience*, those not taking part in the enactment but witnessing it; the *director*, the person trained in psychodramatic theory and technique orchestrating the drama and facilitating the group; the *auxiliaries*, those people chosen to play roles in the drama with the protagonist; and the *stage,* where group members take space for developing their individuation.

Psychodrama is a powerful action oriented technique that allows for group members to act out their needs in a challanging yet safe environment. Information about training and certification may be obtained by contacting: The American Board of Examiners in Psychodrama, Sociometry and Group Psychotherapy, P.O. Box 15572, Washington, D.C. 20003-0572.

REFERENCES

Blatner, A. (1988). *Foundations of psychodrama*. New York: Springer.
Fox, J. (1987). *The essential Moreno: Writings on psychodrama, group method, and spontaneity by J.L. Moreno, M.D*. New York: Springer.
Hale, A. (1985). *Conducting clinical sociometric explorations* (revised ed.). Roanoke, Va: Royal.
Moreno, J. L. (1951). *Sociometry, experimental method and the science of society*. New York: Beacon House.
Moreno, J. L. (1953). *Who shall survive? Foundations of sociometry, group psychotherapy, and sociodrama* (2nd ed.). New York: Beacon House.

IMAGERY IN CONJUNCTION WITH ART THERAPY

Valerie Hookham, M.S.W.

The Halterman Center
Madison County Hospital
London, OH 43140

Art Therapy goes hand in glove with mental imagery. The artwork is after all, a two or three dimensional representation of the client's image. Beverly-Colleene Galyean (1983) says:

> It helps to follow imagery work with a verbal and/or non-verbal mode of expressing what we've experienced. We find that drawing, painting, writing poems, dancing, moving, singing, chanting, sculpting...are quite good ways of helping us remember and learn from our imagery work. (p.29)

Thus, expressive therapies enhance a client's understanding and integration of his or her images. I will describe a sampling of techniques to physically manifest a client's images, thereby making them easier to work with.

Experiential therapy is a gateway to the emotions and, in my experience, is much more likely to achieve catharsis than more traditional insight-oriented therapy. The client's imagery can then be given back to "cement" the experience. Experiential therapy works well for individuals who have experienced verbal, sexual or emotional abuse, especially in childhood. It is contraindicated for overtly psychotic (hallucinating) individuals. I have used it successfully even with non-integrated multiple personality disorders. A specific example might illuminate these points.

IMAGING WITH ART: A SPECIFIC EXAMPLE

If someone is "stuck" in treatment (especially if it is an intellectual person), art can be a way around the intellect into emotion. Bob, one such person, was in his early 30's. His mother died when he was young. His father placed him (not the other children) in an orphanage, took him out for a year, then returned him to the orphanage. As can be imagined, Bob had difficulty attaching to others, particularly women.

Bob had four years "clean and sober" following treatment for chemical dependency. He was working as a counselor to other chemically dependent people while finishing college. He felt some degree of discomfort due to organizational changes at his job and decided to come to a week long workshop at our agency. His facilitators gave Bob an assignment to draw several pictures of his life and his recovery from addiction. He returned the next day with several rather sterile looking pencil drawings. As Bob was unable to say much about the drawings without returning to his highly intellectual state, his facilitators decided to have him act out one of his drawings, using the other participants in the room. He picked a person to play each figure in this drawing, naming them as he went along. Some represented particularly cruel nuns from the orphanage where he grew up, some were other people whom he had known in childhood. One of the figures turned out to be his conception of God or Christ. It turned out in the drawing (as in life) that his anger toward the nuns was blocking the expression of his spirituality which, as the book *Alcoholics Anonymous* points out, is so critical to an addict's recovery. Thus, he was

Mental Imagery, Edited by R.G. Kunzendorf
Plenum Press, New York, 1990

literally surrounded in the externalization of his image. Using the drawing, he was able to express his rage (abreaction) appropriately with the nuns and experience a direct connection with a "Higher Power". He reported a vast feeling of relief after this experience.

As this was taking place one of the facilitators went to the board and changed his drawing into the logo of Alcoholics Anonymous, which had been *the* positive spiritual influence in Bob's life, up to now. Transforming this symbolic drawing helped to "anchor" the experience as a positive one for Bob. Bob started with a mental image, then *drew* his imagery, acted it out, and in the process, transformed it.

A GENERAL EXAMPLE

The "Child Within" is a useful concept for working with clients who were traumatized in childhood. Whitfield (1987) describes it thus:

> Our Child Within is expressive, assertive, and creative. It can be childlike in the highest, most mature, and evolved sense of the word. It needs to play and to have fun. And yet it is vulnerable, perhaps because it is so open and trusting. It surrenders to itself, to othersand ultimately to the universe. And yet it is powerful in the true sense of power. It is healthily self-indulgent, taking pleasure in receiving and in being nurtured. It is also open to that vast and mysterious part of us that we call our unconscious. It pays attention to the messages that we receive daily from the unconscious, such as dreams, struggles and illness. (pp. 10-11)

"Child Within" is variously described as precious child, inner child, high self or true self. All are synonymous. The concept is a useful one for clients as it teaches them that no matter now much they might have been traumatized as children, there is a healthy part of them. The "Child Within" concept can also help to teach self care, i.e. give that child the love she deserved but never received.

Here is one way to begin to access memories of the child within. This exercise works especially well in a group. Materials needed are finger paints and finger paint paper, paper towels and water (to thin the paint, if desired). It works well with clients of all ages and levels of functioning and tends to be regressive in nature, which of course, aids its purpose in building an intrapsychic connection with the child within.

Sit in a comfortable position. Loosen any tight clothing. See if you are willing to make an agreement with yourself that for the next 45 minutes you'll let all your troubles, issues or problems go. You might even picture yourself piling them to the side of you. They'll be there waiting for you if you want to pick them up again. As you sit, begin to pay attention to your breathing. Allow yourself to breathe deeply and fully...............

Imagine that your mind is like a movie screen or a slide projector screen with different images flashing across it. Allow the images to come and go at random knowing that you don't need to hold onto any image or to push it away.............

As you view the images in that movie screen, that slide projector screen, begin to allow images of you as a child to emerge. You might see images of you as a toddler, pre-schooler, in grade school or as a teenager. The images might come from pictures, from stories that you've heard about yourself, from memories of favorite clothes or toys that you had...........Allow all the images of you to flash across the screen........

Then, see which image comes up most frequently or that you feel most drawn to.....Allow that image to come into as sharp a focus as you can.....See if you can see how you wore your hair.....What kind of look you had on your face.....What kind of shirt or dress you wore.....What did you have on your feet? Were your knees skinned?.....See that image of you as clearly as you can.....

You notice that this child, this *you,* is coming towards you....It has something for you. It could be something that's been lost to you or maybe its something that you never had before that you now need. Allow yourself to accept the gift.........experience it........

Then, I'd like you to come back into the room, OPEN YOUR EYES and paint the gift that you received.....Then paint a picture of the child who brought it to you.

NOTE: This exercise can be followed up with other paintings: e.g., favorite fairy tale during childhood. Once the clients have 3 or 4 paintings, they can stop and have "show & tell" with their pictures, which often provide clues about which issues need to be addressed next in therapy.

Another series of exercises which can be helpful is presented below. Again, they work with various age groups and levels of functioning. The main caution is that the therapist needs to be prepared for the intense emotions which may surface and allow time and space for their safe discharge in the session. Thus, it is *not* recommended to do these at the end of the session.

1. Put on some nonvocal music and instruct the client to allow the music to "move" his or her hand across the page. The type of music isn't critical, though the therapist may choose evocative sounds appropriate to the issues with which the client is dealing, such as playing a tape of a thunderstorm breaking for someone who needs to express anger. Crayons, paper, a cassette tape and a cassette player are all that is needed for this exercise. The resulting drawing often brings up unexpected issues or emotions.

2. Ask the client to make a collage of how he or she felt as a child on one side of a posterboard and how they would like to have felt on the other, and have them bring it to the next session and discuss it. This assignment is useful to begin or further an emotional connection with the "Child Within".

3. Another useful assignment to make the connection with the child within is to have the client close their eyes and imagine where his or her child is at that moment. It is not unusual for a client to see the child in a dark space, such as a hole or basement. A female client with whom I was working imagined that her inner child was in a dark closet with the door ajar. I enlisted one of the other clients to be a role player and had her kneel (to be closer to a child's height) in a dimly lit storage area that happened to be in the room. The door was ajar, consistent with her verbal description. I then asked her to open her eyes and walk in to "get" the child. She expressed fear and physically shook as I walked the length of the room with her. She sobbed as she embraced the role player. She was able to have a tangible connection with the part of her that she's repressed so many years ago. I then did a brief imagery with her where she put the "child" into her heart, thereby internalizing the child construct. This was a reclamation that was critical to her continuing recovery from her compulsive behavior.

4. Many clients have introjected punishment and shame. Since shame is not an endogenous emotion, I often have clients symbolically "give back" the shame. A ritual involving a physical construct is useful in doing this. The client is simply instructed to make his or her shame (it can be three dimensional, collage, sculpture, etc.) and bring it to the next session or group. I keep the assignment somewhat vague to allow the clients own imagery to manifest, rather then his or her wish to please the therapist. Clients return with an amazing variety and diversity of responses. A bulimarexic client returned with a model commode that had actual food decomposing inside as the symbol of her shame regarding her eating disorder. Other clients have brought in "webs" made of black yarn which entangle various objects or garbage bags which contain various secrets of which they are ashamed. If this is done in a group setting, it is often helpful to have each member show the construct to the rest of the group and share his or her shame. Then the group can be instructed to build a group "effigy" to shame, using all their individual constructs. The group is then given the task of deciding how to destroy or dismantle it after they have viewed what they made. Groups have done such things as gone out together to burn their shame or carry it out to the dumpster in the parking lot. Individuals usually report this as being a powerful purging experience.

5. When dealing with unresolved grief and loss, have the client construct a memorial to the deceased. This can be written, as in a eulogy, or multimedia. He or she can "present" it at the next session. This assignment can either function as an entree into grief and loss, or as a capstone to the grieving process, depending on the clients progress heretofore.

All five of these exercises have proven helpful in therapy. Other exercises can be designed according to the therapist's needs.

CONCLUSION

It has been my experience that once the therapist gets over his or her reluctance to use expressive therapy, the client is quite willing to comply, even clients who claim that they are not artistic. I have experienced many stunning examples of creativity from "nonartistic" people. Human beings are capable of much more creative expression than they may believe, in my experience.

The techniques outlined in this article are not meant as "quick fixes". Rather in conjunction with imagery, feedback and a positive therapeutic relationship they are tools to help free the client from the continued pain of past trauma.

REFERENCES

Cruse, S., & Cruse, J. (1989).*Understanding the co-dependency trap*. Rapid City, SD: Nurturing Networks.

Galyeon, B. C. (1983). *Mind sight: Living through imagery*. Long Beach, CA: Center for Integrative Learning.

Halpin, M. (1982). *Imagine that! Using phantasy in spiritual direction*. Dubuque, IA: William C. Brown.

Perlmutter, J. (1982). *Basic group psychotherapy competencies* . Unpublished.

Wegscheider-Cruse, S. (1989). *T.U.M.M.S. Training manual for experiential therapy*. Rapid City, SD: Nurturing Networks.

Whitfield, C. (1987). *Healing the child within*. Pompono Beach, FL: Health Communications. Yalom,

Yalom, I. D. (1975). *The theory and practice of group psychotherapy*. New York, NY: Basic Books.

THE CONFERENCE AS THERAPY

Jacqueline B. Sallade, Ed.D.

Clinical psychologist, private practice
P.O. Box 487
Lewisburg, PA 17837

Conferences come and go, and colleagues attend, present, and return from them, usually little-changed, a line added to the resume, perhaps. In June, 1989, a colleague returned from an imagery conference, specifically that of the American Association for the Study of Mental Imagery. He returned with some data and some techniques, but much more importantly he returned with a degree of personal insight rarely achieved in just a few days. His insights were connected to visual symbols, first mental and later gradually transformed into concrete forms which adorned his office artistically.

My curiosity was piqued. Are imagery conferences therapeutic? Do the participants find such a conference more or equally therapeutic than didactic?

I decided to find out, using the AASMI conference as a case study. My process was to interview a random sample of conference attendees, including keynote speakers, workshop presenters, and other attendees. The interview was brief and open-ended. It went something like this: "I'm studying the conference. May I ask you a few questions? What draws you to an imagery conference? In attending the lectures and workshops, do you benefit in a personal way? If so, can you give me some examples?"

My sample consisted of 26 interviews and more than 40 spontaneous comments shared with me which answered the interview questions without my ever having had to ask them. Both sexes and a wide variety of professions were represented, including clinicians, experimenters, professors, physicians, nurses, businesspeople, students and homemakers. Most comments referred to the present conference, but some referred to past imagery conferences.

I noted the responses and then analyzed the responses for common themes--more a journalistic or sociological format than a psychological study. The results are descriptive and are presented in terms of themes.

THE PRAGMATIC OR EXPERIMENTAL OUTLOOK

Several researchers in the imagery field appreciated the small size of the imagery conference because of the "more intimate, meaningful, heuristic discussions". Along with these researchers were some psychologists working to apply imagery. They expressed "awe over the power of the mind".

They theorized, intellectualized, and looked for applications to business, child-rearing, education, and sports as participant observers, even in very experiential workshops. Sometimes, they expressed skepticism about the depth of acceptance achieved by others in imagery exercises. They looked for "safe" ways to "keep in touch with reality". They "learned to divorce [the self] from many of the topics because [they were] looking at it objectively as a scientist and want to think it not feel it." These scientists, though extremely appreciative of the conference were in the minority in terms of their consistent objectivity They are truly the "students of mental imagery".

Mental Imagery, Edited by R.G. Kunzendorf
Plenum Press, New York, 1990

Less objective but equally interested in applying imagery techniques were many mothers, fathers, sons, daughters, husbands and wives. Participants spoke readily about teaching their children to "bring their dreams forward into their lives", to heal their illnesses with imagery, and to expand their dimensions.

Death imagery was used to empathize and deal with aging parents. For example, a man discussed "parents who are facing their own mortality" and received "insight into how to bridge the topic with them". In an image, he flashed back to puberty when his parents helped him deal with a sensitive topic using literature. He can help them the same way.

The variety of helping professionals at the conference learned techniques for use with clients/patients. As one practitioner put it, "imagery is the most powerful way I know to grow and help others". It was striking that every person who mentioned learning techniques for use with clients/patients went on almost immediately to describe vividly the therapeutic use of those techniques toward the development of the self in a very personal way. As an imagery therapist worded it, "Every time I learn another person's methods, I get something personal." Participants spoke of "getting a new approach to an old problem". That aspect of the conference will be discussed below in the section entitled "Therapy for the Self".

RELAXATION

Not everyone found the conference relaxing. Several participants worked so hard listening, learning, thinking, and imagining that they were enriched but exhausted by the end of the conference. However, there were those for whom a main benefit of the imagery conference was relaxation. These participants, all business people and/or spouses of psychologists "enjoyed the unpressured atmosphere" and used the discussions and workshops as "a relaxation technique" more than a growth experience.

FOCUSING

There were more cancer patients than participants knew. They knew the value of imagery and used it all the time. The conference reinforced their focusing. One young man, a psychology student used the death imagery exercises as a reference point for his own well-developed ideas about death. Last year's imagery workshop left him with unremembered words and information but a feeling of deep roots, leading to "a transformation of ideas into the body", physical and personality healing.

As a nurse put it, she was here "to center", to collect herself. This conference is where she reviewed the tragedies, irritations, conflicts, and joys of her life. She took home books and videotapes, inservice ideas, art therapy and other imagery techniques to use with her children and a great deal of forgiveness and healing of her grief for her deceased relatives. She gained power, purpose, and a feeling of well-being, as if "cleaned out".

A therapist found "mother and father in my body...saw the power and control they still had", resulting in better contact with his own feelings. He felt "focused", "tuned in to myself". He gave as an example being able to remember his dreams.

There was expression of "feeling closer to one's family, even when talking with them on the phone" from the conference. Priorities became clear.

FOCUSING TOWARD THE UNIVERSE--BIG AND SMALL

Theodore Barber spoke in images of ant life, birds, black holes, and galaxies. His imagery opened up the soul, broadening perspectives. Real science is awareness and observation for Barber, not mental narrowing. Imagery is powerful but its power lies in how it is used--"trite or big". "It depends on the person."

Asked whether he has gained personally from imagery conference lectures, sessions or workshops, he emphatically said "no". He is stimulated by his own speaking, open to nature through its images, not necessarily wanting to break out of the big paradigm to a human, present, internal focus, which might "narrow" him. This view was a solitary one among the interviews but not irrelevant, as the power of imagery to focus outward cannot be denied.

THE HEALING IMAGERY OF KEYNOTE SPEAKERS

Two keynote speakers presented particularly potent testimonials to the power of imagery in their own transformations. Anees Sheikh, looking cool and comfortable in his elegant suit, had been depressed and seriously phobic of death. After his own death imagery, he relaxed and developed more intimate, earthly ambitions. He has no regrets. Disappointments do not hurt much. He is at peace.

The pre-death, veiled image presented by Anees Sheikh of leaving a fine, borrowed house forever led to deep audience reaction. For example, one woman, a psychology professor, felt comfortable leaving only with her family. She perceived her image as a therapeutic reminder of her closeness to them.

John Schaffer, a well-known imagery therapist, spoke powerfully of his own inside-the-body trip many years ago. He found his prostrate to be an eight inch green balloon with a cork. He mentally removed the cork and healed himself. Now, he is a master at using imagery with others. Still, in experiential workshops, he becomes the client. He was astounded when, confused by a political quandary, he imagined that he was climbing up his own spine, looked at a fluid pool, then sensed going down to his anus. He knew that he felt humiliated! Then, he imagined bottling this rich-smelling stuff in expensive, French bottles, selling it and making millions. The image resulted in his solving the original political quandary and in making a professional reorientation.

THERAPY FOR THE SELF

Over half of the interviews and most of the spontaneous comments related tales of profound personal insight, growth and transformation. These stories ranged from general outlines which preserved privacy to sharing of the most intimate details. This function of the conference knew no sex, profession, age or experience discrimination. It made no difference whether the person was a novice attending an imagery conference or an experiential workshop for the first time or whether the person was a veteran of many such experiences.

Some novices were quite skeptical, at first. One woman "didn't expect therapy from the conference...but got it all along...resolved some important issues...and was amazed and delighted." An art therapist expected little from light and sound imagery. She found "anger expressed in [her] arms...got yellow and bright" and glowing imagery and was surprised at the "relief" which she felt. The same person "wanted" a "peaceful" animal image and was surprised to find "a cougar with wings who said 'I am your anger but I will leave' (fly away)". Her anger was not to be permanent.

Some of the most experimental participants in terms of professional life portrayed visions of deep healing. One research-oriented man discovered such personality changes in psychodrama that he spoke of being "astounded" by "magic". He felt "liberated in fantasy" and propelled toward career changes. Several researchers examined "things that bother" them, including university politics. From techniques given to whole audiences they "got personal messages and solutions".

Generalities included making "discoveries about [one's] own personal pain and discoveries that affect relationships". People could "think differently", "have a flash of insight...to help find a block or [see] how to direct energy", "feel more loving", and be "more accepting of [their] own anger, excitement, insecurity". They experienced their "own internal psychodrama". They became expressive and assertive.

A specific common theme had to do with parental influences. A clinician "became a child again", found that she had indeed not been happy, contrary to family myth. She "looked at [her] mom and dad's reactions at the time of birth", finding her parents young, naive and possibly drunk. She could empathize with her young, not monolithic parents, gaining deep perspective.

Working through inner emotional pain and wounds happened frequently. A physician from a serious childhood worked with his inner child to play, so he could express childhood joy. Similarly, someone saw herself "playing in a sandbox alone" and realized that she needs more time to play as a child herself. There was an "empowering experience related to a sexual abuse situation by volunteering" in a workshop. Psychodrama uncovered helplessness, fear, and anger from earlier days underneath defensive reactions, paranoia, and the need for god-like intellectual power. When more than one person found the same patterns, despite vastly different life circumstances, the support and empathy felt thick and close.

Often the emotional wounds were mixed with conflict and participants outlined resolutions for the conflict. In a workshop using drawings, an imagery expert drew herself crossing a bridge in a European city from the Bohemian left bank to the fashionable, rich right bank. Torn between integrating two aspects of herself, she suddenly realized that she needed "to join the river and get involved with the energy of the current and not choosing sides".

In imaging his inner mind, a man found a vulnerable small white rabbit; but in working through an interpretation, he found an eagle flying off freely. He was ready to stop trying so hard. Also, in reaction to inner mind imagery, a woman found her heart which peacefully directed her away from passionate extramarital memories toward her family. Likewise, some powerful reactions to higher self imagery included a motherly woman with flowing robes outlining a detailed plan of improvement in family relations. A second reaction to the same higher self imagery was to "forgive" and not allow herself to be controlled, leading to a feeling of self-healing.

The pain was not only emotional but often quite physical. In a session on guided imagery, participants listened to their pain, imaged pain and soothed it, usually understanding or intuiting their own symbolism. For example, fatigue was expressed as a dishrag, lower back pain as "horses pulling a heavy cart up a steep hill" (working too hard), and a sore back as a snake ("because the undulating motion helps with long sitting". Participants shared the results of talking to the image and imagining a solution and finally experiencing a spiritual transformation from the healing ritual. (There were comments that never had some observers seen so many men sharing such personal material.) Participants felt free, "as if truth had been experienced,"a glorious sense of purging". Someone wanted to talk to his pain longer, get to know it, and feel "its warm presence". He then experienced the pain as "it", rather than as "pain".

AFTERCARE--INDIVIDUALS HELPING EACH OTHER

Between and after sessions, participants sought each others' advice, support and help working through the emotions generated in the workshops. Many times, someone would cry at the end of a session, and a small group would gather around that person. Later, there were thank you's.

A professor rose above his conflict over university politics by imagining his heroes who "put up with great suffering to make great changes...toward truth", putting his own situation into perspective and healing his anger. He shared his ideas with one of the keynote speakers who helped him "categorize and reconfirm" what he had done.

After watching implosive therapy tapes, participants monitored their fearful, angry, guilty reactions, which included dissociation, intellectualization, depression, and physical symptoms. Small support groups at lunch worked through the tension for those who did not wait to heal in more formal workshops.

A well-known therapist and keynote speaker took a participant aside after they had a short conversation and worked on her seizure disorder. She felt great and had learned a technique to use permanently.

CONCLUSIONS

The American Association for the Study of Mental Imagery annual conference is a case study of an imagery conference. Although there are interesting didactic lectures on research and paper presentations, there are also more experiential workshops than one may find at a typical conference. The participants self-select for such a conference and come primed for experience. Some are there to obtain information, some to relax, and most to learn techniques to apply in a wide variety of settings. Most, whether they expect it or not, receive therapy.

INDEX